Speech Correction in the Schools

Jon Eisenson
Stanford University

Mardel Ogilvie
Herbert H. Lehman College of the City University of New York

The Macmillan Company, New York

Collier-Macmillan Limited, London

Speech Correction in the Schools

Third Edition

The Macmillan Company
866 Third Avenue, New York, New York 10022
Collier-Macmillan Canada, Ltd., Toronto, Ontario

Library of Congress catalog card number: 70-152870

First Printing

Preface

Speech Correction in the Schools is intended to introduce the reader to the problems and therapeutic needs of school age children whose speech requires attention by persons professionally trained for this purpose. In the third edition of this book we have taken cognizance of developments in the field and of the impact of recent research.

The classroom teacher today almost always can rely on the advice and professional expertise of the speech clinician. Because of the current emphasis upon the language arts, the classroom teacher is very aware of the need to motivate and encourage language learnings. The teacher receives professional help from the clinician in improving the child's ability to communicate. Consequently, the teacher must understand the function and role of the speech clinician; and the speech clinician, those of the teacher. Both are important members of a therapeutic team.

Speech clinicians may have one of several titles. *Speech therapist* is probably the one most frequently used. Sometimes they are known as *speech consultants* or as *language clinicians.* Whatever their title, all these professional individuals are educated and trained in the diagnosis and treatment of persons with communicative impairments.

Similarly, the field may be called by various names such as *speech therapy, teaching of the speech and hearing handicapped, speech pathology, speech correction, treatment of speech disorders or communication disorders.* We are retaining the title of the original edition of this book: *Speech Correction in the Schools.* We recognize that other titles, such as *Teaching the Speech and Hearing Handicapped School Child* or *Communicative Disorders in the School* are appropriate.

Some school systems employ professional personnel who are specialists in the assessment and speech training of children with hearing impairments. These professional workers are known as *audiologists.* Speech clinicians and audiologists are workers in related professions. Their educational backgrounds overlap to a considerable extent. Both the speech clinician and the audiologist are likely to have had formal course work in psychology, particularly in the psychology of speech, mental hygiene, and tests and measurements; they are likely to share a common background in their course work in physiology, speech science, phonetics, and general courses in speech disorders and hearing impairments. Beyond this, the speech clinician is likely to have taken addi-

v

tional specialized and advanced courses in areas such as language development, stuttering, voice disorders, acquired language disorders, or articulatory defects. The audiologist is likely to have had specialized and advanced training in the measurement of hearing, in the physics and physiology of hearing, and in techniques for the education and rehabilitation of children with hearing impairments. The speech clinician and the audiologist who work in school situations should be expected to know how the children whom they will be treating are being educated. They should be particularly aware of the kind of language training each school offers. They must also understand the professional obligations and the multiple functions and roles of the classroom teacher.

The chapters in the first part of the book present the general considerations and the background of knowledge that are basic for the necessary common insights of the classroom teacher and the school speech clinician in relation to the child with defective speech. We begin with a chapter on the classification and incidence of speech defects, and follow immediately with a chapter on speech correction services. The content and sequence of the ensuing chapters are based on the assumption that fundamentals of information about normal speech should precede a discussion about defective speech. So we have included material about speech standards, the mechanism for speech, the production of speech sounds, and the development of language in children.

Some of the problems involved in helping a child to communicate are common both to the classroom teacher and to the speech clinician. Many of these center upon language development. The clinician's task may be more specialized, more individualized than that of the teacher, but both share the basic objective of developing the child's language to the point where he communicates efficiently, proficiently, and effectively. Often the speech clinician's assistance is needed in such problems as articulation or delayed language development. The classroom teacher's larger task and scope, building on the remedial work of the speech clinician, is to motivate, stimulate, and help the child communicate effectively in a variety of situations.

To make the achievement of common objectives possible, the speech clinician must have an appreciation of the language arts program in our schools, and an awareness of how his specialized educational and therapeutic efforts take place in the classroom. The teacher, on the other hand, should have an appreciation of the nature of speech therapy and the work of the speech clinician. He must understand what is taking place in the speech clinician's room, and know what is happening to the child who leaves his (the teacher's) classroom to correct his "cleft palate speech," or to overcome his stuttering, or to learn to produce a proficient *l* and *r*. In brief, a mutual appreciation of each other's professional functions by the classroom teacher and the speech clinician is in the best interests of the child.

The second part of the book deals with the specific speech problems that are found in 5 per cent or more of our schoolchildren. We have tried to present the problems as they affect the child in his overall functioning. In each instance we have explained the nature and cause of the speech disturbance, its implications for therapy, and the therapeutic approaches and procedures of the speech clinician. We have also indicated the role of the classroom teacher in regard to the speech problems of the child and the therapeutic efforts of the speech clinician.

In this edition we have endeavored to revise our materials in keeping with the comments and suggestions of some of our readers who were willing to act as constructive critics. We are grateful for the help we obtained from our colleagues' evaluations, based upon their experiences with the book as a required class text.

J. E.
M. O.

Contents

Chapter 1

Classification and Incidence of Speech Defects

Approximately five per cent of school age children have difficulties in communication related to defects in the manner or control of their oral productions. Such defects may be expressed in deviant speech sounds, in voice (vocal quality, rate, or loudness), in rhythm, in the number or choice of words, or in the way the words are "strung" to make utterances. Some of the children seem to be aware of their defects and may be apprehensive about speaking. Others show a benign indifference to their speech or to the reactions of listeners to them. Classroom teachers and professional workers* are likely to make similar judgments about these children. For example, the teacher and clinician are quite likely to agree that the five-year-old who continues his infantile *wawa* for *water*, or *gogo* for *doggy*, has defective speech sound production. He may, of course, have other indications of infantile language competence which, as we will learn later, may be expressed in his vocabulary or in his syntax. The eight-year-old whose utterances are characterized by frequent starts, stops, sound, syllable, and word repetitions, and of whom his classmates say, "Jackie doesn't get his words out right," also has a productive speech problem. Unconsciously,

---

* The professional workers directly concerned with remediation of language and its oral expression have a variety of titles that include speech correctionist, speech therapist, speech clinician, language clinician, and speech pathologist.

both adults and the child's peers are probably comparing Jackie with other children of his age who, in similar speech situations, speak with relatively greater ease and fluency.

When Helen, a five-year-old kindergartener, says *thay* for *say*, or *thoap* for *soap*, no one is likely to take particular notice. Such substitutions are not at all unusual for a child of this age. However, when Nancy, an eighth grader, uses a *th* for an *s*, even though an indulgent classmate may consider Nancy "cute" and observe "I love to listen to Nancy. I wait for her *th's*," we may conclude that, however cute, Nancy does have a speech defect. Her classmate's observation suggests that Nancy's lisp directs attention to how she is talking rather than to what she is saying, and thus gets in the way of what she is presumably trying to communicate.

Some barriers to communication, often confused with speech defects, do not fall within the province of the speech clinician. They include: 1) nonstandard pronunciations and language usage, 2) regional dialects, 3) poor oral reading, 4) immature articulation and fluency patterns, and 5) a psychological disturbance that manifests itself as a speech symptom. The classroom teacher, usually with the help of other specialists, is responsible for these particular problems. The cooperating specialist may be the speech clinician who helps the teacher plan a program of speech and language improvement.

The eight-year-old child who says, "I din't recognize dat neighbor wid de fedders in her hair—de one who's awiz pretendin'. She's actin' in de Cender play," is not in need of help from the speech clinician. Perhaps half of his classmates and even his parents say *dat* for *that* and *de* for *the*. His observation gives evidence of a fairly sophisticated use of language for his age. His classroom teacher, however, usually plans a program to improve his level of speech and language along with that of the other pupils. Undoubtedly this child communicates effectively at home and with most if not all of his classmates. But time and occasion will arrive when his nonstandard pronunciations embarrass or handicap him. We will discuss this problem in Chapter 3.

A child may have come from a section of the country whose inhabitants speak differently from those in the area where he is now living. The child's teacher and his classmates may be very conscious of the differences in his speech. In fact, at times they may be unable to understand what he is saying. As he lives in his new community, however, the differences will be ironed out because usually he will acquire the speech patterns of his playmates. The teacher can help his adjustment by accepting his speech and by explaining his differences to the members of his class. Regional differences in speech are also discussed in Chapter 3.

Oral reading is difficult for some children because they have difficulty in understanding the meaning of the printed page. As a result, their oral reading is uncommunicative; it is hesitant and hard to understand. The conversation of the same children, however, may be quite adequate. Their main problem in communication is one of oral reading although, as mentioned in the chapter on articulatory defects, reading and speech problems are often related. It has been our experience that as children improve in one ability, they frequently improve in another.

Kindergarten and first grade teachers find that many of their children articulate inaccurately. Pendergast (1966), in a study of 15,000 first grade children, found that slightly more than one fourth of first grade children misarticulated one or more sounds. Physical maturity and environmental stimulation will take care of most of these articulatory difficulties, for the children's inaccurate speech reflects a level in their development rather than a speech defect. The speech clinician can prognosticate with some success which children will need help; ways of prognosticating articulatory development is discussed in Chapter 10. More research in this area will bring about more accurate prognosis.

Similarly, children in kindergarten sometimes exhibit disfluences which are part of the normal development of children. The aspects of language development are discussed in Chapter 7.

In some instances, the major problem is not one of speech but of social adjustment. The child whose voice is consistently thin and weak and who speaks with little or no inflection surely exhibits a problem of voice. This problem, however, may be closely related to the child's concept of herself—she feels she cannot do anything very well. She says, "I feel like a big stupid lug most of the time." Her stooped posture, her halting walk, her untidy dress, her sloppy compositions, her lack of enthusiasm, and her dull, light expressionless voice are all part of a syndrome. In such an instance, the voice is merely the symptom of a personality difficulty. The speech clinician can help only in cooperation with other members of the school personnel.

Communication, Speech, and Language

Newman (1962) makes clear the relationships among speech, language, and communication. He defines communication as a social manifestation that includes all the phenomena and activities associated with interaction, whether linguistic or nonlinguistic. Language is a group phenomenon that is generated and maintained in community living;

a system of signs and symbols that is transmitted from generation to generation; a code or a tool or an instrument of communication. Speech, an individual physical activity, constitutes the manner of communication, as distinguished from the means—language.

We believe that you cannot separate the manner and the means—that they are inexorably interwoven. At this point we will discuss some of the necessary language abilities. You will learn about the development of language in Chapter 7 and about stimulating its development in Chapter 8.

Language Abilities of the Child

Every classroom teacher who teaches in the language arts program makes judgments about his children's language. He categorizes his group into those with superior language, those with poor language, and those with adequate language. The members of the superior group speak clearly and intelligibly, listen critically and with discrimination, comprehend readily, and communicate even fine distinctions of meanings. Members of the inferior group speak unintelligibly and listen inadequately, in that their brains have only limited capacity to process in time, to form patterns, and to retain what is heard; consequently, they do not comprehend readily. When they express themselves, their speech is often characterized by concreteness, lack of generalizations, overly simple syntactic structure, syntactic and morphological errors, and an excessive use of nonverbal clues. In between these two extremes, teachers label speech and language adequate.

What, then, is involved in learning to use language? These abilities include the capacity to listen, to process various types of incoming information, to remember and relate on-going experiences with previous experiences, to recall these experiences in meaningful terms, to express ideas and concepts in an appropriately mature manner for the child's age.

McCarthy and Kirk (1969) developed the Illinois Test of Psycholinguistic Abilities with the following eleven subtests:

1. Auditory reception (auditory decoding)—understanding what is heard.
2. Visual Reception (visual decoding)—understanding what is seen.
3. Auditory vocal association—drawing meaningful relationships from what is heard.
4. Visual motor association—drawing meaningful relationships from what is seen.

5. Vocal expression (vocal encoding)—expressing ideas verbally.
6. Manual expression (motor encoding)—expressing ideas through gesture.
7. Grammatic closure—using grammatical structures automatically.
8. Auditory closure—filling in missing parts which were deleted in the auditory presentation. Example: Tele/one? Bo/le?
9. Sound blending—synthesizing sounds of a word into a word.
10. Auditory sequential memory—recalling a series of digits auditorily.
11. Visual sequential memory—recalling a series of geometric forms visually.

These subtests evaluate these areas of language functioning: 1) decoding (receptive functions), 2) encoding (expressive functions), 3) associations between encoding and decoding, 4) ability to integrate discrete units into a whole, and 5) memory processes.

Types of Speech Defects

The speech clinician must view speech and language as more than an ability to articulate sounds. He must be prepared to examine not only the child's phonological ability but also his channels of communication, the psycholinguistic processes involved in recognizing and understanding what is heard, in expressing ideas and responding either vocally or through gesture, the organizing process involving the internal manipulation of precepts, concepts, and linguistic symbols, and the degree to which habits of communication are organized within the child.

When he discovers the child who substitutes one sound for another or who omits sounds, he must decide whether the articulatory problem coexists with other problems of language. The test just described is one means of measuring the child's competence and performance with certain aspects of language. Ferrier's research (1966) points to the concept that articulatory problems coexist with language deficiencies. He studied forty children of ages 6–8.7 with normal intelligence and normal hearing, but who had articulatory difficulties. The means on the ITPA scores of the group were all below the norms with auditory vocal automatic, auditory vocal sequential, visual vocal sequential, and vocal encoding being the lowest. Ferrier also observed that defective articulation appears to affect vocal encoding performance by reducing the total amount of verbalization. He further notes that these children also performed inadequately on the visual motor channels, although to a lesser extent than on the auditory channels. He gives as possible reasons an effect of verbal ability on the visual motor channels and the degree of availability of names for objects. The clinician does well to investigate performance on other language abilities: morphological and syntactic accuracy, syntactic complexity, vocabulary, and sound discrimination.

Speech defects include: 1) retarded language development, 2) articulatory defects, 3) stuttering, 4) vocal defects, 5) cleft-palate speech, 6) cerebral-palsy speech, 7) language impairment, associated with brain damage, and 8) speech defect due to impaired hearing.

RETARDED LANGUAGE DEVELOPMENT

The child who is retarded in language development may initially also be somewhat delayed in language onset. Although one aspect of oral language competence may be conspicuously deviant, the likelihood is, as we shall learn later, that there is some degree of retardation—of lack of proficiency—in most of the components of speech. Thus, he may be obviously retarded in his speech sound production and appear infantile because of his sound omissions and/or the persistence of infantile pronunciations. However, he is also likely to have a smaller productive vocabulary and use shorter phrases and "simpler" sentences than most of his age peers.

To draw the line between retarded language development and an articulatory defect is sometimes difficult. The sound omission or substitution may well be but a symptom of retarded language development. Other aspects of the child's language must be examined before the label "articulatory defect" is applied. The Ferrier study mentioned previously points to the coexistence of articulatory and language problems. That the term "baby talk" is often used to label an articulatory defect is an indication that more than articulation is defective. Therefore, an assessment of the various language abilities is important.

ARTICULATORY DEFECTS

Among articulatory defects are: (1) the omission of sounds. The nine-year-old boy who says *pay* for *play* and *banket* for *blanket* exemplifies the omission of sounds. (2) The substitution of one sound for another. The ten-year-old who says *wabbit* for *rabbit* and *wun* for *run* illustrates the substituting of one sound for another. (3) The distortion of sounds. An example of a distortion of a sound is the twelve-year-old whose *s* has some of the characteristics of *sh*. A child with an articulatory defect may make any or all of these three errors. When the consonants which occur frequently, such as *s*, are involved and when some sounds are involved and when some sounds are missing entirely, the child's speech may be unintelligible. The child may on occasion either include a sound he usually omits or make the sound acceptably. Frequently he makes a sound accurately in its initial position but makes the same sound inaccurately in its final position or in a blend with another sound such as *bl*. He may substitute an *f* for *th* but at the same time substitute a *p* for *f*. In other words, he is seemingly inconsistent in his articulatory errors. Ordinarily, however, a pattern exists even though the same individual uses several different substitutions or distortions for one sound. The substitution or distortion depends on the position of the sound in the word and its proximity to other sounds. A careful analysis of the child's articulatory errors will often point to a particular pattern for them.

Articulatory defects present one of the most important problems of the speech program, for most speech defects are of the articulatory type. About three fourths of the speech defects in a school population are articulatory defects. Of this group, one half have difficulty with *s*. But many parents do not feel that articulatory defects are serious, for they have become so accustomed to their children's articulatory errors that they do not even hear them. Other parents feel that their children will outgrow their articulatory difficulties. To the older child particularly, however, the difficulty often causes concern. His classmates think that he sounds like a baby and at times may treat him as one.

Other terms commonly included in this category are lisping and lalling. Lisping refers to any defect of any or all of the four sibilant sounds: *s*, *sh*, *z*, and *zh*. For example, the *s* may be whistled, sound somewhat like an *sh*, or have a *th* quality about it. Lalling means a person has difficulties with the *l* and *r* sounds. The child may substitute a *w* for the sounds or he may make them in such a weak manner that they are not readily distinguishable. We have suggested tests for the discovery of articulatory difficulties in Chapter 10.

STUTTERING

The stutterer's speech interferes with the reception of his ideas by his listeners. No stutterer's speech is exactly like another's although a disturbance of rhythm is obvious in each case. Symptoms frequently include blocking on sounds, repetition or prolongation of sounds, repetition of syllables or words, and spasms of the speaking mechanism. One stutterer may speak abnormally slowly, another too quickly. The severity of stuttering varies for the individual stutterer. Almost always some situations exist where stutterers speak with comparative or complete fluency. There may be moments, however, when the fluency is so badly interrupted that both the speaker and the listener are unduly aware of the interruptions.

Although many parents remain quite unconcerned about articulatory difficulties, most parents are too much aware of disfluencies. Some parents diagnose the very young child's normal disfluent speech as stuttering long before the child is aware of any difficulty. In the chapter on the development of language, we call attention to the number of times disfluencies occur in the young child's speech. Adults' concern and anxiety about disfluencies may be communicated to children, who in turn may become concerned and anxious. All of us should think long and carefully before diagnosing disfluent speech as stuttering. This idea will be discussed at greater length in the chapter on stuttering.

A type of rhythmic disorder sometimes confused with stuttering is cluttering. The child who clutters speaks at such a rapid rate that he omits and slurs syllables and pauses in the wrong places. He always sounds as if he is in a hurry.

Stuttering is not always easily discernible, because it is intermittent. If the children in the class are asked to read aloud, a stutterer may read aloud well. Furthermore, he may be able to speak easily to strangers but not to friends. The teacher who knows the child well frequently is the person who first notices a child's stuttering.

VOCAL DEFECTS

Vocal defects have to do with faults of pitch, quality, or intensity. A sixteen-year-old boy speaks at a pitch so inappropriate to his age and sex that it draws attention to itself. A sixteen-year-old girl speaks in a pitch so low that when she answers the telephone she is mistaken for her older brother. Both sixteen-year-olds have defects of pitch. A junior high school girl speaks with nasality and a strident quality. Her voice quality needs improvement. A fourteen-year-old girl speaks so softly that she is almost inaudible to her listeners. She needs to be helped so that she will have enough intensity of voice to make herself heard. Sometimes rate of speaking is also included in this category. In this instance, children speak so quickly or slowly that they are difficult to understand.

These terms are not quite as completely whole in themselves as they may seem. For example, Mary's voice sounds high, light, and barely audible. In her case, attributes of pitch, quality, and intensity are interwoven. Joan's voice sounds too low and husky. In Joan's case, the attributes of pitch and quality are interwoven. Separation of the entities of pitch, intensity, and quality in the diagnosis of voices is often impossible. In Chapter 12 on voice we shall discuss pitch of voice in detail.

Defects of intensity are easily recognizable, for voices are so soft that they do not carry, or so loud that they irritate the listener. Here again, however, the lack of intensity and pitch may be interwoven.

Terms describing quality of voice tend to be more nebulous. Some persons will call a particular voice husky; others will call it hoarse; others will call it guttural; still others may call the voice a pleasant one though a bit throaty. But some of the adjectives describing vocal qualities are quite clear and well defined. Laymen may say that a person with a nasal voice talks through his nose. This term indicates excessive nasal resonance. Laymen portray a person with a denasal voice as always sounding as if he had a cold because his *m*, *n*, and *ng* lack sufficient nasal resonance. Some, however, label this an articulatory defect because it involves consonantal sounds. Furthermore, all of us easily recognize the breathy voice and the falsetto voice.

CLEFT-PALATE SPEECH

In cleft-palate speech, the cleft, slight or extensive, may go through the teeth ridge and the hard and soft palates. It may extend through any one of these, or through the teeth ridge and hard palate, or through both palates. Consequently, the air passes freely between the mouth and the nose. This gives the speech a very nasal quality in unrepaired cleft palates. Even in repaired cleft palates the listener often perceives the voice as nasal. Many of the consonant sounds are distorted. The child with a cleft palate often has difficulty with the plosive sounds *p*, *b*, *t*, *d*, *k*, and *g*, for the child cannot built up enough air to explode these sounds. In addition, the fricative sounds *f*, *v*, *s*, *z*, *th*, *th*, *sh* and *zh* are often defective. The child may use a glottal stop or a nasal snort as substitutions. In severe cases the speech is unintelligible. The combination of physical defect and the symptoms of speech defects make cleft-palate speech quite obvious.

CEREBRAL-PALSY SPEECH

Cerebral palsy is a disturbance of the motor function resulting from damage to the brain before, during, or shortly after the birth of the child. The speech of the cerebral-palsied child may be normal when the muscles of the articulatory and respiratory organs are not affected. But, in about 75 per cent of the cases, the speech is slow, jerky, and labored, and the rhythm is faulty with unnatural breaks. The consonants, particularly those which require precise articulation, are apt to be inaccurate. Language development may be retarded.

LANGUAGE IMPAIRMENT

Language impairment associated with brain damage falls into two large categories. The first category includes the developmental failures and the unevenness of development in the child's ability to understand speech, to speak, and later to learn to read and write. The second category includes the involvements in oral and written functions resulting from brain damage incurred after the individual had learned to use language. These are generally referred to as aphasic language disorders. Some persons would include the first of our categories under retarded language development. The second category is primarily a problem for those beyond school age. We will, therefore, not consider this category in our text.

SPEECH DEFECT DUE TO IMPAIRED HEARING

A speech defect as a result of impaired hearing shows itself largely in articulatory errors, in voice aberrations, and in language problems. The child cannot pattern his own speech on that of others because he cannot hear well enough. Consequently, his sounds are not articulated accurately, and his voice reflects his lack of hearing by being too loud, too soft, or devoid of inflection. Because he cannot hear others, his vocabulary and morphological and syntactic development are impaired. How his hearing is impaired influences his articulation and his voice. This is discussed in Chapter 14.

To help the classroom teacher decide whether his students have speech difficulties we have prepared the following questionnaire. When a preponderance of *yes* answers appears, the teacher should consult a speech clinician.

Analysis of Speech Defects

Retarded Language Development
- Is his speech markedly retarded in relation to that of his classmates?
- Is his vocabulary limited for his age?
- Does he omit and substitute sounds substantially more frequently than his classmates?
- Does he use shorter and simpler sentences than his classmates?
- Does he use fewer phrases and prepositions than his classmates?
- Does he make errors in word order for his age?
- Does he use most pronouns accurately for his age?
- Does he use most tenses accurately for his age?

- Does he use most adjectives, their comparisons and superlatives accurately for his age?
- Does he make most plurals accurately for his age?

Articulatory Defects
- Does the child substitute one sound for another?
- Does he omit sounds?
- Does he distort sounds?
- Is he very hard to understand?

Stuttering
- Is the child disturbed by his disfluency?
- Does he repeat sounds or syllables or words more than his classmates?
- Is his speech decidedly arhythmical?
- Does he block frequently?
- Does he have difficulty in getting his words out?

Vocal Difficulties
- Is the child's voice noticeably unpleasant in quality?
- Is his pitch higher or lower than that used by most of his classmates?
- Is his voice monotonous?
- Is his voice light and thin?
- Is his voice husky?
- Is his voice too loud?
- Is his voice too weak?
- Is his voice difficult to hear in class?

Cleft-Palate Speech
- Is there an obvious cleft of the teeth ridge or palate?
- Does his voice sound excessively nasal?
- Are his *p, b, t, d, k,* and *g* inaccurate?
- Are some of his other consonants distorted?

Cerebral-Palsy Speech
- Does the child have obvious tremors of the phonation and breathing musculature?
- Is his speech slow, jerky, and labored?
- Is his rhythm of speech abnormal?

Language Impairment
- Is the child's comprehension of language markedly retarded?
- Does he seem to be inconsistent in his ability to understand as well as to use language?
- Is there a marked disparity between his ability to understand and his ability to use language?
- Is the profile of his linguistic abilities uneven? (For example, can he read much better than he can spell? Is he surprisingly good in arithmetic and yet quite poor in either reading or writing?)

Speech Defect Due to Impaired Hearing
- Does the child have frequent earaches and colds?
- Does he have running ears?
- Does he omit sounds or substitute one sound for another?
- Does he distort sounds?
- Does he speak too loudly?
- Does he speak too softly?
- Does he frequently ask you to repeat what you have said?
- Does he turn his head to one side as you speak?
- Does he watch you closely as you speak?
- Does he make unusual mistakes in the spelling words you dictate?
- Does he misinterpret your questions or instructions frequently?
- Does he do better when given written instructions than when given oral instructions?
- Does he seem more intelligent than his work indicates?

Incidence and Types of Speech Defects

The teacher may have three children with speech defects in his class one year and none the next. But on the average he can expect at least one speech defective in his classroom almost every semester. Surveys afford somewhat different figures on the incidence. A 1959 report of the American Speech and Hearing Association Committee on Legislation (ASHA, 1959) notes that 5 per cent of our school-age children and 1.3 per cent of children under five years of age have speech problems.

The breakdown is

Estimated Number of School-Age Children per 10,000 with Each Type of Speech or Hearing Problem

Type of Problem	Percentage of Children with Serious Problem	Number of Children with Serious Problem
Articulation	3.0	300
Stuttering	1.0	100
Voice	.1	10
Cleft-Palate Speech	.1	10
Cerebral-Palsy Speech	.1	10
Retarded Speech Development	.2	20
Speech Problem Due to Impaired Hearing	.5	50
Total	5.0	500

A more recent report of the incidence of speech defects is that made by the United States Department of Health, Education and Welfare (Eagle, Hardy, and Catlin, 1968). So that it can be compared with the White House Conference Reports, we have placed the data in similar format.

Prevalence of Speech Disorders in School Age Children per 10,000 with Each Type of Speech or Hearing Problem

Type of Problem	Percentage of Children with Problem	Number of Children with Problem per 10,000
Hearing		
Profound Impairment		
(Deafness)	.12	12
Moderate-Severe Impairment	15–20	1500–2000
Distortion (Dysacusis)	not known	
Speech		
Articulatory Defects		
a. Physiologic	4–6	400–600
b. Organic		
Cleft Palate	1.5–2	150–200
Cerebral Palsy	1.3	130
Voice	10	1000
Retarded Speech Development	5	500
Language Disorders	no formula available	

An examination of surveys of speech defects in school systems reveals that up to 10 per cent of our school population are defective in speech. In most surveys the writers are counting those children with speech that is sufficiently different from normal speech to call undesirable attention to itself in conversation. We may arrive at various reasons for the differences in incidence found in publications. (1) The clinician may have to examine too many children too rapidly, so that he is not being thorough enough in his analysis. (2) Classroom teachers with little training in speech may be reporting. They may be inaccurate in their diagnosis. (3) The basis of judgment varies. What may be a decidedly unpleasant voice to one teacher or clinician may be less offensive to another. One person may include a child with an articulatory defect, another may decide not to include such a child because he feels that the difficulty is due to immaturity, while the other person may consider it a serious defect.

Teacher's Role in Locating Speech Defects

A research study by the Subcommittee (on The Clinician: Professional Definition) of the Research Committee of the American Speech and Hearing Association indicates that in locating children who need speech training, 68 per cent of the speech clinicians use the "referral" method and 64 per cent frequently use the "survey" method. Only 12 per cent use the "class visitation" method frequently (ASHA Research Comm., 1961, p. 16). In the survey method the speech clinician carries major responsibility for finding the speech defective, but in the referral method the classroom teacher plays an important role. Since 55 per cent of the clinicians regularly use reports of classroom teachers to determine the extent of children's disorders and another 40 per cent occasionally use them (ASHA Research Comm., 1961, p. 16), the classroom teacher should be trained to hear and identify symptoms representative of the various speech defects. The training may be accomplished by college courses, in-service courses, or a series of lectures by the speech clinician.

In the light of a study by Diehl and Stinnett (1959), this training seems absolutely essential. Diehl and Stinnett made their study in Kentucky, where no public-school speech clinicians had ever practiced, to find out how efficient teachers are in discovering speech defects. The study concludes: (1) Elementary-grade teachers with no orientation in speech disorders can be expected to locate speech defective children with less than 60 per cent accuracy. They can be expected to fail to identify two out of every five who would be located by trained speech clinicians in routine screenings. (2) The same teachers can, however, be expected to locate severe types of articulation defects with slightly better than 80 per cent accuracy. (3) Teachers appear to have least skill in recognizing a voice disorder in a second-grade child. This study emphasizes the need for the elementary-school teachers to be trained in identifying speech defects, particularly in areas where the speech clinician does not conduct a survey and where the classroom teacher is responsible for referring those children who need speech therapy to the speech clinician.

A similar study by James and Cooper (1966) investigated how successfully classroom teachers who were given the aid of a written statement defining and describing speech handicaps could identify speech-handicapped children, and determined the relationship of the teachers' ability to identify speech-handicapped children with the type and severity of the speech disorder. The experiment involved 30 third-grade teachers who had no training in speech correction, and 718 children were screened. The speech clinician found 242 children with speech difficulties; the teachers referred only 98 of them. The teachers were least accurate in their referral of children with voice disorders and most accurate in their referral of stutterers. They referred 87.5 per cent of the severely disordered, 51.9 per cent of the moderate, and 28.7 per cent of the mild. Their percentage of accuracy of referral varied from 10.1 for voice, 41.4 for articulatory defects, and 80.0 for stutterers. This study supports the findings of the Diehl and Stinnett study in that the teachers were most remiss in discovering voice difficulties and that teachers do locate the severe difficulties more than 80 per cent of the time.

The findings of these studies are also supported by Prahl and Cooper (1964). They compared teacher referrals with the results of screening by a speech clinician, and reported that the percentage of accurate referrals rose as the severity of the disorder increased. They suggest two alternative interpretations: either teachers consistently fail to identify a large percentage of speech-handicapped children, or clinicians are unnecessarily severe in their judgments of defective speech and have consequently lost perspective of what constitutes a "speech problem."

The second of these interpretations needs to be examined. If the *s* deviation is such that no teacher, parent, or classmate detects it, is it a problem? Certainly, it does not seriously interfere with communication and in most instances the speaker is unaware of the "handicap." If the *r* is weak but its weakness is not discernible to anyone but the clinician, does a speech problem exist? The answer must be, "Only in the ears of the clinician."

The classroom teacher does not ordinarily do audiological testing.* A research study by the Subcommittee (for Diagnosis and Measurement) of the Research Committee of the American Speech and Hearing Association indicates that audiological testing is accomplished by a variety of specialists. Diagnostic audiological testing is done in public school systems by the following persons in order of decreasing frequency: speech and hearing clinicians (24 per cent), nurses (22 per cent), physicians (15 per cent), school audiologists (13 per cent), health department personnel (4 per cent), and other personnel (7 per cent) (ASHA Research Comm., 1961, p. 54). Practically all public schools have provided for audiological screening, usually no less frequently than every fourth year of a child's school attendance, although in a small percentage only those children referred for the purpose are screened audiologically (ASHA Research Comm., 1961, p. 57).

---

* See Chapter 14 for a more detailed discussion.

Types of Speech Defects
the Classroom Teacher Can Handle

The child with defective speech needs the help of each of his classroom teachers. The teacher knows the child well and is with him for longer periods than any specialist. Frequently he is well acquainted with the child's parents. At times parents will understand the teacher and listen to him with more attention than they will give to the specialist.

As mentioned previously, articulatory defects are most frequent. Most often no oral or dental malformation is associated with the difficulty; it is the result of faulty learning. In some of these cases the teacher with training can help the child to listen to the sound, make it accurately, and incorporate it into words. For example, a particular teacher can successfully manage Johnny's *tree* for *three*. He aids Johnny in hearing that he is substituting a *t* and *d* for *th* and *th̄*, teaches him to make these two *th* sounds accurately, and to incorporate them·into words and conversational speech.

The teacher, however, must be careful in dealing with an articulatory defect. The teacher should be sure that his evaluation of the problem is accurate and that his chosen approaches are likely to produce the desired results. One of the authors once observed a college freshman who consistently used the two *th*'s for *s* and *z*. When her error was called to her attention, she said, "But I can do it right." Whereupon she made what was for her, because of her jaw formation, a very difficult coordination of *s*, almost touching the tip of her tongue to the teeth ridge behind her upper teeth. A teacher had taught her to place the tip of her tongue on the upper gum ridge. The teacher's suggestion for correction was so difficult for the girl that it was almost impossible to accomplish. If the jaw and teeth are so formed that the child needs to be taught compensatory movements, the teacher should refer the child to a speech clinician for help.

The teacher shows good judgment in refusing to accept primary responsibility for the correction of the speech of the stutterer or for serious voice problems. Children with such problems need the assistance of a speech clinician. If the teacher has had no preparation in the handling of speech difficulties, he should refer even the less serious cases such as a lingual protrusion lisp (*th* for *s*) to the therapist. Frequently, in turn, the speech clinician refers the student to another specialist in the field of medicine or psychology. The teacher, however, does have definite responsibilities when a speech clinician is part of the school staff. Often, as noted, the teacher must be able to identify those children who need speech help. Furthermore, to be able to work effectively with a clinician, the teacher must understand the nature of speech therapy and must know how and when he can reinforce the work of the clinician. The teacher's role as a member of the language team is discussed in the next chapter.

References and Suggested Readings

American Speech and Hearing Association Committee on Legislation, "Need for Speech Pathologists," *ASHA*, I (December, 1959), 138–139. (Gives statistics on prevalence of speech defects.)

———, "Services and Functions of the Speech and Hearing Specialists in Schools," *ASHA*, IV (1962), 99–100. (Delineates the services and functions of the speech and hearing specialists in public schools as distinct from those of other teachers.)

American Speech and Hearing Association Research Committee, "Public School Speech and Hearing Services," *Journal of Speech and Hearing Disorders*, Monograph Supplement 8 (July, 1961).

Anderson, V., *Improving the Child's Speech*, rev. ed. New York, Oxford University Press, 1961, Chap. 3. (Tells how to recognize speech disabilities.)

Berry, M., and J. Eisenson, *Speech Disorders: Principles and Practices of Therapy*. New York, Appleton-Century-Crofts, 1956, Chap. 3. (Describes the traits of the speech defective.)

Darley, F. L., *Diagnosis and Appraisal of Communication Disorders*. Englewood Cliffs, N.J., Prentice-Hall, Inc., 1964. (Discusses the five basic communication processes important in the appraisal of a subject's communicative disability: symbolization, respiration, phonation, articulation-resonance, prosody.)

Diehl, C. F., and C. D. Stinnett, "Efficiency of Teacher Referrals in a School Testing Program," *Journal of Speech and Hearing Disorders*, XXIV (February, 1959), 35–36.

Eagle, E. L., W. G. Hardy, and F. Catlin, *Human Communication: The Public Health Aspects of Hearing, Language, and Speech Disorders*. NINDB Monograph 7. U.S. Department of Health, Education and Welfare, Public Health Service, National Institute of Health, National Institute of Neurological Diseases and Blindness, Bethesda, Md., 1968. (Gives prevalence of speech and hearing disorders, and defines hearing handicaps in terms of *db* losses.)

Ferrier, E. E., "Investigation of ITPA Performances of Children with Functional Defects of Articulation," *Exceptional Child*, XXXII (May, 1966), 625–629.

Frostig, M., and P. Maslow, "Language Training: A Form of Ability Training," *Journal of Learning Disabilities*, I (February, 1968), 105–115. (Describes developmental functions, language deficits, influence of education. Talks about a program for training language abilities.)

James, H. P., and E. B. Cooper, "Accuracy of Teacher Referral of Speech-Handicapped Children," *Exceptional Child*, XXX (September, 1966), 29–33.

Johnson, W., et al., *Speech-Handicapped School Children*, 3rd ed., New York, Harper & Row Publishers, 1967, Chap. 1. (Defines the various types of speech defects.)

Johnson, W., F. L. Darley, and D. C. Spriesterbach, *Diagnostic Methods in Speech Pathology*. New York, Harper & Row, Publishers, 1963.

Lee, L. L., "Developmental Sentence Types: A Method for Comparing Normal and Deviant Syntactical Development," *Journal of Speech and Hearing Disorders*, XXXI (November, 1966), 311–330. (Shows how two children failed to follow a normal pattern of development in terms of syntax and were failing to produce a certain type of syntactical structures.)

McCarthy, J. J. and K. A. Kirk, *Illinois Test of Psycholinguistic Abilities*, rev. ed. Urbana, Illinois., Institute for Research on Exceptional Children.

Newman, J. B., "The Categorization of Disorders of Speech, Language, and Communication," *Journal of Speech and Hearing Disorders*, XXVII (August, 1962), 287–289. (Reviews the relationships among speech, language, and communication from a linguistic viewpoint.)

Pendergast, K., "Articulation Study of 15,255 Seattle First-Grade Children with and Without Kindergarten," *Exceptional Child*, XXXII (April, 1966), 541–547.

Prahl, H. M., and E. B. Cooper, "Accuracy of Teacher Referrals of Speech-Handicapped School Children," *ASHA*, VI (October, 1964), 392.

Spriesterbach, D. C., "Speech—An Index of Maturity," *Childhood Education*, XXVII (February, 1951), 260–263.

Van Riper, C., *Speech Correction: Principles and Methods*, 4th ed. Englewood Cliffs, N.J., Prentice-Hall, Inc., 1963, Chap. 2. (Describes the types of disorders of speech.)

Wood, N. E., "Identifying Speech Disorders in the Classroom," *School Life*, XXXXV (March, 1963), 6–8. (Categorizes speech defects in terms of problems of phonation, fluency, articulation disorders, and language disorders.)

Problems

1. Visit a lower-grade classroom and try to screen the children into the following categories: a) those who have speech that will meet their social and classroom needs; b) those whose speech is faulty but likely to improve with maturation; c) those who need speech improvement help; d) those who have more serious defects that require the attention of a speech correction specialist.

2. Visit one of the sessions held by a speech clinician. Indicate the problem of one of the children and the kind of help he received.

3. Visit a kindergarten and a fifth-grade class. Indicate whether articulatory errors decrease or increase and whether disfluencies in the children decrease or increase in the two grades.

4. Answer the questions on pages 10–12 in reference to five particular children. Try to choose one child whom you suspect of having a speech difficulty.
5. Read one of the following references and report on it to the group: Diehl and Stinnett, 1959; James and Cooper, 1966; Newman, 1962; Wood, 1963.
6. Visit a session held by a speech clinician. Indicate in two specific ways how you could reinforce the work done in this session in the classroom.

Chapter 2

Speech and Language Clinical Services

The responsibility of the classroom teacher is as a member of the language team, for the trend toward providing special help for the speech-handicapped is continuing at an accelerating rate. Irwin states that before 1940 only nine states had legislation which permitted recognition of the special needs of the speech-handicapped child by "promoting interest and financial support for the speech-handicapped child in the public schools" (Irwin, 1959, p. 127). In contrast, she notes that in 1959 39 states had special education laws which allowed the extension of services to children with speech problems (Irwin, 1959, p. 142). The expansion is further shown in the requirements for state certification as a public-school speech therapist. In 1955 Irwin (Irwin, 1955(a)), records that 15 states had certification requirements approaching those of basic certification in the American Speech and Hearing Association. She further indicates that in 1959 32 states seemed to have certification plans approximating those of the Basic Speech Certification in the American Speech and Hearing Association (Irwin, 1959). Both the growth of permissive legislation concerning the speech-handicapped and the upward trend in certification requirements augur well for the work of speech correction. As the children's needs for speech clinical work are being met by clinicians, the classroom teacher can turn his attention to reinforcing the work of the speech clinician and to the language program of the school.

21

Organization of Speech Correction Services

Speech programs within schools differ in their administration and organization in many ways. Sometimes the teacher refers the speech-handicapped child to the clinician; at other times the principal, parents, school nurse, psychologist, or guidance director refer him; also, at times, the clinician makes a clinical survey. The clinicians' case loads may vary from 50 in some cities to 300 in others. The clinician meets the child for as short a period as 10 minutes or as long a period as 50 minutes. He may work with each child individually or in groups varying in size from three to 18. The groups are homogeneous or heterogeneous in terms of the speech difficulty and in terms of age.

IDENTIFICATION OF SPEECH- AND HEARING-HANDICAPPED

Clinicians locate children with speech problems primarily by means of surveys and through teacher referrals. However the particular problem is handled, it takes time. Speech screening usually takes from one to three weeks of the clinician's time each year. Teachers often do give a kind of preliminary speech test, but they do not give hearing tests. Although audiological screening is provided in almost all schools, it is under the supervision of nurses most frequently and of speech and hearing clinicians next most frequently (ASHA, 1961, p. 57).

CASE LOAD

A 1961 survey of the American Speech and Hearing Association (ASHA, 1961) gives norms as to numbers in case load, kinds of defects within it, and grade level of the participants. A mean current case load of 130 children was reported by 1,462 clinicians. The average number of children seen weekly is 111, while the average number of children worked within the course of a year is 130. One fourth of the clinicians, when asked to specify what factor seemed to limit their case load, reported that the state law established this limitation; 23 per cent indicated that the number of children with speech problems established their case load; and 45 per cent stated that the size of their case load was left to their own discretion (ASHA, 1961, p. 34). Of the case load, 81 per cent is comprised of children with articulatory problems; 6.5 per cent, of children who stutter; and 4.5 per cent, of children with delayed speech. The remainder, including children with organic and voice disorders, constitutes only a small percentage of the case load (ASHA, 1961, p. 38). About three fourths of clinicians work primarily with children in kindergarten, grade 1, and grade 2. Only 2 per cent work strictly at the high-school level (ASHA, 1961, p. 35).

INDIVIDUAL AND GROUP THERAPY

Approximately nine tenths of the children who are subjects of speech therapy receive the therapy in groups. National averages indicate that clinicians each week see about 10 children individually and 101 children in groups of four or five (ASHA, 1961, p. 38). Most of the clinicians meet both individuals and groups twice a week although a substantial percentage meet them only once a week. Of those responding in this study, 57 per cent indicate that their group sessions last from 25 to 34 minutes while 29 per cent indicate that their sessions last from 15 to 24 minutes. The periods of individual therapy are shorter; 40 per cent devote 14 to 24 minutes to individual sessions; 36 per cent, 25 to 34 minutes (ASHA, 1961, p. 38–39).

Sommers in 1962 (Sommers, 1962) found that 50 minutes of group therapy for articulatory problems was generally as effective as 30 minutes of individual therapy in a special summer program. In 1966 he and others (Sommers, 1966) found that in the correction of articulatory defects group therapy was as effective as individual therapy, regardless of the severity of speech defectiveness or the grade levels of the children involved. In this later study, Sommers used 12 experimental groups of 40 children who were given the McDonald Deep Test of Articulation before and after a period of eight and one-half months of speech correction. These 12 groups provided for the investigation the following sources of variation: a) therapy—half of each group of 40 received group therapy; the other half received individual therapy; b) severity—half of each group had "mild" articulation problems; and half had "moderate" articulation problems; c) grade—four of the groups were from grade two, four from grade four, and four from grade six. The average size of the groups was 4.5 with the largest group containing 6 and the smallest 3.

WORK OF THE CLINICIAN

The speech clinician identifies those children who are speech- and/or hearing-handicapped, diagnoses and evaluates their problems, and then plans, schedules, and conducts a program to handle those problems. He confers with parents concerning their children's difficulties. In addition, he may offer in-service courses to teachers and may serve as a consultant for those classroom teachers who carry on a program of speech and language improvement for those children whose speech and language skills are inadequate in terms of pronunciation, vocabulary, syntax, decoding, encoding, and associative and sequencing functions. Because school curricula revolve around verbal skills, such programs help children to be more successful in their school environment. Chapter 8 deals with these aspects in some detail.

The American Speech and Hearing Association (ASHA, 1964, p. 191) has summarized the responsibilities of the speech correctionist. The association recognizes that the important area of teaching the broad language-arts skills is the responsibility of the professionally trained classroom teacher. It further recognizes that the area of speech improvement appropriately includes the speech clinician working in a consultative relationship with the teacher. Finally, the association views the special services that must be given to the child with speech disorders as being the responsibility of the clinical speech specialist.

The largest part of the clinician's working week is spent in therapy; the mean number of hours spent in therapy as reported by 705 clinicians is 23.09 hours. The distribution of the rest of the clinician's working time is: traveling, 2.68 hours; conference, 2.53 hours; writing reports, 2.12 hours; preparing lessons, 3.23 hours; and other duties, 1.55 hours (ASHA, 1961, p. 15).

LIMITING THE CASE LOAD

A frequent problem in schools is a case load that is too large for the clinician's program. He may find to his dismay that although his therapy schedule cannot effectively accommodate more than 100 cases, he has 182. The situation allows a variety of possible approaches:

1. He can give a little help, in large groups, to all 182.
2. He can train the classroom teachers to take care of the less severely handicapped.
3. He can limit his case load to 100.

The first alternative, to give some therapy to all the handicapped, does not seem feasible, because a small amount of training usually results in a small amount of improvement, and marked success requires effectively treated students. Feasibility of the second alternative depends on many factors: the speech background of the classroom teachers; the availability and ability of the clinician to train the teachers; the size of the various teachers' classes; their schedule and that of the clinician; and the attitudes of the administration and the teachers to the problems of the speech-handicapped. In a few instances, the clinician may be able to give the necessary training to some of the teachers.

Usually, however, he will choose the third alternative of giving training to approximately 100 students. But he must make his selection of the 100 students on the basis of valid principles. Disgruntled parents whose children have been deprived of speech therapy may demand an explanation. So may those parents whose children have been asked to take it. The reasons for selection should be arrived at thoughtfully and carefully and in consultation with the administrative officers of the school.

Such factors as the severity of the handicap, ability to benefit from training, and placement in grade and school are all important. In discussing case selection most authorities agree that children with voice problems, those with speech difficulties that are related to organic involvements, and those who stutter should be enrolled in the speech therapy program. Many authorities believe that the child with a speech defect that is a cause of concern to him, his parents, or his teacher, or which seriously interferes with communication, with interpersonal relationships, or with school progress ought to be included in the program. That the words "seriously interefere with communication" means something different to speech clinicians and classroom teachers is obvious from the research reported in Chapter 1 on page 14.

Most writers cite ability to benefit from training as an important factor in selection. They suggest that measures be used to prognosticate articulatory improvement, such as the child's ability to produce a sound in a nonsense syllable, or to discriminate the correct production of misarticulations from acoustically similar sounds. They also suggest other measures dependent on standardized tests: intelligence tests, language tests, sound discrimination tests.

Some clinicians emphasize therapy in the upper grades rather than the lower grades; others emphasize helping children in kindergarten, first, and second grades, as noted on page 22. A rationale can be made for both positions.

It is important that the speech clinician base his selection of cases on a logical, appropriate rationale and that he use this rationale in defending his inclusion or omission of a child from his case load. When teachers and administrators have been involved in working out this rationale, a parent, concerned about the omission of his particular child, is more likely to accept the decision gracefully.

When classroom teachers have not participated in the discussion of the rationale for placing children in speech therapy, the principles should be carefully explained to them. They will be better equipped to explain the principles to disgruntled parents however, when they have been included in the discussion that led to the formulation of the principles.

Although the administration and organization of speech therapy programs may differ, the clinician always keeps the classroom teacher informed of what he is doing. The teacher, in turn, reinforces the learning acquired in speech sessions. Almost always both the clinician and the teacher confer with the parents. Both teacher and clinician often consult with the school health authorities. In other words, a team approach is appropriate. The composition of the team may vary somewhat, but typically the classroom teacher, the clinician, the school health personnel, and the school psychologist make up the team. Its members meet to discuss the problems of the handicapped children and to work out programs for particular children. At times they invite other specialists such as an otologist, an orthodontist, a neurologist, or a psychiatrist to join the group.

Roles of the Members of the Team

THE CLASSROOM TEACHER

Surely the classroom teacher knows the child better than any member of the team, for he is with him all day. Because he is interested in all of the child's development, he sees the child's speech as part of his total development. Of the members of the team, he in all likelihood has the most opportunity to understand the child. He knows how the child acts on the playground and in class. He recognizes the child's ability to lead, to be a good student, to build bird houses, or to throw a baseball. Furthermore, he usually has more contact with the parents than any of the other members of the team. Consequently, he is the one most intimately acquainted with the child.

The ideal classroom teacher for the speech-handicapped child is a good teacher for both the child with normal speech and the one with defective speech. First, and most important, he accepts the child with a handicap, whether it be speech or physical, and helps his classmates accept him. When the teacher controls his feeling of sympathy and accepts the handicapped child with his difficulty in a matter-of-fact manner, the child and his classmates are likely to adopt the same attitude. Second, the teacher makes sure his classroom invites oral communication. When the children plan their work together, when they like to play with each other, they talk and listen. As they go on purposeful trips, as they act in a play, or as they build a bookcase, they have worthwhile discussions. Their classroom, with its interesting bulletin board, with its busy work corner, invites conversation. Chapter 8 contains suggestions on how to stimulate speech activities. Third, the teacher fosters good human relationships among the children. When a warm friendly feeling exists in the classroom, when youngsters like each other and their teacher, when the teacher helps to build a positive concept of self in the child, when activity is stimulating, speaking is both necessary and enjoyable. As children participate in decisions, as they realize that they are the most important part of the school program, they have a feeling of belonging to their school group. Last, the good teacher is a cooperative person. He reinforces the learning taught by other teachers. He contributes factual information about the child to other colleagues when it will prove useful.

In addition, the classroom teacher who is to be successful in helping the child with handicapped speech must have certain other qualifications more directly related to speech: (1) His own speech and voice must be worthy of imitation. These factors will be discussed in Chapter 4. (2) He must have a discerning ear so that he can hear the articulatory and vocal errors his children are making. (3) He must have an accurate knowledge of how the American-English vowels and consonants are made. The chapter on the production of speech sounds covers this area. (4) He must be able to plan a program of speech improvement for all his children. Whereas only 5 per cent have need of speech correction, almost all students have need of speech improvement. This need is explained in Chapter 8. (5) He should have enough knowledge of communicative disorders to reinforce the teaching of the clinician. He must, therefore, be able to understand the latter's aims, objectives, and procedures. In this book the chapters on the various speech defects contain this material. (6) He should be able to pick out those students in his class who need speech help. The chapter on the definition of speech defects includes some of this information.

The teacher can cooperate in other ways too. For example, classroom teachers can help students above the first grade to carry the responsibility of watching the clock for the time when they are to go for speech help. Frequently, the teachers write the time on the blackboard on the day the child is to go for help. Through some means, the teacher should help the child to get to the clinician at the scheduled time.

THE CLINICIAN

The clinician must appreciate that he is a working member of an educational team. As such, he must have a professional awareness and attitude, and must get along with his students, their parents, and the school personnel. In addition, he must be able to gain the help of other school personnel, set up his program effectively and cooperatively, and report on its progress capably and efficiently.

Professional Status and Attitudes. Part of being a good teacher is maintaining professional status and attitudes. Now that the study of speech disorders has attained a professional status, the clinician should be aware of it. The first factor in awareness is gaining the necessary training. The American Speech and Hearing Association lists the requirements for the certificate of clinical competence. If the speech clinician is working in the schools, it is preferable that he meet the requirements upon his employment. If he does not, he should take work in summer school to meet them as quickly as possible. A second factor is the clinician's relationship to other professions. He must recognize the delimitations of his field from those of the doctor, psychologist, psychiatrist, dentist, and physical therapist. He should neither criticize these workers nor make even a hint of a diagnosis in a field other than his own. The third factor is the knowledge of his own limitations. When he does not understand a voice case or when he has difficulty with a parent, he must seek help from someone who knows more than he. Professors in universities, experienced workers in the field, and administrative officials of a school are all glad to help the young clinician.

Because the clinician is working with individuals and with small groups, he must be particularly careful to maintain a professional and workmanlike attitude and to allow no undue familiarity between him and his students. He should be friendly but at the same time keep the necessary professional distance. He should not respond emotionally to a child's problem, for his attitude must remain objective. He undoubtedly wants a permissive atmosphere for his speech correction work; however, he should set limits and hold strictly to these limits. His permissive attitude should not mean a laissez-faire attitude. The failure of the clinician to establish limits and to hold to them may cause the classroom teacher to be justly critical. Some language and some activities should be discouraged. A cartoon in the *New Yorker* (August 19, 1961) points to such a situation. A mother, very erect and very proud, is walking with a six-year-old in hand who is nonchalantly puffing a cigarette. Two long-nosed females say, "I think there's such a thing as being *too* permissive."

Human Relationships. Another part of the clinician's being a good teacher is in his ability to get along well with others. He will need to have good personal relationships with members of the community, with teachers, and with the parents of his children. In other words, he must be able to work with people effectively. The success of his program depends to some extent on how well the members of the community receive it. He must be able to explain his program to the men of the Rotary Club or the Lions Club. Such people are already sympathetic to the handicapped child, but the clinician must be able to make them understand that the speech-handicapped child can receive help. Furthermore, he must motivate them to think that their community must offer such help. One specialist talked to a club in the town about the kind of help being given to three children with quite different difficulties. His presentation was persuasive.

The clinician needs the cooperation and help of the classroom teachers. In turn, he must appreciate the teachers' work. One clinician made it his duty to visit a classroom when he had some free time because of the absence of a child in his case load. His few warm words of appreciation to the teacher at the end of the visit aided in building a good relationship between the two.

The support of the parents of the handicapped children is as important as that of the classroom teacher. One father remarked recently, "I'll only live in this town three years, but I'll always be thankful for Davy's speech help. Suppose I'd happened to be in a place where there was no help." Sincere appreciation by parents is an asset in firmly establishing and maintaining a speech correction program. The conferences with parents and the home visits are most important. The clinician must be able to gain the confidence of the parents so that they will cooperate for the good of the child and the success of the program.

Parent Counselling. Many speech clinicians meet regularly with the parents of the children they service. In one area of an inner city, the clinician meets frequently with the parents of her children in groups of about 25. Their discussions have ranged from helping the child to build a strong self image to the verbalizing of feelings of guilt and anger by the parents. Members of this group talked frankly about their relationships with their youngsters and about their own needs and feelings, which were often reflected in their children's attitudes and behavior. As they discussed these problems with each other and with the clinician, they were better able to understand their own feelings and the feelings their children had about themselves and about their parents.

One parent lived in fear that his son, a stutterer, would become a dope addict. He kept repeating, "I try to set him straight." When questioned, he acknowledged that the reason for his fear was the boy's anger, which was often expressed in "beating up" his younger brother and other kids on the block. He began to understand why the boy felt angry and to be able to communicate this understanding to him. Even though the boy's behavior was unacceptable, the father *did* accept the fact of his anger, even when it was unprovoked. As the boy perceived his father's understanding and acceptance of his feelings, he began to communicate. The father, who had communicated mostly nonverbally, to reprimand, began to communicate verbally, and particularly at times such as when the boy was elated at his success in writing poetry. The father previously had looked on this activity as a foolish waste of time. Admittedly, the severity of the stuttering did not diminish, but the boy became a happier and much more communicative member of his family and of his school community. The other parents in the group, mostly mothers, were instrumental in helping the father to look at himself and his son realistically and honestly.

Webster (1966) says that parent conferences provide parents with three vital aids:

1. Important information about the child's specific disorder.
2. Opportunities for parents to experiment with tools for promoting better communication: a) trying to understand the child's feelings and verbalizing this understanding, b) trying to accept the child's feelings, even when the behavior is unacceptable, c) allowing the child time with his parents when they can concentrate on communicating, d) giving the child a chance to communicate at times when he feels success and satisfaction, and e) attempting to communicate with the child on his own level.
3. A chance to verbalize frankly about vital issues in their relationships and the forces that motivate them.

In-service Courses. In some schools, the clinician will not only treat the children but willl also lead discussions and give lectures or-in service courses so that the teacher can reinforce the work given in correction sessions. He will give the teachers the necessary training to diagnose the speech difficulties of the children in their classrooms. He will send out mimeographed bulletins to help them understand the various speech handicaps of their children. He will explain to them the relationship of speech and language difficulties to academic achievement, such as reading, and to behavior problems. He will report to them research that relates the study of speech disorders to classroom teaching.

As he talks to teachers and parents, he will use nontechnical terms. He will not say that Mary has dysphonia and that Johnny has a lall; rather he will explain that Mary's voice is hoarse and that Johnny substitutes *w* for *r* and *l*. Parents particularly are wary of specialists' terms; therefore, both the classroom teacher and the clinician will not talk about "cases," "clinicians," or "clinics."

In-service courses, lectures, and discussions are but one avenue of cooperation between the clinician and the classroom teacher. The clinician will explain to the teacher the kind of difficulty a particular child has, what he and the child are doing about it, and what the child's chances of success in controlling the difficulty are. In short conferences or notes, he tells the teacher what words and phrases the child has learned to say or what kind of behavior he has exhibited during speech help. For example, one clinician aided a child in preparing to read aloud a report he was to give before a meeting of the parents of his class. Another noted that William could now say his own name correctly and that he could also pronounce the name of the street he lived on: Maple Street. The teacher commended William's accomplishment.

Preparing Schedule. Last, the clinician must serve as a teammember in preparing his schedule of correction classes and in making his reports. Many variables make the preparation of a correction schedule difficult. The clinician may want to place students homogeneously in terms of defect and age, to work with certain cases in the morning, or to cut across several classes and age levels for stuttering groups. In addition, he usually has to work around the schedules of the classroom teachers and other specialists; for example, the classroom teacher may not wish a child to lose certain fundamental work that is usually given at a particular time. Because so many of the school personnel are involved, their cooperation and that of the administration is essential in working out a schedule. Consultation with the teachers and the administration helps to insure the prompt and regular attendance of the speech-handicapped children. The resulting schedule should be placed in the hands of the administrator and the teachers involved. All the members of the team should adhere to the schedule except for necessary absences.

When assigning students to the speech correction classes, the clinician should notify the parents. In this activity, the advice of classroom teachers is important, for most teachers meet with the parents at least once a semester. With the advice and consent of the supervisor or principal, the clinician or director of speech and hearing services sends a letter such as the following to the parents of children to be enrolled in speech correction classes:

Dear Mrs._____:

A recent test shows that your son can profit from work in speech. I have, therefore, scheduled him to work with me twice a week during which time I shall try to teach him to speak more clearly.

I shall be glad to have your help. You can, I am sure, give me information and advice that will make my work with your son more effective. Won't you come to see me next week when I have planned conferences with parents? Would Tuesday at 3:00 be a possible time? If it is not, please call me between three and five on Friday at Forest 6–7000, extension 7, and we can arrange another time.

Sincerely yours,

Before enrolling a child in speech therapy class, the clinician should make sure that the child is not receiving help from a speech and hearing center or from a private individual. Speech instruction from both a school and another source usually are not advantageous to the child, although overanxious parents often believe that the more help received the better, and consequently enroll a child for private help without informing the school. Local centers and school personnel should cooperate to do what is best for the youngster. In some instances the child is better treated at a center; in other instances, he is better treated at school. A school administrator may coordinate the work by approving the child's taking therapy from an outside source and by excusing him from school therapy. A signed slip is then sent to the outside source. The superintendent or another official should also request information on the amount and kind of therapy being given the child by outsiders. The work between the agency and the school should be related.

Records. Clinicians keep records for several reasons: (1) The clinician wants to know as much as he can about each child. From interviews with the child, teachers, and parents, he acquires information about the child's interests, personality, medical history, and intellectual attainments that can be helpful in handling the child. When such information is recorded, the next clinician has a basis for understanding the child. (2) The clinician needs to know what has been done with a child prior to his arrival and how effective the therapy has been. (3) Teachers, administrators, and other school personnel need to find out what has taken place in the speech correction program. (4) Administrators frequently want reports so that they can justify the program to their governing bodies. (5) State departments of education often require reports to serve as a basis for financial aid to the local community.

According to the American Speech and Hearing Association, clinicians maintain the following kinds of reports for individual students. Numbers indicate the percentage of 705 clinicians who stated that they kept records for each student:

Record	*Percentage*
Case history	73
Record of phonetic improvement	71
Reports of conferences	69
Daily log	33
Weekly or monthly progress reports	41
Semester or annual reports	21

Source: ASHA, 1961.

The school case history is much simpler than the case history kept in a speech and hearing center. The following form suggests the kind of case history that might well be kept in a school.

CENTRAL VALLEY ELEMENTARY SCHOOL

Speech History

Date_____

Name of Student_____Address_____

Name of Guardian_____Address_____

Telephone Number_____

Date of Birth_____Sex____Homeroom____Homeroom Teacher_____

Speech Difficulty_____

Father: Age_____Education_____

Occupation_____Speech defect, if any_____

Health_____

Mother: Age_____Education_____

Occupation_____Speech defect, if any_____

Health_____

Brothers and Sisters:

Names	Ages	Speech defect, if any
_____	____	_____
_____	____	_____
_____	____	_____
_____	____	_____

Physical Condition: Weight_____Height_____

Abnormality in Mouth, Throat, Nose, or Teeth Structure_____

_____

Motor Impairment_____

Defect in Hearing_____

Defect in Vision_____

Serious Illnesses_____

Mental and Educational Development:

I. Q._____Test_____

Scholastic Achievement_____

Scholastic Interests_____

School Attendance_____

Some districts prepare more detailed forms for all students. The February, 1969, issue of the *Journal of Speech and Hearing Disorders* tells about the development of a standard case record form by a group of clinicians and supervisors in the Los Angeles area who found transfer of information among school speech clinicians inefficient. This form includes the usual obvious identification data such as name and address and material on spontaneous speech and language including dialect, length of responses, vocabulary, grammar; on articulation, on fluency; on voice; on intelligibility; on the speech mechanism; on communicative responsiveness; on general health history; on observed physical behavior; more detailed identification data including case identification, years of therapy, type of class, grade level, test results from such tests as WISC, Binet, Peabody, and CIMM, reading scores, arithmetic scores, an articulation record, and a hearing test record. Such a detailed source of data accumulated over years can supply answers to many questions, including queries about case selection, prognosis, dismissal criteria, associated learning difficulties, and related family and health conditions.

Other reports frequently made by clinicians include results of speech testing, results of hearing testing, schedules of schools and classes, therapy progress reports, and final reports (ASHA, 1961, p. 42). Geraldine Garrison suggests the following reports for her staff: a case history when the speech difficulty is the result of a physical, psychological, social, or educational condition, and a short record when the speech difficulty is minor; a brief report including nature of difficulty, progress, attitudes, attendance, and cooperation of parents, for the child's cumulative record; a report to the principal indicating the progress of each child; a report to the classroom teacher about his students' progress; a report to parents; and a report to superintendents (Garrison, 1960, p. 23).

The report to the superintendent may well include:

1. Number of students who have received clinical help during the term, including breakdown for each type of speech or hearing problem.
2. Number of students receiving clinical help at the end of the term.
3. Number of students dismissed during the term with reasons for their dismissals.
4. Number of students added during the term.
5. Number of conferences with parents.
6. Number of conferences with students.
7. Number of home calls.
8. Number of referrals—broken down specifically.
9. Number of meetings with parent group—broken down specifically.

Facilities. Space in schools is being utilized as never before. Because of the demand for space, clinicians can find themselves in nurses' outer offices, under stairwells, in locker rooms, and, more fortunately, in well-equipped, especially planned "speech rooms." When the clinician is asked to plan such a room for a new building, he may wish to put in writing his needed facilities. A committee of ASHA has listed room requirements, including lighting, heating, ventilation, necessary furniture, storage facilities, and equipment in the April, 1969, issue of ASHA (ASHA, 1969).

Competencies of Speech Clinicians. All of these duties point to the need for a certain level of competence of the speech clinician. A bulletin published by the United States Government (Mackie and Johnson, 1957, p. 48–50) suggests the following requisites for competence of speech clinicians in the public schools:

1. The speech correctionist must understand the various types and causes of speech defects and be able to apply specific diagnostic and remedial procedures to individual children.
2. The speech correctionist must have a broad understanding of human development and specific knowledge of how speech disorders affect such development in children. He must understand the needs of both typical and atypical children.
3. The speech correctionist must be able to establish rapport with the child and to help him deal with social and emotional problems which he may have as a result of his speech condition or which may be slowing down therapy. Closely related to this competency is the one that he will be able to develop a teaching atmosphere free from pressure and conducive to good mental health.
4. The speech correctionist must understand the general principles of education—curriculum, methods, philosophy, and organization—and should be able to integrate and correlate his speech correction work with the total program of the school.
5. The correctionist should be able to apply survey and referral systems and to develop, plan, and coordinate an effective schedule for a speech correction program in several schools that is acceptable to pupils, teachers, and parents.
6. The correctionist should be skillful in working as a team member and should be able to coordinate the resources of the school and community for the good of the child.
7. The speech correctionist should have a knowledge of the facilities for obtaining information and evaluations concerning the child's

physical, social, emotional, and intellectual status, be able to interpret the information obtained so as to further the speech correction program, and be skilled in reviewing and writing reports and case histories.

8. The speech correctionist should have the ability to help parents understand their child's speech problems and personal attitudes.
9. The speech correctionist should have a knowledge of professional literature and research studies.

PSYCHOLOGIST

The psychologist helps the teacher, the clinician, and the parents to understand the child. The results of his testing program may help all three in handling the child. For example in one case a psychometric test showed a child to be far brighter than the teacher, clinician, or parents had thought. In another case, the administration of the Children's Thematic Apperception Test revealed a definite adjustment difficulty for the child. Because of the information and advice given by the psychologist, both the teacher and the clinician were able to treat these children more wisely.

In still another case, the counseling services of the psychologist were of inestimable value. A stutterer was determined to become a lawyer. The choice definitely appeared to be his own. But the psychologist discovered in talking with him that the choice was really his grandfather's. The boy was deeply interested in science and mathematics. As a result of conferences with the psychologist and the boy's parents, the boy changed his high-school major from social science to science and mathematics. The pressure to major and to do well in social studies, about which he was not enthusiastic, was removed.

A mother and father, both college graduates, set high academic standards for their boy—who was struggling through an academic high-school course. The psychologist helped the parents to understand their son and his academic problems—and in the process to better understand themselves. The boy is now doing very well in a general course. He spent some of his free time selling Christmas cards, which until recently was a forbidden activity. The suggestions and advice of the psychologist are particularly helpful in the adjustment of children such as these.

The psychologist's services may be of a more general nature. The problem may be one of social adjustment. Some children with speech difficulties need help in becoming a vital part of a group. According to a study by Marge (1966), sociometric results have indicated that there is a trend for the speech-handicapped child to hold a lower social position than that of the normal-speaking child in certain social inter-personal relationships. In the areas of study and work activity and of desirability as a dinner guest, the speech-handicapped child has a significantly lower social position than his normal-speaking peers.

MEDICAL PERSONNEL

When a speech defect is the result of an organic or psychological difficulty, the health authorities contribute to solving the speech problem by arranging for appropriate medical treatment. They talk the health problem over with the parents and frequently refer the child to medical specialists. For instance, the nurse's home visits may be the beginning of a sound health program for the child. At times the need for the help of other specialists is obvious. For example, when the results of the audiometric examination reveal a hearing loss, the child is referred to an otologist. The child with a cleft palate will be under the care of an oral or a plastic surgeon and an orthodontist. A stutterer with a serious adjustment difficulty may require psychiatric help. The situation where many specialists work together for the benefit of the child is ideal.

As the specialists work together, an appreciation for and an understanding of the work of the others comes about. Inevitably, some overlapping takes place. The speech clinician, for example, surmises that certain problems of the speech-handicapped child need investigation by the psychiatrist, psychologist, or doctor. The pediatrician, on the other hand, is concerned that a child has developed a stutter and recognizes that the child's speech difficulty needs treatment. The psychologist, in examining the speech-handicapped child, may uncover a deep-seated personality problem that the psychiatrist must handle. Each specialist is learning from those in other fields, and each is primarily interested in helping the child to develop into an effective and well-functioning human being.

References and Suggested Readings

Ainsworth, S., "The Speech Clinician in Public Schools: 'Participant' or 'Separatist'?" *ASHA*, VII (December, 1965), 495–503. (Explains point of view of speech clinician, his responsibilities to the schools, professional responsibilities, and implications for training.)

Allen, E. Y., et al., "Case Selection in the Public Schools," *Journal of Speech and Hearing Disorders*, XXXI (May, 1966), 157–161. (A group of authorities answer two questions: "What guidelines do you use in determining which children to enroll?" and "What tests of articulation have you found appropriate and predictive for children in primary grades?")

American Speech and Hearing Association, "Public School Speech and Hearing Services," *Journal of Speech and Hearing Disorders*, Monograph Supplement 8 (July, 1961.)

———, "The Speech Clinician's Role in the Public Schools," *ASHA*, VI (June, 1964), 189–191. (Details the functions and responsibilities of the speech clinician in the school setting.)

———, "Recommendations for Housing of Speech Services in the Schools," *ASHA*, XI (April, 1969), 181–182. (Describes room, equipment, furniture, and storage space for the speech correction room.)

Beckman, D. A., "Role of the Elementary-School Speech Therapist," *Today's Speech*, XIV (February, 1966), 2–4.

Black, M. E., "The Origins and Status of Speech Therapy in the Schools," *ASHA*, VIII (November, 1966), 419–425.

Breinholt, B. A., "New Look in Speech Education: Goals and Techniques for Programming," *Exceptional Child*, XXII (February, 1956), 194–196. (Explains the importance of the community in developing a successful speech program.)

Chipman, S., "On Receiving Your First Appointment as a Speech Correction Teacher," *The Speech Teacher*, IV (September, 1955), 173–175. (Gives advice about human relationships with teachers and supervisors.)

Edney, C. W., "The Public-School Remedial Speech Program," in W. Johnson et al., *Speech-Handicapped School Children*, 3rd ed., New York, Harper & Row, Publishers, 1967, pp. 433–501. (States the problems of the school speech therapist and makes sound suggestions for their solutions.)

Flower, R. M., E. Leach, C. R. Stone, and D. E. Yoder, "Case Selection," *Journal of Speech and Hearing Disorders*, XXXII (February, 1967), 65–70. (Gives rationale for selecting cases for remedial speech work in an institution for the mentally retarded.)

Fossum, E. C., "Cooperating with the Speech Correctionist," *Journal of Education*, CXXXVI (March, 1954), 182–184. (Explains the services of the clinician including surveys and in-service institutes for classroom teachers. Talks about the counseling of parents and cooperation with physicians.)

Garrison, G., *Speech and Hearing Services . . .A Design for Program Development*. Hartford, Conn., State Department of Education, Bulletin 92, 1960. (Suggests policies and procedures which will help in: 1) determining need for such a program, 2) organizing, conducting, and improving services, and 3) clarifying procedures to be followed in securing state funds for speech and hearing services in Connecticut. Contains samples of many forms needed in providing speech and hearing services.)

Irwin, R. B., "Speech Therapy in the Public Schools: State Legislation and Certification," *Journal of Speech and Hearing Disorders*, XXIV (May, 1959), 127–143. (Reviews state legislation and certification requirements for speech therapists in each state.)

———, "State Programs in Speech and Hearing Therapy: Certification," *The Speech Teacher*, IV (November, 1955), 253–358.(a)

————, "State Programs in Speech and Hearing Therapy: Legislation," *The Speech Teacher*, IV (March, 1955), 101–109.(b)

————, "State Programs in Speech and Hearing Therapy: Organization and Administration," *The Speech Teacher*, V (March, 1956), 125–131. (Studies case loads, patterns of organization, and the cost of therapy.)

Lilly, D., et al., "Annual Review of Journal of Speech and Hearing Research, 1967," *Journal of Speech and Hearing Disorders*, XXXVI (November, 1968), 303–317. (Reviews research concerning case selection and articulatory testing.)

Lillywhite, H. S., and R. L. Sleeter, "Some Problems of Relationships Between Speech and Hearing Specialists and Those in the Medical Profession," *ASHA*, I (December, 1959), 127–131. (Suggests sound, specific ways in which the speech clinician can cooperate with the medical profession.)

Luper, H. L., and S. H. Ainsworth, "Speech Correction Rooms in the Public Schools," *Exceptional Child*, XXII (October, 1955), 24–26. (Indicates space, acoustic treatment, and special furnishing needed for the speech correction room.)

Mackie, R. P., and W. Johnson, *Speech Correctionists: The Competencies They Need for the Work They Do*. Washington, D.C., U.S. Government Printing Office, Bulletin 19, 1957.

Marge, D. K., "The Social Status of Speech-Handicapped Children," *Journal of Speech and Hearing Research*, IX (June, 1966), 165–177.

Martin, E. W., "Client-Centered Therapy as a Theoretical Orientation for Speech Therapy," *ASHA*, V (April, 1963), 576–578.

Matis, E. E., "Psychotherapeutic Tools for Parents," *Journal of Speech and Hearing Disorders*, XXVI (May, 1961), 164–170. (Suggests help for parents of speech-handicapped children.)

Monsees, E. K., and C. Berman, "Speech and Language Screening in a Summer Headstart Program," *Journal of Speech and Hearing Disorders*, XXXIII (May, 1968), 121–126. (Describes screening test which is the result of a study of the characteristics of language of the culturally disadvantaged.)

Peins, M., "Client-Centered Communication Therapy for Mentally Retarded Delinquents," *Journal of Speech and Hearing Disorders*, XXXII (May, 1967), 154–161. (Lists purposes and goals of therapy emphasizing two-way communication. Describes therapy programs in terms of ten mentally retarded delinquent adolescent boys.)

Powers, M. H., "What Makes an Effective Public-School Speech Therapist," *Journal of Speech and Hearing Disorders*, XXI (December, 1956), 461–467. (Includes material on professional relationships, personal characteristics, and professional attitudes and ethics.)

Pronovost, W., "Case Selection in the Schools: Articulatory Disorders," *ASHA*, VIII (May, 1966), 179–181.

Prahl, H. M., and E. B. Cooper, "Accuracy of Teacher Referrals of Speech-Handicapped School Children," *ASHA*, VI (October, 1964), 392.

Rees, M., and G. L. Smith, "Some Recommendations for Supervised

School Experience for Student Clinicians," *ASHA*, X (March, 1968), 93–103. (Suggests criteria for scheduling, qualifications of college supervisors, supervisions, evaluation, and experiences of student clinicians.)

Sommers, R. K., et al., "Effects of Various Durations of Speech Improvements upon Articulation and Reading," *Journal of Speech and Hearing Disorders*, XXVII (February, 1962), 54–61.

———, "Effectiveness of Group and Individual Therapy," *Journal of Speech and Hearing Research*, IX (June, 1966), 219–225.

Stern, J., "Speech Correctionist, Classroom Teacher, Parents, and the Child with a Speech Defect," *ASHA*, I (November, 1959), 84. (Discusses cooperation among speech clinicians, parents, and classroom teacher.)

Van Hattum, R. J., "The Defensive Speech Clinicians in the Schools," *Journal of Speech and Hearing Disorders*, XXXI (August, 1966), 234–240. (Talks about the basic issues in training the school speech clinician, and suggests solutions.)

Van Riper, C., "Success and Failure in Speech Therapy," *Journal of Speech and Hearing Disorders*, XXXI (August, 1966), 276–278. (Suggests that the therapist ask two questions, "What is it that this person needs?" and "What is it that he needs from me?")

Webster, E. J., "Parent Counseling by Speech Pathologists and Audiologists," *Journal of Speech and Hearing Disorders*, XXXI (November, 1966), 331–340. (Tells how to help parents modify the circle of poor communication with their children.)

Webster, E. J., W. H. Perkins, H. H. Bloomer, W. Pronovost, "Case Selection in the Schools," *Journal of Speech and Hearing Disorders*, XXXI (November, 1966), 352–358. (Helps to develop criteria for choosing children who need speech correction services.)

Weiner, P. S., "The Emotionally Disturbed Child in the Speech Clinic: Some Considerations," *Journal of Speech and Hearing Disorders*, XXXIII (May, 1968), 158–166. (Discusses the problem of whether the emotionally disturbed child should be accepted in a speech clinic.)

Zinner, E. M., "Role of the Speech Correctionist as a Colleague on the School Health Team," *Journal of School Health*, XXXIII (May, 1963), 193–195.

Problems

1. Outline the kind of program for speech-handicapped children that your state provides. How does this program compare with that of one of your neighboring states?
2. Read and report on one of the following references: Allen et al., 1966; American Speech and Hearing Association, 1964; Black, 1966; Breinholt, 1956; Chipman, 1955; Fossum, 1954; Luper and Ainsworth, 1955; Martin, 1963; Powers, 1956; Pronovost, 1966; Sommers, 1962; Van Hattum, 1966; Webster, 1966.

3. Indicate how the services for the speech and hearing-handicapped in your town are organized. What do you think can be done to improve this program?
4. What are the professional requirements for a school speech therapist in your state? How do these compare with the requirements in one of your neighboring states?
5. Does your state provide additional financial help to schools that have speech correction programs? Does your school superintendent consider the financial assistance sufficient?
6. Compare the requisites for competence needed by the speech clinician with those you believe the classroom teacher needs.

Chapter 3

Standards
of Speech

In the first chapter we indicated that some students communicate with their fellow students and their teacher quite adequately even though the speech patterns of some of these students are nonstandard. We noted that helping students attain established speech patterns lies within the realm of the classroom teacher rather than of the speech clinician. This chapter deals with the concept of speech standards and the role of the teacher in helping students eliminate nonstandard speech.

In discussions of pronunciations, neighbors, friends, storekeepers look to the teacher as an authority. Rarely a week goes by when a teacher is not asked to arbitrate an argument about the pronunciation of a word. Comments heard during these discussions vary:

- "Jane's affected. She says *tomahto*. Why doesn't she say *potahto*?"
- "One of my students criticized me for saying *ketch* for *catch*."
- "That conductor always says *krick*. I wish somebody would tell him it's *creek*."
- "You pronounce *orange* funny. You say *ahrange*."
- "I distinguish between the verb and the noun when I use *rise*. I say the *rice* of civilization."

All these queries and complaints are trivial. Even though a person says *tomahto*, his speech is not necessarily affected. Those who live in the North Central section of America usually do say *ketch*. In the United States as a whole *krick* is used almost as commonly as *creek*. *Awrange* is common in some areas; *ahrange* in others. If you live in Eastern New England, the New York City area, the Middle Atlantic area, or the South, you probably say *ahrange*. If you live in the Southern Mountain area, you are more likely to say *ahrange* than *awrange*. But if you live in another part of the country, you usually say *awrange*. Few of us, and probably no recent dictionaries, distinguish between the noun and the verb form for *rise*.

Interest in pronunciation arises because pronouncing words acceptably is essentially a social skill. The true test of a social skill is whether the act is performed without apparent effort and in a manner that draws no attention to its execution—that is, the act is completely habitual. Because of this social skill, cultivated, educated persons tend to sound alike. Their speech is characterized neither by nonstandard pronunciation nor by usage that suggests self-consciousness or affectation. Educated people with different regional dialects find that their speech patterns are not a handicap. Although the educated American from Georgia speaks somewhat differently from the educated American from Boston, their pronunciations and intonation patterns provide interesting and desirable variety. These individuals are speaking the prestigious dialect of their particular community.

The Classroom and a Prestigious Dialect

What can be a handicap in both a social and a learning situation is a social dialect that is not prestigious in the local community. For example, Ozark, Pidgin, Appalachian, or various Negro dialects spoken by poorly educated persons can be handicapping in a community other than their own. These people possess what in the eyes of many leaders of a larger community are nonstandard features. Consequently, in certain social circles the nonstandard features hinder communication. The candidate for District Attorney who says "tooim" and "dis" and "dat" detracts from his "source image" or "ethical appeal" with some of his audience even though what he has to say has real and significant import to the community.

We believe, therefore, that it is usually best for children to acquire the more prestigious dialect. Although we do not believe it to be "more correct," we do believe that in the United States the fact of speaking a community's prestigious dialect brings with it positive values, both socially and economically. We also believe that children should be given the opportunity to learn the prestigious dialect, just as they are given the opportunity to learn other acceptable modes of behavior in today's society.

Here we should note that some writers who believe that teachers should not confuse the middle class' social stigma of a particular dialect with its linguistic capacities as a linguistic tool are not particularly concerned with presenting children with the option of learning the "prestigious" dialect. They consider the sum total of dialectal variations as self-contained, systematic, ordered systems different from but neither communicatively more or less effective than what is considered "standard English." They believe that a nonstandard dialectal system with its logical and consistent rules is an effective code for expressing ideas and concepts. Because of this point of view, they would not believe teaching standard English to be as desirable as we do.

Language and culture and language and one's self-concept are entwined. If in Hawaii pidgin is part of an individual's culture and of his image of himself, it should not be ridiculed but accepted. However, to learn a different dialect, one that seems to be demanded by another culture, should also be possible. That the high-school student may want to speak pidgin with his friends is surely understandable and often desirable, but that he be able to speak a type of standard English in certain other circumstances seems equally understandable and desirable.

Every young child must develop language to express his ideas and feelings; for this purpose he should use whatever language feels most comfortable. In a few instances, the young child's language may necessarily be almost entirely pantomimic. But it is better that he communicate through gesture than not at all. Eventually he can be weaned from his pantomimic language to spoken (oral) language. In other instances, the child's language may possess many nonstandard features. In still others, it may be the prestigious dialect of the community. But every young child must first speak in sentences, so that he is developing his particular linguistic potential; furthermore, in his early years he does better with his native tongue than with a superimposed one.

In discussing when to start teaching standard English, Loban writes:

> The strategy is merely that the pre-school stage and kindergarten are much too early to press him to be concerned about using standard dialect continuously. Such teaching only confuses small children, causing them to speak much less frequently in school. Usually from grade three and after, the children's daily recitation should adhere to standard English, but in the early years the teacher would accept "him a good dog." At this stage the teacher would be more interested in eliciting from the child, "him a good dog but with three fleas"; indeed, the teacher would be very much interested in such qualification and amplification (Loban, 1968, p. 595).

William Stewart and other linguists believe that the Negro dialect is a viable tool for communication, that the speaker can use it to communicate abstractions, and also that it is based on a different linguistic system from standard American English. Bailey illustrates this last concept:

> Specialists in Creole linguistics believe that the verb system of the Negro speakers of non-standard English is much more like that of the English-based Creoles than of standard English, and that unless teachers understand that this is a valid system with its own grammatical rules, they cannot intelligently guide the children into an acquisition of the new system that is so much like their own that the possibility of linguistic interferences increases at every turn. The Creole languages express the possessive relationship, the number distinction in nouns and verbs, the past tense in verbs, and the cases of pronouns by different means from the Indo-European languages, in which such relationships are indicated by suffixation of some kind. Grammatical relations in the Creoles are largely expressed by juxtaposition of words, by the aid of special function words, or by the stress and pitch patterns (Bailey, 1968, p. 573).

This difference from American English may well persist in children's speech because of the dominance of the language that the child first learned. Therefore, when the child systematically omits the final *t* and *d* for the past tense as in *I like her* for *I liked her* and *I lug the box* for *I lugged the box*, he may well be using a morphological system that is different from those of children speaking American English. The teacher's acceptance of this as one mode of communication is important although at some point he must attempt to help the child build a second mode of communication.

TEACHING THE PRESTIGIOUS DIALECT

In the early years of the child the teacher provides for the building of this second mode through a series of listening experiences. For instance, she can introduce children to dialects quite different from their own. Robbie Burns' Scots dialect has a lovely lilt to which children enjoy listening. The teacher can then translate the dialect into American English. Thus, at an early age, the child begins to ascertain dialectal differences. The teacher can focus attention on the contrasting features of two different dialects.

Loban suggests talking over social language discrimination in grades five, six, or seven:

> Eventually the time comes when the teacher must talk over with these pupils the facts of social language discrimination, and that time, to my

way of thinking, usually is grade five, six, or seven. Teachers differ on the ideal age for introducing the concept, but I see no point in telling children this earlier. Before they can really see the value of learning standard English, pupils need to understand the social consequences the world will exact of them if they cannot handle the established dialect. Grade five, six, or seven, therefore, would be the point at which the concept would be discussed, although parts of the total concept might be sketched in earlier as answers to questions children ask. At this grade level I would select most carefully teachers who do not have snobbish attitudes about language, the scholar-linguist-humanists whom the school could most safely entrust with the important task of explaining sociological truth to these children, aged 11 and 12 (Loban, 1968, p. 519).

We have already indicated some of the problems of teaching the established speech patterns. Others exist. You yourself may feel that according to the democratic idea, you should go beyond being accepting of the child's native language into encouraging him to continue to use it through his school life. Or you may feel that you are helping children to spurn those with whom they are growing up. When, however, you are teaching standard American English as a second language, your children can use it as a necessary tool of communication when they have to. Even a popular magazine such as *Newsweek* advocates this procedure. Part of an article, "A Guest in Ghetto America," includes a statement describing the attitude of Warren Saunders, who runs Chicago's Better Boys' Foundation, whose pet project is nonstandard English and whose pet peeve is teachers who are forever upbraiding the kids for the way they talk.

> "If I tamper with a person's first language," says Saunders, "I'm suggesting that all he has been and felt in the past is bad." The ghetto dialect has a discernible structure and idiom of its own. Example: "My sister gone" means that she is away but will soon be back; "My sister be gone" means that she's gone away, perhaps for good. Not that Saunders thinks children shouldn't be taught proper English; emphatically, they should, but they should be told it is another, and very useful, way of speaking (Elliott, 1969, pp. 42–43).

Definition of Standard English

We have already talked about "prestigious" speech and "established" speech. According to Webster's *Third New International Dictionary*, standard English is defined as "the English that with respect to speaking, grammar, pronunciation and vocabulary is substantially uniform though not devoid of regional differences, that is well established by usage in the formal and informal speech and writing of the educated, and that is widely recognized or acceptable wherever English is spoken or understood."

On the other hand, "substandard" usage ("nonstandard" is not defined) is defined by Webster's *Third* as "conforming to a pattern of linguistic usage existing within a speech community but not that of the prestige group in that community in choice of word (as *set* for *sit*), form of word (as *brung* for *brought*), pronunciation (as *twicet* for *twice*), construction (as *the boys is growing fast*) or idiom (as *all to once* for *all at once*). The older child who says, "*Awri I din't*" is using nonstandard speech and is calling attention to his lack of education and a culture different from the common middle and upper class culture.

Onflowing Speech

Words, almost never spoken singly, are usually part of a phrase or a sentence. As your friend asks, "Are you going to buy a red or blue dress?" you may respond, "Red." Even here, however, you are apt to respond with, "A red dress" or "I need a red one to match my shoes and purse." Speech moves or flows onward from word to word within a phrase. In onflowing speech an assimilative process is always at work and the sounds of syllables of different words may be linked as "Aredress," [ərɛd:rɛs] for *a red dress. What is* usually becomes "Whats" or "Wats" [hwɑts] or [wɑts].

These words and phrases are made up of individual speech sounds, each represented by a symbol of the IPA. The phrases have been written as you might hear a speaker uttering them. The study of sounds and their combination is a tool needed in studying both the normal and the abnormal speech of children. You will find a discussion of speech sounds and their representation in Chapter 6.

CHANGES IN LANGUAGE

Styles of pronunciation change. Many of these changes are obvious. We do not pronounce the *k* in *know, knight,* and *knee.* These words began to lose their *k* sound in the seventeenth century and completed the loss in the eighteenth century. *K* does remain in the Germanized pronunciation of such proper names as *Knag* or *Knode.* The seventeenth-century poet Alexander Pope rhymed *join* with *thine.* We know that *join* was then pronounced *jine.* Furthermore, he rhymed *obey* with *tea. Tea* was then pronounced *tay.* Changes may occur in the pronunciations within families from one generation to the next. A father and mother may say *erster* for *oyster* and *boin* for *burn*. Their daughter, however, pronounces *oyster* and *burn* the way most of the rest of us do. Here some outside influence, perhaps that of the child's playmates or her teachers, brings about the change.

ASSIMILATION

Language is always changing as words, meanings, and pronunciations are added or discarded. Part of the change in pronunciation is the result of the influence of adjacent sounds. *Assimilation*, the modification of pronunciation, has usually occurred over the decades in the direction of simplicity and economy of effort. For instance, the past tense of *flip* is *flipped*. The final sound is not a [d] but a [t]. [p] is an unvoiced sound that influences the unvoicing of the sound [d] that follows. [t] is made like [d] except that it is unvoiced. In other verbs where the final sound of the verb in its present tense is voiced, the [d] of the past tense is preserved. For instance, the final sound in *begged* is [d] because [g] is a voiced sound; the same is true of plurals. The final sound in *taps* is [s] but in *tabs* is [z]. The [b], which is voiced, influences the [s] to become [z]. *Captain* sometimes becomes *Capm* [kæpm]. [p] is made with both lips and this position influences [n] to become [m]. But the nasal characteristic of the [n] is maintained. [t] is dropped entirely, however. In *horseshoe* [s], too, is completely lost; [ʃ] takes over [s].

Some assimilations are widely used; others are not. *Nature* and *picture* are commonly pronounced *nacher* and *pikcher*. Almost all of us take these pronunciations with their assimilations for granted. Almost none of us attempt to say *natyer* or *pictyer*. The same kind of change occurs when we say *wonchu* for *won't you*. Some persons are loathe to accept the assimilation in *wonchu* although they themselves use the same kind of assimilation in *nature*. The following lines of Ogden Nash represent this type of assimilation:

> What would you do if you were up a dark alley with Caesar Borgia
> And he was coming torgia.

Assimilation is illustrated by what has occurred in derivatives of words with the Latin prefix *cum*. The [m] remains in *complicate* and *comfort*, has become [n] in such words as *conspire* and *consign*, and is *ng* [ŋ] in such words as *congregate* and *conquer*. In *complicate* and *comfort*, [m], [p], and [f] all involve the lips. In *conspire*, *consign*, and *contain*, [n], [s], and [t] all involve the tip of the tongue and the gum or alveolar ridge. In *congregate* ['kɑŋgrɪˌget] and *conquer* ['kɑŋˌkɚ], the *ng* [ŋ], [k], and [g] all involve the back of the tongue and the soft palate.

DISSIMILATION

Dissimilation is a change where a sound is dropped or changed from the original to make it less like its neighbor. Making two identical or closely similar articulatory movements within a brief time span proves difficult; therefore, to omit or change the sound is easier. The modern English word *turtle* is the result of the change of the final *r* in the original *turture* to *l*. A present-day example is the loss of the first *r* in *library* or in *February*.

STRONG AND WEAK FORMS

Another example of change in onflowing speech is the use of weak rather than strong forms. The following are examples: When a child reads the word *to* in a list of words, he pronounces it as he does *two* or *too*. But when he reads *to* in the sentence, "I want to do it," the vowel in *to* is no longer a long $\overline{oo}$ but a short $\breve{oo}$ or even the schwa [ə], the sound in the last syllable of *sofa*. The *to* pronounced like *two* is the strong form while the *to* pronounced like [tə] is the weak form. When we say, "We live in Apartment 2A," we pronounce the *a* to rhyme with *day*. But when we say, "We live in a house," the *a* is the same sound as we use in the last syllable of *sofa*, the schwa. The *a* that rhymes with *day* is the strong form; the one that is the schwa is the weak form. The *a* in *and* in a list of words is pronounced with a short *a*, but the *a* of *and* in the phrase *Mary and John* is likely to be the schwa. The first *a* is the strong form; the second *a*, the weak form. Ordinarily we use the weak forms of pronouns, prepositions, articles, auxiliaries, and conjunctions in conversation, except where we stress a particular word. For example, when we want to stress that *both* Mary and John are going, we may use the strong form of *and*. In strong forms, the vowel is stressed; in weak forms it is unstressed.

Influence of Spelling on Pronunciation

Until the fifteenth or sixteenth century spelling, changing frequently, kept pace with changes in pronunciation. As we look at the following extract from the Prologue to *The Canterbury Tales*, we realize how different our spelling is today. This excerpt is representative of Middle English.

THE PRIORESSE:

Ther was also a nonne, a Prioresse,
That of hir smylyng was ful symple and coy;

Hir gretteste ooth was but by Seint Loy;
And she was cleped Madame Eglentyne.
Ful wel she soong the servyce dyvyne,
Entuned in hir nose ful semely, ...

For the last four or five hundred years spelling has remained relatively constant while pronunciations have changed. Spelling today, therefore, does not closely approximate the pronunciation of words. For example, the *t* sound in *castle* and *whistle*, the *b* sound in *limb* and *comb*, the *w* sound in *write*, the *s* sound in *island*, and the *l* sound in *calm* are not pronounced. The *ĭ* [ɪ] sound is variously spelled as *o* in *women*, *y* in *myth*, and *i* in *linen*.

The discrepancy between sound and spelling has caused some persons to ask that the writing conform to the sounds. Thus, over the years, many attempts have been made to change spelling to reflect the spoken word. Before George Bernard Shaw died, he specified in his will that a considerable sum of money be used for spelling reform. Such systems are frequently proposed, then abandoned. The same discrepancy has caused others to try to make the sound conform to the spelling. Some people today try to pronounce both *p* and *b* in *cupboard* and all the sounds in *indict*. Although the *t* in *often* was dropped, it is creeping back. The same is true of the *l* in *almond*. Some of our American pronunciations as distinguished from British pronunciations show that we have placed some value on spelling. For example the name *Anthony* in Britain is pronounced with a *t* for the *th* and *secretary* in British English usually has three syllables as compared to our four syllables.

Influence of Dictionaries on Pronunciation

Long before dictionaries existed, people understood the words that others pronounced. Today, however, lexicographers record pronunciations. One of the dictionary's functions is to describe the pronunciation of a word, not to dictate or prescribe it. The early lexicographers based their recording of pronunciations not only on the pronunciations of the cultured people of the time, such as statesmen and actors, but also on their own idiosyncrasies. Daniel Webster, however, realized that pronunciations must be based on the pronunciations of the people. Mencken says of Webster:

He was always at great pains to ascertain actual usages and in the course of his journeys from State to State to perfect his copyright on his first spelling book he accumulated a large amount of interesting and valuable material, especially in the field of pronunciation. . . . He proposed therefore that an American standard be set up, independent of the English standard, and that it be inculcated in the schools throughout the country. He argued that it should be determined not by "the practice of any particular class of people," but by "the general practice of the nation . . ." (Mencken, 1946, p. 9).

Today, lexicographers do try to record accurately the pronunciations of the educated, cultured members of our country and to keep the recordings current.

A pronunciation given in a dictionary is a generalization of the way many persons say a word. The recording of this generalization differs from dictionary to dictionary. Dictionaries frequently record more than one pronunciation. In some instances, the first pronunciation is the one held to be more widely used; in others, the editor makes no attempt to show which pronunciation is the more prevalent. At least one dictionary indicates pronunciations current in regional areas. Most do not. Some dictionaries record the pronunciations using diacritic markings; others record them with phonetic symbols. Some adopt for representation the style of formal platform speech; others include informal pronunciations. The teacher should read the introduction to a dictionary to learn what its levels and procedures are. He should also note its date to determine whether the pronunciations recorded are current.

Dictionaries are useful in assisting us to pronounce unfamiliar words. When students come across a word like *esophageal*, the dictionary is an excellent source of information for pronunciation. But for the usual, everyday words, students do better to train their ears to listen rather than to find the pronunciations in the dictionary, for we learn pronunciation largely through imitation. The person desiring to improve his pronunciation must listen to the speech of the educated, cultivated members of his community who have had certain social advantages. In addition, he must listen to himself (often with a recorder) so that he knows how his speech differs from theirs. If a student looks up *duty* in the dictionary, he may find the *y* sound before the *u*; however, careful reading of the introduction of the dictionary usually indicates that the word is pronounced both with and without the *y* sound. Surely to listen and to perceive the differences is more helpful than to use the dictionary. Furthermore, dictionaries give pronunciations of a word as it is used individually. When we speak, however, we rarely speak in single words, but rather in phrases or sentences. The same words used in different phrases with different rhythm, tempo, intonation, and meaning intended by the speaker do not sound alike. For instance, dictionaries usually include the strong forms (stressed ones), not the weak forms (unstressed). The student, whether in elementary or in secondary school, should learn to use the weak forms both in speaking and in reading aloud.

Speech Styles

The particular speaking situation influences the speaker's speech patterns. Martin Joos (1962) notes that people use a wide variety of speech styles—varying from the most intimate to the most formal and that they automatically shift to whatever is appropriate to the social situation. When children play ball in an open field, they speak more loudly than usual, more quickly, often in shorter phrases and with a quite different choice of language from when they are playing a word game upon which they are concentrating to recall unusual words. As they speak together in the classroom, they are likely to speak more formally, in longer phrases, and be more careful of their pronunciations than they are when they call to each other on the playground. In a school assembly, the child who introduces the speaker speaks still more formally—more slowly, with more stresses, with more careful choice of language. Thus, the continuum goes from very informal speech, often with many nonstandard pronunciations, to formal speech with few nonstandard pronunciations. Labov notes that when subjects in his research answered questions that they formally recognized as part of an interview, their speech was careful. He explains that the situation was not as formal as a public address and was less formal than the speech that would be used in a first interview for a job, but was certainly more formal than casual conversation among friends or family members (Labov, 1966, p. 92).

Cultural Differences

Voice and pronunciation characteristics exist on all kinds of local cultural and subcultural levels. The influence of the social group on both voice and pronunciation is important. When you hear "She roars like a fishwife," you know exactly what the speaker is implying. Similarly, the influence of the social group on pronunciation is strong. When the child grows up in an environment where all the children say "acrost" for *across* and "elem tree" for *elm tree*, he probably uses the same pronunciation. Vance Packard notes a difference in upper and middle class vocabulary. The middle classes sit on a davenport, wear a formal gown or tuxedo, and greet a newcomer with "Pleased to meet you," whereas the upper classes sit on a sofa, wear a long dress or a dinner jacket, and greet a new friend with "Hello" (Packard, 1961), page 124). Similarly, certain speech patterns often suggest certain social classes.

Regional Differences

We have spoken about "prestigious" pronunciations and have indicated that pronunciations, voice, and vocabulary differ in varying speech situations. We have talked about the influence of particular social cultures and subcultures. Another difference exists—that of region. Kenneth Goodman points out that socially acceptable speech varies from region to region and that no dialect of American English has ever achieved the status of some imaginary standard which is correct everywhere and always. He writes:

> It is obvious that a teacher in Atlanta, Georgia, is foolish to try to get her children to speak like cultured people in Detroit or Chicago . . . cultured speech, socially preferred, is not the same in Boston, New York, Philadelphia, Miami, Baltimore, Atlanta, or Chicago. The problem, if any, comes when the Bostonian moves to Chicago, the New Yorker to Los Angeles, the Atlantan to Detroit. Americans are ethnocentric in regard to most cultural traits, but they are doubly so with regard to language. Anybody who doesn't speak the way I do is wrong. A green onion is not a scallion. I live in Detróit not Détroit. I can carry my books to work but not my friends. *Fear* ends with an *r* and *Cuba* does not. Such ethnocentrisms are unfortunate among the general public (Goodman, 1967, p. 41).

The educated person from Boston has little difficulty understanding the educated person from Atlanta. The backwoodsman from Minnesota with little education may, however, have difficulty understanding the mountaineer from Tennessee with little education. Differences in speech among the educated are not as wide as those among the uneducated, even though admittedly there are discernible differences in the speech patterns of educated persons of different areas.

Early texts dealing with phonetics list three main regional zones: Southern, Eastern, and General American, with General American being spoken by about four fifths of the population. The work of linguistic scholars, however, now defines geographical divisions more precisely. Thomas (1958, p. 216) reports that the geographical divisions in American speech are most clearly defined along the Atlantic coast. There he notes Eastern New England, the Middle Atlantic area, and the

South. He adds to these areas the New York City area which he says is anomalous because its speech resembles both the Middle Atlantic and Southern types and because this type was never reflected farther west. He further includes the North Central area, Western Pennsylvania, with Pittsburgh as its cultural and economic center, the Southern Mountain area, including most of the mountain settlements of some Southern states, Central Midland, the Northwest, and the Southwest coastal area.[1]

The differences among the areas are, however, not too numerous. A New Englander and a Southerner may say *bahn* for *barn*, whereas an Ohioan is likely to pronounce the *r* in the same word. A New Englander approaches *pahth* for *path*. The Ohioan is likely to use the same vowel in *path* that he uses in *cat*. In the South the *o* in *glory* is usually the same *o* as in *tote;* whereas in some other regions, it may be the *aw* sound in *law*. The vowel in the word *scarce* in the North Central and Eastern areas may be either the vowel found in *hate* or the one in *let;* in the South, for the word *scarce* the vowel in *hat* is heard frequently. In *greasy* and the verb *grease*, the New Englander uses the *s* sound whereas the Southerner uses the *z* sound.

Improving Pronunciation

The first question is *what* to improve. Teachers are not concerned with regional differences, nor with pronunciations that are widely accepted. They are concerned with those characteristics that tend to generate the impression that speech is not prestigious, that it contains many nonstandard pronunciations. These nonstandard deviations, unlike articulatory defects, which are definitely speech difficulties, are not the responsibility of the speech clinician but of the classroom teacher. The ten-year-old boy who substitutes *f* and *v* for the two *th*'s and says *acrost* for *across* is in need of help from the teacher to understand and sometimes to eliminate his nonstandard speech.

Nonstandard Speech

Nonstandard speech may include: 1) substitution of one sound for another, 2) omission of sounds, 3) addition of sounds, 4) transposition of sounds, and 5) distortion of sounds.

---

[1] See map in C. K. Thomas, *Phonetics of American English* (New York, The Ronald Press Company, 1958), p. 232, or in A. J. Bronstein, *The Pronunciation of American English* (New York, Appleton-Century-Crofts, 1960), p. 46.

SUBSTITUTION OF SOUNDS

Nonstandard pronunciation frequently involves the substitution of one sound for another; for example, one consonant may be substituted for another. A common substitution is that of *d* for *th*, as *dem* and *dose* for *them* and *those*. The teacher must remember, however, that many substitutions are made by educated people. For example, many educated speakers pronounce *when*, *where*, and *what* with an initial *w*, though others do use the *wh* sound. Other substitutions frequently used by the educated are *ingcome tax* for *income tax*, *grampa* for *grandpa*, and *pangcake* for *pancake*. The substitution may involve vowels rather than consonants, as when *boyd* is substituted for *bird*. In some areas, this substitution is fast disappearing—perhaps partly because of the humor associated with it. Stories like the following give a social impetus to drop the substitution:

> The child said to the teacher, "Look at the boid on the windowsill."
> The teacher remonstrated, "You mean *bird*."
> To which the child replied, "Choips like a boid."

Many vowel substitutions are so widely employed that they have become acceptable. *Git* for *get* is heard so frequently that many speakers would not even notice the substitution. Other vowel substitutions are regional. Many Midwesterners use the same vowel in *merry*, *Mary*, and *marry*. Again these substitutions are so widely used that almost no one would notice them. On the other hand, as *milkman* becomes *mulkman*, as *been* becomes *ben*, the substitution may distract from the message.

OMISSION OF SOUNDS

In informal speech most of us omit many sounds even though they are included in the orthographic representation of the word. For example, the word *clothes* is frequently pronounced *cloz*, omitting the *th* sound. Both the *American College Dictionary* and Webster's *New Collegiate Dictionary* accept these variants. Before a teacher insists on the inclusion of a sound, we recommend that he consult a good, recent dictionary. The following are some of the omissions that probably do not occur in formal speech: *bout* for *about*; *Bufflo* for *Buffalo*; *kunt* for *couldn't*; *ask* for *asked*; *mosly* for *mostly*; *simily* for *similarly*; *reconize* for *recognize*.

ADDITION OF SOUNDS

Sounds are frequently added or inserted. Historically we have added sounds; for instance, *against* was once *agens*. Although dictionaries for years did not recognize the *t* in *often* or the *h* in *forehead*, some dictionaries now include both of these pronunciations. Many, many speakers pronounce *mince* as if it were *mints* or *dance* as if it were *dants*. The insertion of the excrescent [t] makes for easier, more economical pronunciation by all, including the educated. But some additions and insertions are less common in the speech of the educated. Examples of these are: *athaletic* for *athletic*; *anywheres* for *anywhere*; *oncet* for *once*; *drownded* for *drowned*; *wisht* for *wish*; *pursh* for *push*.

TRANSPOSITION OF SOUNDS

Children frequently and adults sometimes transpose sounds. Here again, dictionaries record that educated persons use some of these transpositions. Kenyon and Knott list both *children* and *childern* and *hundred* and *hunderd*. Transpositions rarely used by educated persons include: *prespire* for *perspire*; *plubicity* for *publicity*; *modren* for *modern*; *revelant* for *relevant*; *I akst him* for *I asked him*; *pernounce* for *pronounce*; *tradegy* for *tragedy*; *patrin* for *pattern*; and *osifer* for *officer*.

DISTORTION OF SOUNDS

Sometimes a child approximates a given sound but distorts it. He may make an *s* so that it cannot be readily distinguished from an *sh*. The problem arises as to how liberal to be in accepting distortions. The first part of the diphthong of *now* is normally a back sound. Many Americans, however, raise the tongue on the first part of this diphthong so that it is in the same position as the vowel in *cat*. Many Americans raise the tongue on the vowel sound in *hat* nearly to the position of the vowel sound in *met*. The teacher must make a value judgment on whether to motivate the child to change the pronunciation of the diphthong in *now* and the vowel in *cat*.

Establishing Prestigious Dialects

As noted earlier, some children need to learn to speak standard English as a second language. The work of Roger Shuy suggests methods for this. Other children need to be made aware that to speak well is a social advantage. For this second group, the teacher leads a discussion by asking such questions as: What do we mean by "speaking well?" Who speaks well? Are there various degrees of speaking well? Should we always speak equally well? When do we need to speak particularly well? Where do we need to speak particularly well? How can we help each other to speak well?

As children talk about effective speech, they will not only list
"correct" pronunciation, pleasant voices, saying the sounds "correctly," but they will also include other factors such as sounding
friendly, making oneself clear to others, and having others respond
favorably. One child said that speaking well was really a way of getting
along well with others. This idea, at first rejected by the children, provided the basic impetus for the children's speech work. A teacher can
help children to realize that our speech today is a living, changing
medium of communication. Children are interested in the idea that
pronunciations have changed, that meanings of words have changed,
and even that grammar has changed over the centuries.

As children talk about who speaks well, they are really setting up
standards against which to compare their own speech. They usually
include some of the educated members of the community, some of the
well-known broadcasters. Analyzing what makes the speech of a
particular broadcaster effective is helpful. Such talk encourages children to listen to the pronunciations of broadcasters and, as a result,
often to be critical of their own pronunciations. Many times they
imitate some of the pronunciations of broadcasters. One teacher
employs a very interesting device to teach the influence of varying
speech situations on those involved in them. She uses puppets dressed
in various ways—as a king, a queen, a bedraggled beggar. As the
children manipulate the puppets, they speak as they think the characters would. This device serves as a basis for a discussion of how people
in various walks of life speak differently.

The question, "Why do we need to speak well?" is provocative.
Some students frankly feel little need to speak well; they say that
nobody seems to have trouble in understanding them and that the
quality of their speech makes no difference in their relationships with
people. Other youngsters, on the other hand, consider good speech a
valuable asset. One boy said that when he collected for his newspapers
he talked carefully. He said he thought his customers might not consider him a good salesman if he spoke carelessly. He also made the
point that his attempts at good speech and good manners paid divi-
dends in terms of tips. He ended by admitting that he enjoyed speaking
well and being courteous to his customers.

This topic leads naturally into a discussion of the places where acceptable speech is important. Children usually agree that whatever their
jobs are going to be, they will have to speak well. This objective is not
immediate. Therefore, children must think of present situations where
they need good speech. One child said that while he works in his
father's shoe repair shop, he must wait on customers with good manners
and with good speech so that they will feel right toward him and
understand easily.

In this discussion the teacher's own voice and pronunciations are important. Unconsciously, the child thinks of how his teacher sounds as he speaks. As children feel warm and friendly toward their teachers, they imitate them. They wear similar clothes, walk like the teacher, and talk like him.

Feedback

Having been motivated to speak well, what does the child do about it? Authorities who discuss change often emphasize the need for three functions: 1) scanning, 2) comparing, and 3) correcting.

In *scanning*, the child receives information through sensory channels about how his speech mechanism is performing and about the result of the performance, the utterance. In addition, he feels what part of his speech mechanism works on what other part and is aware of such a factor as the nasal emission of [m]. The child must be taught to scan effectively so that he can examine the product of his speech mechanism carefully.

In *comparing*, the child must match his speech patterns against the standard he desires to achieve. He examines the dominant features of an utterance and matches what he says against what he wishes to say. Because there is obviously not time to match every sound before uttering the next sound, he compares key features of entire patterns of sounds rather than individual sounds.

Ogilvie and Rees use the comparison of the expert typist: As you watch an expert typist, you can understand the comparison of the back-flow of message against a standard pattern. The typist places her fingers on the eight designated keys and proceeds to hit the necessary keys to type the words that correspond to the pattern she is following. In her almost automatically controlled typing, a discrepancy between her pattern and her copy can take place. She discovers the error through her "feel" that she has hit the wrong key or through her visual inspection of her typed copy. The "feel" is all important for speed in typing. The expert typist often knows through "feel" that she is about to make an error; she may then correct it before it actually occurs, thereby maintaining her rhythm and speed. But when the error has occurred, she confirms her impression of error through visual inspection and proceeds to correct the error. In this instance, the rhythm has been broken. Thus the corrector function becomes involved. In speech improvement the discrepancies between the desired speech patterns and the actual speech patterns (error signal) are what determine the amount and kind of improvement. Here, too, correcting is involved (Ogilvie and Rees, 1970, p. 16).

The third function, then, is *correcting*, based on information obtained through the child's scanning and comparing. As an adult, you are aware of this function. When you unconsciously mispronounce a word, you correct the mispronunciation by stressing a different syllable. When you utter a sound incorrectly, you change your mechanism to what feels and sounds right. You vary your utterance until no difference exists between the pattern you are producing and the one you want to produce (zero error signal). The child becomes aware, with your help, of what speech patterns need to be changed, finds for himself patterns he wishes to produce consistently, and adjusts his mechanism through hearing, feeling, and seeing so that it produces the desired patterns. Then he proceeds to practice until the control is automatic.

The expert typist as she started to learn to type found her control far from automatic. She probably began with *a-s-d-f-space semicolon-l-k-j-space* and practiced until an almost automatic "feel" took over. Just as in typing, an almost automatic "feel" for control of speech is learned. In early childhood, you compared the self-hearing of your own utterances with those around you; as you matched fairly well, those around you rewarded you. The kinesthetic and tactual messages from your placement and from the operation of parts of the articulatory mechanism became vivid and satisfying. Soon the kinesthetic and tactual feedback was so well established that the auditory feedback became secondary. You came to rely almost entirely on the "feel" of the movements of the speech mechanism rather than on hearing.

In helping the child to change his speech patterns, you are helping him to substitute conscious control for automatic control. He must match the auditory feedback from his mouth with the auditory patterns of someone else—either you or a tape. He adjusts his mechanism by hearing, seeing, feeling. You make use of yourself, of tapes, or of other speakers as models.

Having helped the child to find a pattern as a model, having helped him to make the necessary corrections, you then encourage him to work toward automatic control. Learning to type is often slow and clumsy. Learning to speak differently is also often slow and clumsy. In both instances practice is essential. You supply the child with phrases, poetry, limericks, ditties. You teach him to "feel" himself going through the necessary motions. Eventually the control does become automatic.

Improving Voice

UNACCEPTABLE VOCAL QUALITIES

The teacher is concerned that a student's voice serves his communicative purposes as well as it can. The student's voice problems may be serious. We will discuss the more serious difficulties of voice in Chapter 12. When a child has a consistently hoarse voice, the teacher may assume that the difficulty calls for specialized help. Many times, however, children's voices are adequate for communicative purposes but they would be more effective if improved. In such instances the teacher works for improvement. He takes into consideration four aspects of voice: volume, pitch, quality, and rate of speaking. (See Chapter 12 for correcting significant vocal difficulties.)

LOUDNESS

The child's voice should not be too loud or too soft. He should be able to adjust the loudness of his voice to the demands of the room in which he is speaking. Florence always spoke rather quietly. In the classroom children heard her fairly well although sometimes they had to listen carefully. But when she was to act as mistress of ceremonies in the auditorium, she discovered that the children in the back of the room could not hear her. She had to learn to adjust the volume of her voice to the size of the larger room. She further learned that speaking more slowly and articulating more clearly helped her to be heard. Harry, a ten-year-old, seemed to be yelling. He rarely spoke quietly. He seemed afraid that his classmates would not heed him and felt that when he spoke loudly they listened more attentively. He came from a family where he who spoke loudest received the most attention. With the teacher's direction he came to realize that he was more effective as a personality and easier to listen to when he spoke more softly.

PITCH

The child's voice should be appropriate to his age, sex, and physical maturity. It should express the meaning and emotion of what he desires to communicate. The material on pitch, pages 304–305, is important in consideration of children's pitch. No child's habitual pitch should be changed without careful diagnosis of his pitch difficulty. Many changes can safely be made, however. Mark's voice tended to be monotonous, for he spoke on one pitch level. Although he was a lively youngster, he had acquired the habit of speaking with little inflection. The school psychologist felt that his monotonous speech was a carryover from a time when he had had many adjustment problems. These problems were no longer evident, but the monotonous voice was. The teacher helped him to make his voice more lively.

QUALITY OF VOICE

Quality of voice refers to the tone that distinguishes one voice from another. The tone differs because of the way the resonating system acts to modify it and because of the particular way in which vocal cords vibrate. The quality may be clear, pleasant, resonant; or it may be breathy, muffled, or nasal. The changing of a consistent quality of voice is discussed in the chapter on voice. Quality, however, is also used to help express a person's feelings and emotions. The teacher can help the child to use a quality of voice that does express his feeling. One child, partly because of personality difficulties, always spoke as if he were angry. With the teacher's help, the child began to realize that his attitude toward life tended to be negative rather than positive. With the guidance of the school psychologist and with such classroom work as creative dramatics, the boy changed his tone from one of almost consistent anger to one of friendliness.

RATE OF SPEAKING

Few children speak too slowly. A large number of them speak at too fast a rate. Some are in a hurry to get their words into the conversation. Others tend to run fast, to work fast, and to talk fast. They need to realize that their listeners miss part of what they are saying because of their speed. One fourteen-year-old boy sang very well. In fact, he was the best boy vocalist in his school. But when he spoke, he ran his words together and overassimilated sounds so that his listeners missed at least half of what he was saying. The speed with which he spoke affected even the quality of his speaking voice. It became muffled. Yet when he sang he articulated very clearly and the quality of his voice was excellent. As he heard the contrast between his singing and speaking voices on a recording, he diagnosed his own difficulty and proceeded to do something about it.

Teaching the Improvement of Voice

Discussing voice and its part in communication makes children aware of their own voices. Children talk about the kinds of voices they like. Almost inevitably the discussion goes on to how voice reflects personality. They ask themselves whether certain voices suggest friendliness and kindness or whether they indicate that the person is bored and irritated. They talk about the control of pitch, volume, and speed. The next step is for the individual child to use a voice that expresses the meaning and feeling he intends to express. A recording of voice is an excellent motivation for children to change their voices.

LOUDNESS

Almost all children have to be reminded to speak loudly enough to be heard in a classroom. Inability to hear a child justifies interrupting him. One teacher said that he did not like to interrupt Jimmy to ask him to speak louder, because Jimmy was so interested in what he was telling. Jimmy was interested, but at least sixteen children in the room were squirming and at least six were talking with one another. They resented the teacher's admonition to them to listen. An early interruption, casually asking Jimmy to speak so that all could hear, might well have avoided the discourtesy on the part of his audience. Children need to know that rate of speaking and clear articulation are related to ability to be heard. When the teacher insists on each child's speaking loudly enough to be heard, communication is easier. In some instances, the child's speaking too softly may be related to his feeling of insecurity in the room or of general insecurity. The teacher must do what he can to make sure the social atmosphere of the room is conducive to speaking and being heard. If the child is generally insecure, help should be given to modify this situation.

PITCH, QUALITY, AND RATE

Children learn that the rate of speaking and the pitch and quality of their voices show how they feel about what they are reading or saying. Some teachers use puppets or creative dramatics very effectively for this purpose. One child holds the angry puppet who tells the others off. Another holds the sad puppet who speaks slowly of the misfortunes of others. Another holds the gay puppet whose speech is merry. The teacher helps the child to use the pitch, quality, and rate that are most expressive for his particular puppet. The teacher can use creative dramatics for the same purpose. Through setting up particular situations, children realize the importance of pitch, quality, and rate of speaking in their interpersonal relationships. They learn that the expression of different moods and of different meanings requires differences in pitch, quality, and rate.

One teacher uses a single phrase, asking that the children think of as many ways as possible of conveying different meanings with it. One of her phrases is, "Why, Joe and Jill were half an hour late." Children express happiness, sorrow, anger, sarcasm, or sympathy at Joe and Jill's being late. Sometimes they build a story around a particular child's rendition of the phrase.

References

ALLEN, H. B., *Readings in Applied English Linguistics*. New York, Appleton-Century-Crofts, 1968. (Contains an excellent discussion of the standards of pronunciation and grammar.)

———, et al., "Webster's Third New International Dictionary: A Symposium," *Quarterly Journal of Speech*, XLVIII (December, 1962) 431–440. (Evaluates the dictionary from the linguistic point of view.)

BAILEY, B. L., "Some Aspects of the Impact of Linguistics on Language Teaching in Disadvantaged Communities," *Elementary English*, XLV (May, 1968), 570–578. (Reports the findings of linguistic research as related to the teaching of English in schools that serve the disadvantaged. Includes phonology, grammar, language programs. Contains many examples of the speech of the disadvantaged.)

BARATZ, J. C., "Language and Cognitive Assessments of Negro Children: Assumptions Are Research Needs." Washington, D.C. ARIC Ed. 020518, 1968.

BRONSTEIN, A. J., *The Pronunciation of American English*. New York, Appleton-Century-Crofts, 1960 (Chap. 1 gives the nature of standard speech and explains levels of speech; Chap. 3 talks about regional variations.)

EISENSON, J., *The Improvement of Voice and Diction*, 2nd ed. New York, The Macmillan Company, 1965. (Chap. 10 discusses changing speech patterns.)

ELLIOTT, O., ed., "A Guest in Ghetto America," *Newsweek*, LXXIII (June 9, 1969), 42–43. (Talks about speech in the ghetto area.)

EVERTTS, E. L., ed., *Dimensions of Dialect*. Champaign, Ill., National Council of Teachers of English, 1967. (Contains a series of articles about social dialects.)

GOLDEN, R. L., *Improving Patterns of Language Usage*. Detroit: Wayne State University Press, 1960. (Stresses the importance of speech improvement as self-improvement.)

GOODMAN, K. S., "Dialect Barriers to Reading Comprehension," in E. L. Evertts, (ed.), *Dimensions of Dialect*. Champaign, Ill., National Council of Teachers of English, 1967. (Discusses regional variations.)

JOOS, M., "The Five Clocks," Publication 22, Indiana University Research Center in Anthropology, Folklore and Linguistics, April, 1962. (Discusses a wide variety of speech styles, from the most intimate to the most formal.)

KENYON, J. S., and T. A. KNOTT, *A Pronouncing Dictionary of American English*. Springfield, Mass., G. and C. Merriam Company, 1944. (Provides an excellent source for the pronunciation of American English words.)

LABOV, W., *The Social Stratification of English in New York City*. Washington, D.C.: Center for Applied Linguistics, 1966. (Indicates the different pronunciations of certain sounds in different strata of society in New York City.)

LEFEVRE, C. A., "Language and Self: Fulfillment or Trauma?" *Elementary*

English, XLIII (March, 1966), 230–234. (Decries the ancestral, puritanically rigid adherence to the black and white syndrome of correct and incorrect English.)

LOBAN, W., "Teaching Children Who Speak Social Class Dialects," *Elementary English*, XLV (May, 1968), 592–599. (Tells how to add a second language, to teach a prestigious dialect, established usage, and pronunciation.)

McDAVID, R. I., Jr., "Variations in Standard American English," *Elementary English*, XLV (May, 1968), 561–564. (Considers regional differences.)

MENCKEN, H. L., *The American Language*, 4th ed. New York, Alfred A. Knopf, Inc., 1946.

OGILVIE, M., and N. REES, *Communication Skills: Voice and Pronunciation*. New York, McGraw Hill, Inc., 1970. (Chap. 1 discusses effect of voice and pronunciation on communication; Chap. 8 discusses speech standards.)

PACKARD, V., *The Status Seekers*. New York, Pocket Books, Inc., 1961. (Talks about social aspects of various classes.)

SHUY, R. W., "Detroit Speech: Careless, Awkward, and Inconsistent, or Systematic, Graceful, and Regular?" *Elementary English*, XLV (May, 1968), 565–569. (Shows the distinction between language differences and value judgments about these differences. Talks about collecting the features of pronunciation, grammar, and vocabulary which set off different social groups, races, age groups, and sexes from each other in Detroit. Tells how to gather this information, and analyze it and evaluate its impact on the teaching of English.)

SHUY, R. W., ed., *Social Dialects and Language Learning*. Proceedings of the Bloomington, Indiana Conferences, 1964. Champaign, Ill.: National Council of Teachers of English, 1965.

STARKWEATHER, J. A., "Vocal Communication of Personality and Human Feelings," *Journal of Communication*, XI (June, 1961), 63–72. (Reports research dealing with voice as one facet of nonverbal communication.)

THOMAS, C. K., *An Introduction to the Phonetics of American English*, 2nd ed. New York, The Ronald Press Company, 1958. (Chap. 22 describes speech areas; Chap. 23 discusses standards of pronunciation.)

VENEZKY, R. L., "Nonstandard Language and Reading," *Elementary English*, XLVII (March, 1970), 334–345. (Contains selected references on specific dialects.)

Problems

1. Visit a classroom. List either (a) the articulatory errors you hear, or (b) the characteristics of the voices that are ineffective in the classroom situation.
2. Indicate the ways in which the teacher of a classroom you have visited helped the children to speak with more pleasant and more effective voices.

3. Find a list of frequently mispronounced words. Look up ten of them in three different recent dictionaries. Note the agreement or disagreement on how to pronounce these words in the dictionaries you consulted.
4. Read the introductions to two unabridged dictionaries. Tell how the information might prove helpful in your use of the dictionary in the classroom.
5. Listen to your favorite newscaster. What are the characteristics of his voice that made you think him effective?
6. Using the word *insane*, indicate synonyms that might be used in formal, informal, and substandard speech.
7. As far as possible, list the influences of parents, school, community, and education upon your own speech.
8. List five sentences, phrases, or words in which assimilation occurs. Indicate the assimilation that may occur.
9. List the voicing and unvoicing errors, if any, made by one child.
10. Would you accept the following omissions or transpositions in the pronunciation of the following words?
    goverment for *government*
    childern for *children*
    liberry for *library*
    English (without the *g*) for *English* (with the *g* sound)
    Support your "decision."

Chapter 4

The Teacher or Clinician as a Communicator

In this chapter we will talk about the teacher's and clinician's roles as communicators of their ideas and feelings to their students, as recipients of their students' ideas and feelings, and of the resulting interaction. Teaching *is* communication. Children regard the communicator who imparts meanings and feelings with sensitivity, clarity, and fairness, who in turn receives the children's messages with understanding, thoughtfulness, and appreciation, and who, as a result, interacts positively, as a capable teacher or clinician.

In print, the teacher's suggestion, "Let's tidy up this room," carries a minimal sense of the communicative situation. What motivates the remark? Miss Fearful, glancing apprehensively at the clock, finds the arrival of an unknown supervisor imminent. Consequently, she is anxious and concerned, for she doesn't want this supervisor to observe apparent confusion. Her "Let's tidy up" conveys this concern. Miss Let's-Get-Going may be casually saying, "We've done as much as we can with this project today. Let's clean up and get on to other things." Miss Tidy Perfection may be saying, "I loathe, hate, and detest mess." The rate of speaking, the stress, the pitch, the tone of voice, the accompanying gestures all bring meaning to the symbol, "Let's tidy up this room," and make the attitude of the teacher apparent.

The responses may take various forms: As a result of the request, Miss Fearful's children may quickly, quietly tidy up. Miss Fearful in her anxiety wanted this kind of control. Or her children may say: "But we're not through." "Why?" "Now?" "Right away?" "Must we?" "I've got to finish my sky." This feedback to the teacher may convey her students' resentment at what seems a sudden autocratic action or curiosity as to "What's bugging you?" Or the children may balk with, "No!" "We don't want to," or may sit inert. This feedback says to her, "Your students are rebelling." How does Miss Fearful handle the rebellion? She may repeat the request; she may reason with the children; she may scold—or even threaten. Thus, the cycle commences again.

In print, the remark of the speech clinician, "Let's try again," also carries minimal meaning. Miss Bored-to-Death may be saying, "You'll never learn." Miss Supportive may be saying, "You're coming along fine. One more try." Miss Authoritarian may be saying, "Drill is important. Say the phrase once more."

The responses here, too, may take various forms. Miss Bored-to-Death's child may respond with, "Time to go back to class," reflecting the clinician's apathy. Miss Supportive's child, responding to her warmth and concern, may try to do still better. Miss Authoritarian's child may also try to do still better, recognizing the clinician's interest in him behind her "bossy" manner. Or the child may resent her particular style and remain stubbornly silent.

Each teacher or clinician has attempted to manipulate or control the learning environment through her message to her receivers, who in turn have reacted according to their feelings, which are often the direct result of the teacher's or clinician's attitudes. Furthermore, her encoding or expressing of her message has been skillful or not as measured by its influence on her children's attitudes toward her and toward what she wants done. The listeners' reactions in turn have depended both on their attitudes and on their decoding or receiving skills—the skills involved in understanding the message of the teacher or clinician. The teacher or clinician gets feedback, positive, negative, or somewhere in between, through words, vocal attributes, physical gestures, and facial expressions. The attitudes of the children become very clear. The communication in a teaching or clinical situation is like that in any other situation except that the teacher or clinician has a high degree of control over the message, its content, structure, and treatment, over the use of the channels of hearing, seeing, touching, smelling, and tasting, and even over the receivers themselves.

The following diagram based on the Berlo model represents the teaching* communicative act.

---

* We believe that the clinician is a teacher in that he wishes to affect attitudes, skills, and often to instill knowledge.

Teacher (Source)	Message	Channel	Receiver
Knowledge	Educational	Seeing	Knowledge
Attitudes	Purpose	Hearing	Attitudes
Social Milieu and	Structure	Touching	Social Milieu and
Background	Treatment	Smelling	Background
School Cultural		Tasting	School Cultural
Environment			Environment
Communication Skills			Communication Skills
	Feedback		

Adapted from model in D. K. Berlo, *The Process of Communication.* New York, Holt, Rinehart, and Winston, Inc., 1960.

The Teacher or Clinician as an Encoder (Source)

The factors involved in the teacher's or clinician's ability as a speaker are: (1) his knowledge, (2) his attitudes and the effect of his own self-concept on them, (3) his own social milieu and background, (4) the cultural environment of his school, and (5) his communication skills.

KNOWLEDGE

Everyone agrees that teachers should be knowledgeable. When the teacher has read widely, thought deeply, inquired judiciously, observed keenly, listened carefully, and appraised completely, he has extensive knowledge and, consequently, a fund of ideas from which to draw. The ideas need not be derived from books, travel, or learned individuals, for some ideas are original. For instance, the teacher may find a picture from which an exciting bit of theater can grow, or discover a cartoon that motivates discussion, or invent a game for auditory discrimination. Or perhaps he may make up a story that is sheer nonsense but well suited to his group. The teacher is a person with wide knowledge and a creative urge, who will continue to acquire a liberal education throughout his life. Similarly the clinician must be knowledgeable. He must know both the theory and practice of his field. He must be able to diagnose accurately, to know when to refer, when to handle the child himself. He must know whom to consult. He must have at his hand tests which will help him diagnose. He must be able to plan a program to help the speech and hearing handicapped. His competencies are discussed in Chapter 2. Undoubtedly this intellectual development is significant, but the teacher or clinician must also believe that particular knowledge is important, that it can be communicated to others, and that it will affect the lives of others.

ATTITUDES AND THE TEACHER'S SELF-CONCEPT

Effective teaching involves human beings interacting positively. The teacher who believes his students capable of learning behaves differently from the one who believes them incapable. Furthermore, the teacher who feels he is an able teacher will try very hard to teach his children. Teachers who do not feel they are able give up. The teacher, therefore, should possess a positive self-concept a "fully functioning self," or a "high-level wellness." Since the speech clinician is interacting with either an individual or members of a small group, his impact is deeply felt. He must believe that his students are capable of learning to communicate and that he is capable of teaching them to communicate. He should not believe that a particular child cannot and will not respond to therapy. Like the teacher, he should possess a positive self concept. Combs and Snygg say this kind of teacher is characterized by four general qualities:

1. They tend to see themselves in essentially positive ways. That is to say, they see themselves as generally liked, wanted, successful, able persons of dignity, worth, and integrity.
2. They perceive themselves and their world accurately and realistically. These people do not kid themselves. They are able to confront the world with openness and acceptance, seeing both themselves and external events with a minimum of distortion or defensiveness.
3. They have deep feelings of identification with other people. They feel "at one with" a large number of persons of all kinds and varieties. This is not simply a surface manifestation of "liking people" or being a "hail-fellow-well-met" type of person. Identification is not a matter of polished social graces, but a feeling of oneness in the human condition.
4. They are well informed. Adequate people are not stupid. They have perceptual fields which are rich, varied, and available for use when needed (Combs, 1965, p. 70).

Studies support this point of view: Christenson (1960) found that vocabulary growth was significantly greater under a teacher whose pupils rated him high on a "warmth scale." Lippert and White (Lippert and White, 1958) discovered that authoritarian patterns of leadership resulted either in apathetic withdrawal, which would hinder oral language practice, or in aggressive resistance, which would channel oral language into narrow destructive uses. Research by Ryans (1961) indicates that teachers who are understanding and friendly yet organized and stimulating encourage their pupils in productive and confident participation.

Rosenthal and Jacobson (1968) note that the reason usually given for the poor performance of the child from a different culture is simply that he is a member of a disadvantaged group. They point out that there may be another reason: that the child does poorly in schoool because that is what is expected if him. His shortcomings may originate not in his different ethnic, cultural, and economic background but in his teacher's response to that background. Their study, therefore, was devised with this concept in mind: that one person's prediction of another person's behavior somehow comes to be realized. The prediction may, of course, be realized only in the perception of the predicter. But it is also possible that the predictor's expectation is communicated to the other person, perhaps in quite subtle and unintended ways, and so has an influence on his actual behavior.

They therefore set up a situation whereby teachers would expect certain pupils to show superior performance. The school was one where most of the children came from lower-class families where the parents were receiving welfare payments, had low incomes, and/or were Mexican in origin. The children were tested with instruments that measured verbal ability and reasoning ability at the beginning and end of the school year. The teachers were told early in the term that certain children were "spurters" who were in reality chosen at random. The results showed that children from whom teachers expected greater intellectual gains showed such gains. The teachers were also asked to describe the classroom behavior of their pupils. The children from whom intellectual growth was expected were described as having a better chance of being successful in later life, and as being happier, more curious, and more interesting than the other children.

The most obvious explanation for these results is that the teachers spent more time with these particular students. But no evidence for this explanation exists. The authors believe that the explanation seems to lie in a subtle feature of the interaction of the teacher and her pupils. Her tone of voice, facial expression, touch, and posture, may be the means by which—probably quite unwittingly—she communicates her expectations to her pupils. Such communication may help the child by changing his conception of himself, his anticipation of his own behavior, and his motivation in his cognitive skills.

The Teacher's or Clinician's Social Milieu and Background

A teacher has usually been brought up in a middle-class home; his colleagues and friends generally come from a similar background. But the teacher or clinician may be working with students from either upper- or lower-class homes. The modes of communication in the various social classes differ. Schatzman and Strauss (1966) in a study involving a sampling from 340 interviews of white subjects, 21–65 years old, living in Arkansas, compared the oral communication of a group low in income and educational opportunity with one that was decidedly higher in income and educational opportunity. They pointed out differences—not merely in success or failure of communication, or correctness or elaborateness of syntactical structure and vocabulary usage—but in: a) number and kinds of perspectives used in communication, b) ability to take the listener's role, c) the handling of classification, and d) framework and stylistic devices which order and implement the communication.

For example, the description of the catastrophic event by the members of the lower class was a straight, direct narrative of events, whereas the description by members of the higher class was not confined to so narrow a perspective. It involved another person, class of persons, an organization, an organizational role, even the whole town. The members of the higher class described the behavior of others and even included sequence of events as others saw them.

The teacher or clinician needs to be aware of the differences between the mode of communication of his social class and that of the class of his students.

Cultural Environment of the School

The students, the faculty, the school administration, and the locale all contribute to the environment of the school. Some schools have rich, stimulating environments: As you enter the school building, you see pictures drawn by inspired young artists, poems written by imaginative young writers; you hear music, other than the ordinary, emanating from a classroom; you feel your muscles tense as you watch young dancers portraying a riot. In this school, children from all social classes have anticipating, eager looks. Or the school can have a well-ordered, tightly-run-ship look: The poems are beautifully handwritten. The floors are barren of even a scrap of paper. The students look like models from the children's fashion section of the newspaper. Almost everyone moves in an orderly fashion.

These are but two examples of school environments. Just as individuals have different life styles, schools can display a variety of postures, of moods, and of collections of culture. But these affect the communicative processes of the students, of the teacher and of the clinician.

Clinicians who travel from school to school often have a "favorite" school, the style of which makes clinical speech work profitable. A school with a humanitarian principal, with teachers interested in every child from the gifted to the retarded, with pride in the achievements of each student, with a somewhat permissive attitude but with boundaries firmly established, with an attractive speech room adequately equipped falls into the category of one clinician's "favorite" school. The principal casually commends the clinician on the ability of a once silent child to communicate with others. A teacher sends a note indicating that one child's mother is ill in the hospital; another, that a child has completed an unusually attractive poster. This school's style fosters effective clinical work.

Communicative Skills of the Teacher or Clinician

The teacher's or clinician's ability to encode his message so that his receivers accept it as he intended is important. His choice of words and of syntactic complexity, his illustrations, his analogies, his ability to make information exciting, to make a point clearly, to persuade, to adapt what he has to say so that his charges understand and respond—all these are facets of this ability.

The teacher's or clinician's voice and pronunciation can be an asset or a liability to purposeful, satisfying communication. When effective interaction between the teacher or clinician, his message, and his students takes place, the teacher or clinician seems to have confidence in himself, his ideas, and his teaching. His voice revealing this confidence is "clearly audible, with a steady rhythm, with a rate slow enough for comprehension but varied so as to express enthusiasm and vigor, with an appropriate pitch and intonation pattern, and with a strong resonant quality" (Ogilvie and Rees, 1970, p. 6). The voice of the warm, friendly teacher or clinician, flexible in pitch and loudness, indicates that he has heard his children's comments, values their worth, and anticipates a reaction.

The teacher or clinician may well tape-record a classroom discussion or a clinical session and then listen to his voice to discover what kind of communicative instrument he possesses. When it gives an impression contrary to what he intends, the teacher does well to consult the school speech therapist who can often make suggestions for improvement. For example, one teacher spoke much too rapidly. When she lengthened her vowels and continuant consonants and took more time for pauses, her students were able to perceive a new and different voice quality—seemingly less nasal, less staccato, and much more pleasant. When the clinician finds his own voice inadequate he needs to put into practice his own theory.

Just as the voice may add or detract from the teacher's or clinician's message, so may his pronunciations. Your patterns of pronunciation should not distract your students. If you possess a regional dialect unlike that of those whom you are teaching, your pronunciation may at first be distracting. When your pronunciation represents educated speech, however, the absolute differences are few, and it is rarely found distracting. Just the same, you may perhaps want to adopt some of the pronunciations of the region in which you are working.

Message

In teaching, the message is usually motivated by the teacher's desire to impart knowledge, to change or confirm an attitude, and/or to instill certain skills—all of which involve behavioral responses on the part of his students. The teacher himself may present information or may use discussion techniques to foster its acquisition. Sometimes the teacher expects the children to make no value-judgements based on knowledge. For instance, the scientific principles of the flight to the moon are facts that can be understood in lesser or greater scientific detail depending upon the scientific sophistication of both the encoder and the decoder. On the other hand, the teacher may expect the children to make value-judgements that are based on knowledge, as when, having come to understand the present system of electing the President of the United States, the children then debate that system's merits. The teacher deciding whether to involve his students in making particular value-judgements may ask himself such questions as: Are my students mature enough to handle this problem? Am I trying to instill my particular bias in them? Is my sole purpose the protection of the status quo? How essential is involvement in the problem for these students?

Many times the acquisition of knowledge and its resulting value-judgements changes or strengthens attitudes; it may even motivate the formulation of completely new ones. As high-school students learn more about language patterns they may become much less certain of accepting wholeheartedly a pronunciation like *status* with a long *a* rather than *status* with a short *a*. They begin to listen for variant acceptable pronunciations and to understand why they hear many pronunciations that differ from the ones they normally use and believe "correct." As they study language they open their minds to the values of accepting descriptive rather than prescriptive attitudes toward pronunciation. The teacher's skill in leading discussion, his source image (involving the respect with which his students regard him), and his ability to bring facts to light influence his children's acceptance or rejection of attitudes. At other times, the particular environment, the cultural backgrounds, and the social milieu are subtle but dominant influences on certain attitudes. The speech clinician plays an important role in influencing attitudes of the speech handicapped child. For example, he helps the stutterer to accept his stuttering. His own attitude about speech difficulties is reflected in the children's attitudes about them and in the teachers' attitudes. As a result, teachers can become more accepting of the speech handicapped child.

The teacher usually has a set of skills that he wishes his students to acquire. He may make sure his students understand the prerequisites of the skills, may demonstrate them, and may then provide opportunity for practice. Similarly, the clinician almost inevitably wants his children to acquire certain skills. He first motivates the child to accept change as desirable, proceeds to explain and demonstrate the needed change, and then provides interesting drill material to effect the change. Finally he gives opportunity to use the changed communication in conversation. The ability of the teacher or clinician to decode, and to demonstrate the skills, the ability of the children to encode, and their mental and motor readiness to try the skills are all important in their acquisition. But equally important is the teacher's or clinician's ability to make those skills seem desirable, for the group's attitude in accepting or rejecting their desirability influences their acquisition.

In any of the three purposes, the acquisition of knowledge for knowledge's sake, the making of value-judgments, and the acquiring of skills, the teacher or clinician is interested in the "how" of teaching. He uses what is commonly called "motivation"—either extrinsic or intrinsic, for he cannot expect his students to react as sponges, soaking up knowledge, or as robots, automatically performing skills. The students must be an intimate part of the process. Affect plays an important role here.

Every message from the teacher has some kind of structure. The structure may be tight, as when the teacher makes his aim clear and then proceeds in a developmental fashion to accomplish it. It is less tight when the teacher presents examples, encourages the students to give examples, and then guides the students to draw inferences leading to the accomplishment of the aim of the lesson. The lesson may have a loose structure, as when it consists of guided conversation used to open avenues of possible investigation or activity. But every lesson possesses some kind of structure.

Similarly every clinic session has a purpose. It may be to improve the child's ability to discriminate between plosive and fricative sounds, to encourage the child to be objective about his stuttering, to decrease stuttering symptoms, to improve expressive language in terms of opposites as *hot* and *cold*, to improve ability to hear a particular defective sound. The structure may be tight or loose. In working with some aspects of language development, the structure may be loose as exemplified in the conversation about the Christmas tree noted on pages 265–266. In other aspects, as when the clinician is teaching the child to build concepts about trucks and their various uses as exemplified on page 244, the structure may be as tight as a developmental lesson.

Channel

Children usually receive the messages in the classroom through seeing and hearing. They receive, interpret, and evaluate the ideas presented by the teacher and by their classmates. Because the classroom is traditionally a verbal community, listening is particularly important. The child must listen carefully rather than attend to his own affairs. As the message conveys graciousness, the child listens courteously. As it conveys information, he listens thoughtfully and carefully; as it conveys persuasion, he listens critically.

The teacher or clinician does well to remember that learning can be reinforced through channels other than hearing—that looking at a picture showing a boy, a bigger boy, and the biggest boy, pantomiming answering the phone or the actions of a bully, feeling a smooth stone as contrasted with a rough stone, or tasting a bitter lemon and a sweet orange all add another dimension of communication to the purely verbal one. Not all modalities are integrated. Often a student possesses a primary modality such as pantomimic action—that is a favored one. The teacher or clinician then does well to make use of this particular modality—to further communication—to further the acquisition of knowledge, attitudes, and skills.

Receiver (Decoder)

The child's knowledge, his attitudes, including the effect of his own self-concept, his own social milieu and background, his cultural environment provided by the school, and his communication skills all affect his ability to understand. These factors also affect the teachers' or clinicians' responses, which are directly motivated by feedback from the children.

KNOWLEDGE

The basic understandings which the child brings to school with him either facilitate or hinder his acquisition of further understandings. Some children bring to school understandings far beyond their years. For example, a seven-year-old when asked, "What does *secure* mean?" responded with: "When the bad guy is put in prison, he's secure; he can't get out." After a pause, she added, "When my brother glues two pieces of his airplane together, they're secure." Other children bring less understanding. Another seven-year-old, when asked the same question, responded with: "Scure ... Scure ... Scure ... Sewer ... Sewer. Jackie Gleason. The guy in the sewer."

The gap between these two seven-year-olds represents a gap in knowledge already acquired—probably not only in the meaning of this word but in the meaning of many more words and, furthermore, in ideas and concepts.

SOCIAL MILIEU AND BACKGROUND

The child's own social milieu and background may make his decoding easier or more difficult. He may have been brought up in a home full or devoid of books, music, trips, and stimulating conversation. Or his particular milieu may have certain inbred attitudes. In his study, "Communication Processes Among Immigrants in Israel," Eisenstadt lists among reasons that immigrants disattached themselves from formal elites:

1. Growing disillusionment about the elites' ability to assure them of various amenities and rights accruing to them in a new social system.
2. Doubts as to the elites' prestige position within the new social system.
3. The feeling of attachment to the old ways blocks their achievement of full status within the new society (Eisenstadt, 1966, p. 587).

Similar feelings existing in ethnic groups in today's schools directly influence communication in the classroom.

ATTITUDES

The child's self-concept affects his ability to communicate. The teacher's or clinician's influence is important, for his evaluation of the child affects the child's self-concept. Davidson and Lang (1960, p. 107–108) found that children's perception of their teachers' feelings correlated positively and significantly with their self perception. Furthermore, language and self-concept are inexorably entwined: Language is an inherent part of the classroom culture—for it is a tool that the child uses in his thinking, in his communicative acts, and in his social intercourse. Erwin and Miller (1963, p. 107–108) say that language is the greatest force for socialization that exists, and that at the same time it is the most potent single factor in the development of individuality. Language reflects self and self reflects language. Affect related to attitudes engendered by environment and by the teacher influences both the development of a positive self-concept and language. The emergence of the development of language in and out of the classroom may signify emergence and growth of self.

CULTURAL ENVIRONMENT OF THE SCHOOL

The school environment has an effect on the verbal behavior and on the emergence and growth of self. When the school teaches material that has personal meaning for the student, when it helps the child to become personally involved with ideas, with the school's program and with other children, the child will become more effective in communication. As the curriculum is rich in motivating acquisition of knowledge and skills, as it develops imagination, as it adapts to its students, language ability improves.

COMMUNICATION SKILLS

Lastly, the child must be learning to participate in this verbal environment—recognizing purposes of communication, achieving these purposes effectively, listening to and responding to others in a communicative situation. He learns to express himself in different ways in different situations, to gauge the particular language needs of a particular situation. Consequently, he needs to find his own identity, to bring his image of himself close to reality. The classroom should ideally be a place where each child can find a sense of personal worth in his life through communication, and can feel he is contributing to the society of the classroom. Eventually, he needs to recognize standard and nonstandard usage so that his decoding can be encoded by all members of society—inside and outside the classroom.

Thus, the amount of knowledge, the attitudes, the social milieu and background, the school's cultural environment, and the communication skills of the teacher, the clinician, and the students will influence the effectiveness of the communication activity. The message may have different purposes tied to the students' behavioral consequences, different structures, different treatments. It may not only be heard, but seen, touched, smelled, or tasted. The receivers' attitudes about both the teacher and the clinician, the message, and the channel influence the success or failure of the communicative processes. The teacher and the clinician are made aware of these attitudes through feedback. Feedback is a way of monitoring a system which signals correct and incorrect operations, sometimes even before the incorrect operation occurs. This permits and facilitates correction. The teacher and clinician will recognize its importance for they can most accurately communicate when they are truly responsive to the reactions of their students.

References

BARNLUND, D. C., *Interpersonal Communication Survey and Studies*. Boston, Houghton Mifflin Company, 1968. (Contains a series of studies related to the problems of interpersonal communication.)

BERLO, D. K., *The Process of Communication*. New York, Holt, Rinehart and Winston, Inc., 1960.

BURKE, W. S., "Leadership Behavior as a Function of the Leader, the Follower, and the Situation," *Journal of Personality*, XXXXIII (March, 1965), 60–81.

CHRISTENSON, C. B., "Relationships Between Pupil Achievement, Pupil Affect-Need, Teacher Warmth, and Teacher Permissiveness," *Journal of Educational Psychology*, LI (June, 1960), 169–174. (Indicates the effect of warmth of the teacher upon vocabulary development.)

COMBS, A. W., ed., *Perceiving, Behaving, Becoming: A New Focus for Education*. 1962 ASCD Yearbook. Washington, D.C., Association for Supervision and Curriculum Development, 1962. (Gives a concept of teaching based on Rogerian psychology.)

COMBS, A. W., *The Professional Education of Teachers*. Boston, Allyn and Bacon, Inc., 1965. (Chap. 6 describes the self of the effective teacher; Chap. 7 explains the purposes of teachers.)

DAVIDSON, A. H., and G. LANG, "Children's Perceptions of Their Teachers' Feelings Toward Them," *Journal of Experimental Education*, XXIX (December, 1960), 107–108.

DeCECCO, J. P., *The Psychology of Language, Thought, and Instruction*. New York, Holt, Rinehart and Winston, Inc., 1967. (Contains readings on language, thought, and culture, language and social class, language and learning, and language and problem solving.)

DeVito, J., *The Psychology of Speech and Language: An Introduction to Psycho-linguists*. New York, Random House, Inc., 1970, Chap. 4. (Deals with communication theory.)

Eckroyd, D. H., *Speech in the Classroom*, 2nd ed. Englewood Cliffs, N. J., Prentice-Hall, Inc., 1969. (Covers the development, uses, and techniques of effective speech in terms of both teacher and student.)

Eisenson, J., J. J. Auer, and J. V. Irwin, *The Psychology of Communication*. New York, Appleton-Century-Crofts, 1963. (Chaps. 9, 11 deal with communicative process; Chaps. 14, 15 deal with factors in group discussion. Chaps. 19, 20, and 21 deal with personality and speech.)

Eisenstadt, S. N., "Communication Processes Among Immigrants in Israel," in A. G. Smith, ed., *Communication and Culture*. New York, Holt, Rinehart and Winston, Inc., 1966, pp. 576–587.

Erwin, S., and W. Miller, "Language Development," in *Child Psychology*, 62nd Yearbook of National Society for Study of Education. Chicago, University of Chicago Press, 1963, pp. 107–108.

Lippert, R., and R. K. White, "An Experimental Study of Leadership and Group Life," in D. D. Maccoby, ed. and others, *Readings in Social Psychology*. New York, Holt, Rinehart and Winston, Inc., 1958.

Nichols, R. G., "Do We Know How to Listen? Practical Helps in a Modern Age," *The Speech Teacher*, X (March, 1961), 118–124.

Ogilvie, M., and N. Rees, *Communication Skills: Voice and Pronunciation*. New York, McGraw Hill, Inc., 1970, Chap. 1. (Notes the effects of voice and pronunciation on communication.)

Rogers, C. R., *On Becoming a Person*. Boston, Houghton-Mifflin Company, 1961. (Makes the perceptual viewpoint of psychology clear.)

Rosenthal, R., and L. F. Jacobson, "Teacher Expectation for the Disadvantaged," Scientific American, CCXVIII (April, 1968), 3–7.

Ross, R. S. "Fundamental Processes and Principles of Communication," In K. Brooks, ed., *The Communication Arts and Sciences of Speech*. Columbus, Ohio, Charles E. Merrill Books, Inc., 1967, pp. 107–128. (Explains communication perception process.)

Ryans, D., "Some Relationships Between Pupil Behavior and Certain Teacher Characteristics," *Journal of Educational Psychology*, LII (April, 1961), 82–90.

Schatzman, L., and A. Strauss, "Social Class and Modes of Communication," in A. G. Smith, ed., Communication and Culture, New York, Holt, Rinehart and Winston, Inc., 1966, pp. 442–455.

Problems

1. Visit three classrooms. In terms of the communication model cited in this chapter, analyze the communicative situation.
2. Visit two classrooms. Indicate what you consider to be the effect of the teachers' voices on their students.

3. Visit a speech correction clinic. Indicate what channels were used in the therapy procedures. What other channels might have been used and how?
4. Describe the "culture" of the elementary school that you attended.
5. Listen to any teacher. Give the indications of the kind of self-concept you think he possesses as indicated by his verbalizations.
6. Visit a classroom from a lower socioeconomic area. Describe how you would have to modify your middle-class values in teaching this group— both in terms of language and in terms of social customs.

Chapter 5

The Mechanism for Speech

Voice Production

The human voice-producing mechanism functions in a manner roughly comparable to that of a musical wind instrument. The wind or horn instruments employ: (1) reeds or the lips of the blower as vibrators or noisemakers; (2) air blown over or through the reeds as the source of energy to set the reeds in vibration; and (3) an elongated tube to reinforce the sound produced by the "vibrating" reeds. The human voice-producing mechanism employs laryngeal folds (vocal bands) for vibrators, air that might otherwise have served only normal respiratory purposes for a source of energy, and the cavities of the larynx, pharynx (throat), mouth, and nose as reinforcers or resonators. These cavities, if we include the trachea or windpipe, may be directly compared to a curved, elongated tube of a wind instrument. The human "elongated tube" is considerably more modifiable than that of any wind instrument, however, and so is capable of producing a wide variety of laryngeal tones that may be modified in respect to pitch, quality, loudness, and duration. The arrangement of the parts of the voice mechanism is indicated in Figure 1.

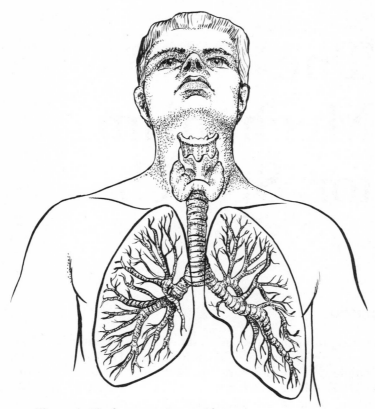

Figure 1. The larynx, trachea, and lungs.

THE LARYNX

The larynx, commonly referred to as the voice box, is located in the neck between the root of the tongue and the trachea. The outer and largest part of the larynx consists of two shield-shaped cartilages fused together along an anterior line. Together, these fused shields are known as the thyroid cartilage. The reader may locate the larynx at this point by running his index finger down from the middle of his chin toward his neck. His finger should be stopped by the notch at the point of fusion of the cartilages.

From each side of the larynx, folds of muscle tissue lined by mucous membrane appear as transverse folds that constitute the vocal bands. The upper pair of folds (the paired ventricular or false bands) are relatively soft and flaccid, and not as "movable" as are the true bands below.

In normal breathing, the true vocal bands are separated in a letter V arrangement. To produce voice, the vocal bands must be brought together (approximated or adducted) so that they are close and parallel (see Figure 2).

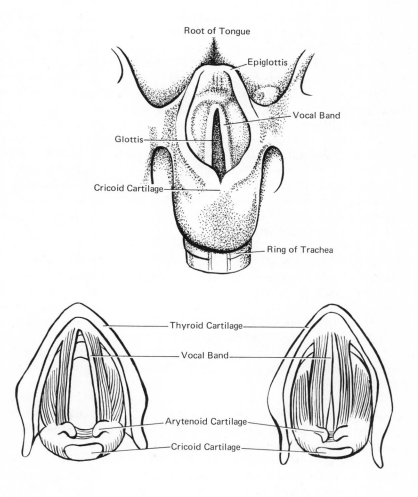

Figure 2. The larynx from above and behind. Below, the vocal bands, in position for breathing (left) and for vocalization (right).

The Vocal Bands. The vocal bands or vocal folds* are small, tough strips of connective tissue, which are continuous with comparatively thick strips of voluntary muscle tissue. Viewed from above, the vocal bands appear to be flat folds of muscle with inner edges of connective tissue. In male adults the vocal bands range from about $\frac{7}{8}$ inch to $1\frac{1}{4}$ inches; in adult females they range from $\frac{1}{2}$ inch or less to about $\frac{7}{8}$ inch.

The opening between the vocal bands is called the glottis. In normal phonation (vocalization) the breath under pressure meets the approximated vocal bands and forces them to move apart. As a result, a stream of air flowing with relatively high velocity escapes between the vocal bands, which continue to be held together (approximated) at both ends. The reduction in pressure beneath the bands, together with the reduced air pressure along the sides of the high-velocity air stream, aided by the elasticity of the bands themselves brings about recurrent closures after successive outward movements of the bands. Thus vocalization is maintained. If the action or position of the vocal bands fails to produce a "complete" though momentary interruption in the flow of air, the result is a kind of noise or voice quality we identify as breathiness or hoarseness. Figure 2 indicates the position of the bands as they are approximated and ready to be set into motion by the pressure of the air beneath them.

Loudness. The loudness of the voice is directly related to the vigor with which air is forced from the lungs through the larynx, though not to the total amount of air that is expended. Pressure and velocity depend, in part, upon the size of the glottal opening and the length of time the glottis is open. Loudness is, in effect, a result of the pressure of the released pulsations produced by the movements of the bands. Vocal tones are reinforced in the larynx, in the tracheal cavity immediately below the larynx, in the cavities of the throat and mouth, and in the nasal cavities.

Pitch. The fundamental pitch of a vibrating body varies directly with its frequency of vibration. Thus, the greater the frequency, the higher the resultant pitch. Vocal pitch is a product of factors related to the condition of the vocal bands. The primary factors are the mass or thickness of the bands, their length, and the elasticity (tension) in relationship to mass and length. In the process of phonation the vocal bands elongate as they increase in tension. By the same process, the

---

* Unless otherwise specified, all references are to the true vocal bands. These may also be referred to as the vocal folds or vocal cords.

bands are reduced in mass per unit area. The overall effect of the modification of mass-tension factors is to produce a higher rather than a lower pitch when the bands are set into motion. In general, the greater the tension, the higher the pitch. If tension is held constant, with greater length or mass, the pitch is lower. If length and mass are held constant, the greater the tension of the vocal bands, the higher the pitch.

Women tend to have higher pitched voices than men because usually they have shorter and thinner vocal bands than men. Our voices become lower in pitch as we mature because maturation is accompanied by an increase in the length and thickness of the vocal folds.

The changes in pitch that we are able to produce under voluntary control take place, as we have indicated, largely by modifications in the degree of tension of the vocal folds. Through these modifications, we are capable of producing tones with ranges of pitch. The ranges may vary somewhat for singing and speaking. Good speakers may have a range of about two octaves. Poor speakers may have narrower ranges. For most nonprofessional speakers it is probably more important to have good control of a one-octave range than poor control of a wider range. For each individual speaker it is important that voice be produced within the pitch range easiest and most effective for him. The range will include the optimum pitch level—the level of pitch at which the individual is able to produce the best quality of tone with least expenditure of effort. This will be considered later on in our discussion of optimum pitch.

The Arytenoid Cartilages. The vocal bands are attached at their sides to the wall of the thyroid cartilage. At the front, the bands are attached to the angle formed by the fusion of the two shields of the thyroid cartilage. At the back, each of the bands is attached to a pyramidal-shaped cartilage known as the arytenoid. The shape and muscular connections of the arytenoid cartilages enable them to move in ways that make it possible for the vocal bands to be brought together for vocalization, partly separated for whispering, or more widely separated for normal respiration. The arytenoids can pivot or rotate, tilt backward, or slide backward and sideways.

The Cricoid Cartilage. The arytenoid cartilages rest on the top of the first tracheal ring. This ring, which has an enlarged and widened back, is known as the cricoid cartilage.

The movement of the vocal bands is brought about by the muscular connections of the bands to cartilages, and by the inter-connections of the cartilages. Two types of action are important for vocalization. One is for the closing and opening of the bands (adduction and abduction) and the other is for changing the length and tension of the approximated bands to bring about changes in pitch.

THE CHEST CAVITY

The larynx, with its intricate structure of cartilages and muscles, provides the vibrator for phonation. The source of energy that sets the vibrators into motion is found in the chest cavity.

The chest (thoracic) cavity comprises a framework of bones and cartilages that includes the collarbone, the shoulder blades, the ribs, the breastbone or sternum, and the backbone. The diaphragm, as may be noted in Figure 3, constitutes both the floor of the thoracic cavity and the ceiling of the abdominal cavity. The lungs and the trachea are within the chest cavity. In the abdominal cavity directly below are the digestive organs, which include the stomach, the intestines, and the liver.

The Lungs. The lungs consist of a mass of air sacs that contain a considerable amount of elastic tissue. The lungs expand or contract, and so are partly filled or partly emptied of air as a result of differences in pressure brought about by actions of the muscles of the ribs and abdomen, which expand and contract the thoracic cavity. When the muscles of the ribs and abdomen and the downward action of the diaphragm expand the chest cavity, air is forced into the lungs by the outside air pressure. When the ribs and the upward movement of the diaphragm and abdominal muscles act to contract the chest cavity, air is forced out of the lungs. Through these actions, inhalation and exhalation take place.

The Diaphragm. The diaphragm is a double-domed muscular organ that separates the thoracic and abdominal cavities. The right half of the diaphragm rises somewhat higher—is more dome-shaped—than the left. When the capacity of the chest cavity is increased, air enters the lungs by way of the mouth, nose, throat, and trachea. In this part of the respiratory cycle—inhalation—the diaphragm is actively involved. The contraction of the diaphragm and its downward action serve to increase the volume of the chest cavity. In exhalation the diaphragm is passive. It relaxes and returns to its former position because of the upward pressure of the abdominal organs. In the modified and controlled respiration necessary for phonation and speech, the muscles of the front and sides of the abdominal wall contract and press inward on

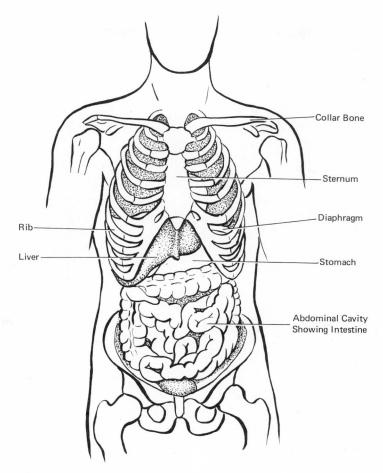

Figure 3. The chest and abdominal cavities.

the liver, stomach, and intestines. These organs in turn exert an upward pressure on the diaphragm, which transmits the pressure to the lungs and so forces air out of the lungs. Throughout the respiratory cycle, the diaphragm remains roughly dome-shaped. The height of the dome, as may be observed from Figure 4, is greater after exhalation than after inhalation.

Although the diaphragm is passive during exhalation, it does not relax suddenly and completely. Because the diaphragm maintains some degree of muscular tonus at all times, pressure upon it produces a gradual rather than an all-at-once relaxation. Gradual relaxation makes

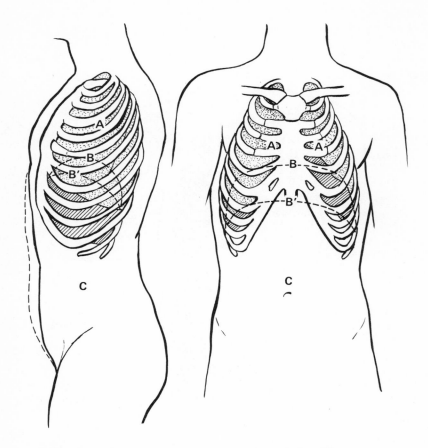

Figure 4. Action of the diaphragm and abdomen in breathing.

A. The chest cavity or thorax.
B. The diaphragm "relaxed" when exhalation is completed.
B'. The diaphragm contracted as in deep inhalation.
C. The abdominal cavity. The abdominal wall is displaced forward as the diaphragm
   moves downward during inhalation.

it possible for a steady stream of breath to be created and used to set
the vocal bands in vibration. Pressure exerted by some of the abdominal
muscles on the diaphragm supplies the extra amount of energy needed
for setting the vocal bands in vibration. Without such pressure, exhalation would be passive, and sufficient only for normal respiratory
purposes.

Breathing for Phonation. Normal respiration for a person without pathology or anomaly of the respiratory mechanism requires no special thought or effort. Breathing for phonation is different from normal respiratory breathing in at least two respects: (1) the ratio cycle of inspiration to respiration is modified so that there is a considerably longer period for exhalation than in casual breathing; (2) a steady stream of air must be created and controlled at the will of the speaker to insure the initiation and maintenance of good tone. This type of air flow is usually most easily accomplished by controlling the abdominal musculature and by using small amounts of air rather than by inhaling large amounts of air. Attempts at deep inhalation tend to be accompanied by exaggerated activity of the upper part of the chest. This type of breathing (clavicular), which Gray and Wise (1959, p. 154) observe, frequently promotes unsteadiness. The result may be a wavering tone and a strained voice quality. Clavicular breathing tends to produce excessive neck and throat tensions, and so prevents free and appropriate reinforcement of vocal tones in the cavities of the larynx and throat. Adequate breath supply is difficult to maintain, and the speaker needs to inhale more frequently than in abdominally controlled breathing.

THE RESONATING CAVITIES

The important resonating cavities for the human mechanism are those of the larynx, throat (pharynx), mouth (oral or buccal cavity), and nose (nasal cavity). To a lesser but not insignificant degree, the part of the windpipe below the larynx also serves as a resonating cavity. The principal cavities may be located by an examination of Figure 5.

The resonating cavities serve two functions in voice production: (1) they permit us to reinforce or build up the loudness of tones without resorting to constant energetic use of air pressure; and (2) through modification in the tension and shape of the cavities of the mouth, the nasopharynx, and the nasal cavity we produce changes in the quality of vocal tones. For example, nasality may result when sound is permitted to enter and be emitted through the nasal chambers. This, however, is not the only cause of nasality as a voice quality.

We have little control over the larynx as a resonating chamber. We have most control over the oral cavity and considerable control over the pharynx. The speech sounds we identify as vowels are produced by modifications in the size and shape of the oral cavity. Those we recognize as consonants are produced as a result of changes of the organs of articulation, the lips included, within the oral cavity.

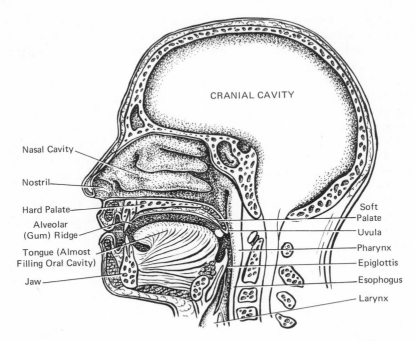

Figure 5. Head section showing principal resonators and organs of articulation.

THE NERVOUS MECHANISM

Primates such as the apes have oral and respiratory mechanisms that approximate and parallel that of human beings, but with one important exception. The exception is that the nonhuman primates do not have a nervous system capable of the fine and specialized perception of those auditory events that constitute the signals and symbols of oral language. Nor do their systems permit, even on a reflexive level, the production of the variety of sounds that is normal for the infant and young child. (See pages 120–122). Most apes are relatively quiet unless they are agitated. The chimpanzee, the subject of considerable study and training for its possible capabilities for acquiring speech, is notably a very quiet animal.* So if we proceed on the assumption that, until proven otherwise, only the human being is capable of oral speech, we ought to consider what is unique about him that is associated with this capability.

---

* Two psychologists, Gardner and Gardner (1969), report success in the training of a chimpanzee to learn the American Sign Language, a gestural system employed by many deaf people in North America.

The Cerebral Cortex. The very special part of the nervous system that endows man with the capability for speech is the cerebral cortex, the outer layer of the brain. The ten or more billion cells of the cortex enable man to perceive, analyze, and synthesize events that come to the cortex through his sensory avenues, and to determine appropriate output in the light of what he has received. Particular areas of the cortex are related to different kinds of intake and output. For the purposes of this chapter there is no need for us to go into detail about cerebrocortical functions. The diagram of the brain (Figure 6) shows some of the areas of specialization in which particular language functions are normally controlled or localized.

Man's cerebral system is significantly different from that of other primates in that the two hemispheres have become functionally

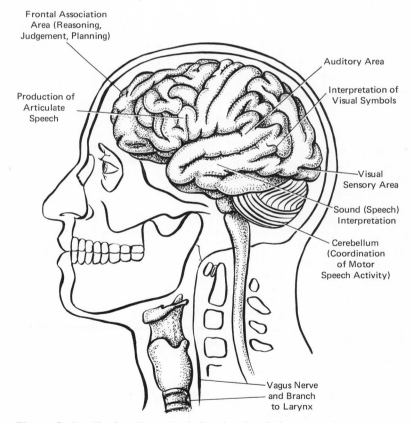

Figure 6. Localization of some brain functions in relation to speech.

different. Most important for us in regard to speech is the recently gained knowledge that the left temporal area of the cortex processes speech events for almost all right-handed persons and for a majority of left-handed persons, while the right temporal cortex processes auditory intake that is not speech, e.g., musical, mechanical, and other environmental noises. By virtue of this specialization we may say that the left brain (cortex) is for speech listening. Because those of us who do not have severe impairment in hearing learn to speak by imitating what we hear, the left brain is also for talking. Damage to the left temporal cortex impairs the capacity for auditory perception of speech and so results in serious delay in the onset and development of language. Damage to a child or an adult who has acquired language will usually result in a breakdown of language function. Fortunately for the child below the age of 12, his cerebrocortical system at this stage seems to have sufficient plasticity for the alternate or nondominant hemisphere to take over the language functions normally controlled by the left or dominant hemisphere. Unfortunately, this is not so for most adults. Impairments of language function associated with brain damage are known as aphasias. We will discuss the aphasic child in Chapter 16.*

References and Suggested Readings

ANDERSON, V. A., *Training the Speaking Voice*, 2nd ed. New York, Oxford University Press, Inc., 1961, Chap. 2.

EISENSON, J., J. J. AUER, and J. V. IRWIN, *The Psychology of Communication.* New York, Appleton-Century-Crofts, 1963, Chap. 4. (An exposition of the nervous mechanism in its relationship to speech production.)

EISENSON, J., and P. H. BOASE, *Basic Speech*, Rev. Ed. New York, The Macmillan Company, 1964. (An introductory consideration of the speech mechanism, including the central nervous system.)

GARDNER, R. A. and B. T. GARDNER, "Teaching Sign Language to a Chimpanzee," *Science*, CLXV, (August, 1969), 664–672. (An expository narration of how two psychologists brought up and trained a chimpanzee to learn a gesture language system.)

GRAY, G. W., and C. M. WISE, *The Bases of Speech.* New York, Harper & Row, Publishers, 1959, Chap. 3. (An advanced and technical consideration of the mechanism of breathing for speech.)

KAPLAN, H. M., *Anatomy and Physiology of Speech.* New York, McGraw Hill, Inc., 1960, Chaps. 6 and 12. (A technical and detailed treatment of the voice and articulatory mechanisms.)

---

* For a discussion of the perceptual functions that underly speech read Jon Eisenson, "Perceptual Disturbances in Children with Central Nervous System Disfunctions and Implications for Language Development," *The British Journal of Disorders of Communications*, I, 1 (1966), pp. 21–32.

Van Riper, C., and J. V. Irwin, *Voice and Articulation*. Englewood Cliffs, N.J., Prentice-Hall, Inc., 1958, Chaps. 10 and 11. (A detailed consideration of the mechanisms for vocalization and articulation.)

Problems

1. What determines the range of pitch of a musical instrument? What part of the violin reinforces the sounds of the vibrators? What are the essential differences between the sounds of a violin and those of a cello?
2. Is deep breathing necessary for most speech purposes? Why should clavicular breathing be avoided?
3. Read pages 344-346 of Van Riper and Irwin, *Voice and Articulation* (Englewood Cliffs, N.J.: Prentice Hall, Inc., 1958). What do these authors recommend as the best techniques to control breathing for vocalization? How do their recommendations compare with those of this text?
4. What are the functions of the resonating cavities in phonation?
5. Over which resonators do we have most control? Over which do we have least control?
6. What is nasality? What is denasality? Is nasal reinforcement always to be avoided?
7. What cavities does the diaphragm separate? What is the shape of the diaphragm during exhalation? How does the shape change during inhalation?
8. What is a syrinx? What are the essential differences in sound-making between birds and most mammals? How does a parrot manage to sound as if he is speaking?
9. Male and female vocal bands overlap in range of length, yet it is usually easy to distinguish the voices of low-pitched females from high-pitched males. Why?
10. What is cerebral dominance? How is cerebral dominance related to language functioning?

Chapter 6

The Production of Speech Sounds

In this chapter we will explain how consonants, vowels, and diphthongs are usually produced. We recognize that the described positions are merely the conventional ones and that, because our mechanism is adaptable, we produce sounds in ways other than the conventional ones. We will further attempt to show characteristics that are shared by a number of sounds, for to recognize likenesses in sounds is important in understanding the development of speech sounds and in the correction of speech sounds. The teacher needs this information to understand children's speech patterns and the clinician needs it to work with children who have articulatory problems.

We are basing this discussion of sounds on the writings and research of articulatory phoneticians who work primarily in the discipline of speech. Such authors include C. K. Thomas, A. J. Bronstein, and C. Wise. Most of you who are using this book will be either majors or minors in speech who have studied phonetics from this viewpoint. Linguists may attack the problems somewhat differently. Acoustic phoneticians may also attack the problems somewhat differently. We include a brief explanation of some of the terms used in acoustic phonetics, because some of the literature in speech correction is based on the study of acoustic phonetics.

Relationship of Spelling to Sounds

It is hardly necessary to impress the readers of this text with the realization that American English, or British English for that matter, does not consistently represent the same sound with the same alphabet letter. The teacher who has had any concern with teaching children to read has on numerous occasions had to explain that many words are pronounced in a manner only remotely suggested by their spellings. Perhaps the teacher has been aware that we have 40 or more sound families in our spoken language. If not, the teacher has surely known that we have 26 letters, many of which represent more than one sound, and some of which, according to given words, represent the same sound. So the child has been instructed to memorize the pronunciation and spelling of such words as *though, enough, through,* and *cough* as well as the varied ways in which the sound *sh* is represented in the words *attention, delicious, ocean,* and *shall.* Vowel sounds, too, have their inconsistencies so that before the child at school is too far along in his career he becomes aware that the sound of *ee* in *see* may be represented differently in words such as *eat, believe, receive, species,* and *even.* Later, he may be able to accept without too much consternation the spellings of words of foreign derivation such as *subpoena* and *esprit.*

PHONEMES

If the teacher has had a course in phonetics, the concept of the phoneme may have been established. A phoneme is a distinctive phonetic element of a word. It is the smallest distinctive group or class of sounds in a language. Each phoneme includes a variety of closely related sounds that differ somewhat in manner of production and in acoustic end results, but do not differ so much that the listener is more aware of difference than of similarity or sameness. So, for example, the *t* of *tin* is different from the *t* of *its, spotted, button,* and *metal,* and of the *t* in the phrase *hit the ball,* but an essential quality of *t* is common in all these words. Despite differences we have a phoneme *t.*

In this text, phonemes will be represented by the symbol of the International Phonetic Alphabet (IPA).

It will be noted that phonetic symbols represent pronunciations as they are made. The same sound and its phonemic variants are represented by a single symbol. This is not the case with diacritic symbols which, for some vowels and diphthongs, require several representations for the same phoneme.

The Common Phonemes of
American-English

Key Word	IPA Symbol
	CONSONANTS
1. *p*at	[p]
2. *b*ee	[b]
3. *t*in	[t]
4. *d*en	[d]
5. *c*ook	[k]
6. *g*et	[g]
7. *f*ast	[f]
8. *v*an	[v]
9. *th*in	[θ]
10. *th*is	[ð]
11. *s*ea	[s]
12. *z*oo	[z]
13. *sh*e	[ʃ]
14. trea*s*ure	[ʒ]
15. *ch*ick	[tʃ]
16. *j*ump	[dʒ]
17. *m*e	[m]
18. *n*o	[n]
19. si*ng*	[ŋ]
20. *l*et	[l]
21. *r*un	[r]
22. *y*ell	[j]
23. *h*at	[h]
24. *w*on	[w]
25. *wh*at*	[ʍ] or [hw]
	VOWELS
26. f*ee*	[i]
27. s*i*t	[ɪ]
28. t*a*ke	[e]
29. m*e*t	[ɛ]
30. c*a*lm	[ɑ]
31. t*a*sk	[æ] or [a] depending upon regional or individual variations
32. c*a*t	[æ]
33. h*o*t	[ɒ] or [ɑ] depending upon regional or individual variations
34. s*aw*	[ɔ]

* If distinction is made in pronunciation of words such as *what* and *watt; when* and *wen.*

Key Word	IPA Symbol
35. *o*bey, s*ew*	[o] or [ou]
36. b*u*ll	[ʊ]
37. b*oo*n	[u]
38. h*u*t	[ʌ]
39. *a*bout	[ə]
40. upp*er*	[ɚ] by most Americans and [ə] by many others
41. b*i*rd	[ɝ] by most Americans and [ɜ] by many others
	DIPHTHONGS
42. s*igh*	[aɪ]
43. N*oi*se	[ɔɪ]
44. c*ow*	[aʊ] or [ɑʊ] depending upon individual variations
45. m*ay*	[eɪ]
46. g*o*	[oʊ]
47. ref*u*se	[ɪu] or [ju] depending upon individual variations
48. *u*se	[ju]

If you wish to memorize the phonetic symbols, it may encourage you to know that sixteen of the consonant symbols are taken from the English alphabet. They are: p, b, t, d, k, g, f, v, s, z, m, n, l, r, h, and w. IPA symbols for vowels, however, vary considerably from alphabetic representations.

MORPHEMES

The speaker combines phonemes meaningfully to produce what the linguist calls *morphemes*. A morpheme is a minimal unit that carries meaning and is made up of one or more phonemes. Lloyd and Warfel note that "written sentences break up into words, but spoken sentences break up into morphemes" (Lloyd and Warfel, 1956, p. 61). When the speaker combines morphemes in meaningful ways, he produces phrases and sentences, or what the linguist calls *utterances*. This example may illustrate: The word *hit* is a combination of the phonemes [h], [ɪ], and [t]. This combination [hɪt] is a morpheme, for it cannot be broken into a smaller form with meaning. The word *lemon* constitutes a morpheme for neither the syllable [lɛm] or [ən] carries meaning. In the plural form [lɛmənz], the added [z] is a morpheme in itself for it is a minimal unit that does carry meaning.

In this chapter, although we are primarily concerned with phonemes, we wish to emphasize the influence of one sound upon another in context. The discussion immediately following will be concerned with how sounds are produced and a description of the parts of the speech mechanism that are employed in articulation.

Articulatory Mechanism

Speech sounds are produced when the breath stream that comes from the lungs by way of the trachea and larynx is modified in the mouth before leaving the body. Breath may be modified by movements of the lips, teeth, jaws, tongue, and the soft palate (roof of the mouth). Most American-English sounds are produced as a result of lip and tongue activity and resulting contacts with other organs of articulation. The front part of the tongue (tip and blade) and the part of the mouth at or near the upper gum ridge is the "favored" area for articulatory contact for American-English speech sounds. The sounds *t, d, l, n, s, z, sh* [ʃ], *zh* [ʒ], *ch* [tʃ], and *j* [dʒ] are all produced by action of the anterior tongue and contact at or close to the upper gum ridge.

If we examine Figure 7 we will note that the upper gum ridge or alveolar process is the area directly behind the upper teeth. Immediately behind the alveolar process is the hard palate. Posterior to it is the soft palate or velum. The uvula is the most posterior part of the "roof of the mouth."

The tongue lies within and almost completely fills the oral or mouth cavity. The tongue, from the point of view of articulatory action, may be considered as being divided into tongue tip, blade, front (mid), and back, as indicated in Figure 7.

The lips act as articulators for the production of the sounds *p* and *b*. The sound *m* is produced with closed lips. The sounds *f* and *v* are usually produced as a result of action involving the lower lip and upper teeth. The various vowel and diphthong sounds are produced with characteristic lip and jaw movement, though the lips do not make any articulatory contacts for these sounds. The production of American-English sounds will be considered later in somewhat greater detail.

Speech sounds may be emitted either through the mouth or through the nasal cavity. In the absence of specific pathology, the speaker is able to determine the avenue of sound emission. Most American-English sounds are emitted through the mouth. The sounds *m, n,* and the con-

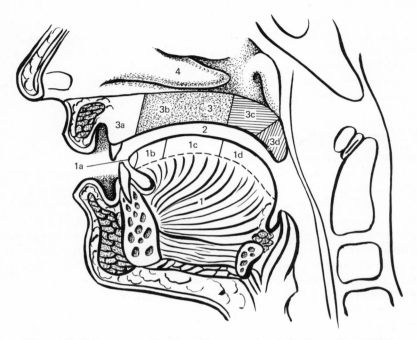

Figure 7. Diagram showing parts of the tongue in relationship to the roof of the mouth.

1. Tongue	3. Palate
1a. Tongue tip	3a. Gum or alveolar ridge
1b. Blade of tongue	3b. Hard palate
1c. Front or mid of tongue	3c. Soft palate
1d. Back of tongue	3d. Uvula
2. Mouth (oral) cavity	4. Nasal cavity.

sonant that is usually represented in spelling by the letters *ng* are emitted through the nasal cavity.

Sounds usually are categorized as: 1) consonants, 2) vowels, and 3) diphthongs. A consonant is a sound that results from the action of articulating agents somehow interrupting the expiring breath, with the vocal bands sometimes vibrating, sometimes not. A vowel is a sound with little or no stoppage of the breath stream, whose quality comes from the vibration of the vocal bands and from the shape and size of the resonating chambers in the throat and mouth. Diphthongs are combinations or rapid blends of two vowels—usually beginning with one vowel and gliding into another.

Consonants

As you say *pat*, *bat*, and *mat*, you hear three distinct words, because the first consonant in each of these three words is different. However, as you say the three words, you find that in each instance you have made the sounds with your two lips. Another likeness exists in [p] and [b]. In these sounds, you have held the sound briefly and quickly released it. [p] and [b] are called *stops*. How, then, do [p] and [b] differ? [p] is made without voice, [b], with voice. How, then, do [b] and [m] differ? Both sounds are voiced but [p] is held and quickly released without nasal emission whereas [m] is continued and is emitted nasally. Thus, the manner of production of [m] results in acoustic features that enable the listener to distinguish it from [p].

From this discussion we can then classify the consonant sounds according to: 1) manner of production, 2) place of articulation, and 3) the vocal component.

MANNER OF PRODUCTION

Stops. When you say the [p] and [b] in *pat* and *bat*, you use your lips but you also make the sounds by compressing the breath and suddenly releasing it. These sounds are therefore called stops. Other stops are [t], [d], [k], and [g].

Continuants. All other sounds are continuants, which in turn are classified as 1) frictionless consonants or semivowels, and 2) fricatives. The continuant [m] which you hear in *mat* is emitted nasally by lowering your velum and by directing the air through the nose. The other two nasal sounds are [n] and [ŋ] as in *sing*. The lateral [l] and the glides are also classified as semivowels. [l] is made with the sound being forced over two sides of the tongue. The glides, [r] as in *run*, [j] as in *yell*, [w] as in *won*, and [ʍ] as in *what*, are made by the movement of the articulatory agents from one position to another. All these sounds are frictionless. Other continuant sounds called fricatives, however, have a frictionlike quality, which is caused by the release of sound through a narrow opening between the organs of articulation. A stream of breath is maintained with some pressure to make the sound continuous. These sounds are [f], [v], [s], [z], [h], [θ] as in *thin*, [ð] as in *this*, [ʍ] as in *what*, [ʃ] as in *she*, and [ʒ] as in *treasure*.

Affricates. Lastly, American-English sounds include affricates or the consonantal blends, as [tʃ] in *check* and [dʒ] in *jump*. Thus each sound achieves some of its characteristic acoustic quality by its manner of production.

PLACE OF ARTICULATION

The classification of consonants just given was according to manner of articulation. Consonants may also be classified as to which articulators are used and the position they are in during the act of sound production. The following is a classification of consonants as to position of articulators:

1. *Bilabial.* Sounds are produced as a result of the activity of the lips. The sounds [p], [b], [m], [ʍ], and [w] are bilabials.

2. *Lip-teeth* (*labiodental*). Contact is made between the upper teeth and lower lip for the production of labiodental sounds. The sounds so produced are [f] and [v].

3. *Tongue-teeth* (*linguadental*). Contact is made between the point of the tongue and the upper teeth or between the point of the tongue in a position between the teeth. The *th* sounds [θ] and [ð] may be made either postdentally or interdentally. Most mature speakers are likely to produce these sounds postdentally

4. *Tongue-tip gums* (*Lingua-alveolar*). The region of the mouth at or near the gum ridge is the "favored place" for the articulation of American-English sounds. The sounds [t], [d], [n], and [l] are produced with the tip of the tongue in contact with the upper gum ridge. The sound [r] is most frequently produced with the tongue tip turned back slightly away from the gum ridge. The sounds [s], [z], *sh* [ʃ], *zh* [ʒ], *ch* [tʃ], and *j* [dʒ], are produced with the blade of the tongue making articulatory contact a fraction of an inch behind the gum ridge.

5. *Palatal.* The sound *y* [j] is produced with the middle of the tongue initially raised toward the hard palate. The sounds [k] and [g] are usually produced with the back of the tongue in contact with the soft palate. In some contexts [k] and [g] may be produced with the middle of the tongue in contact with the hard palate. The reader may check his place of articulation for the [k] in *car* compared with [k] in *keel*. He may also wish to compare the [g] of *get* with the [g] of *got*.

The sound of *ng* [ŋ] is most likely to be produced with the back of the tongue in contact with the soft palate.

In some contexts, the sound [r] is produced with the middle of the tongue raised toward the palate. Some persons produce the [r] of *rose* and *around* in this manner.

6. *Glottal.* One American-English sound, [h], is produced with the breath coming through the opening between the vocal folds and without

modification by the other articulators. The [h] is referred to as a glottal sound.

VOCAL COMPONENT

A third classification of sounds is according to the presence or absence of voice. Consonants produced without accompanying vocal-fold vibration are referred to as *voiceless* or *unvoiced*; those produced with accompanying vocal fold vibration are called *voiced*. The voiceless consonants of American-English speech are: [p], [t], [k], [ʍ], [f], *th* of *th*ink [θ], [s], *sh* [ʃ], and [h]. The voiced consonants are: [b], [d], [g,] [m], [n], *ng* [ŋ], [v], *th* of *th*is [ð], [z], *zh*, [ʒ], [w], [r], y[j], and [l].

A resumé of the multiple classification of American-English consonant sounds is presented in the chart that follows.

Production of American English Consonants

Involvement of Articulatory Agents

Manner of Production	LIPS (BI-LABIAL)	LIP-TEETH (LABIO-DENTAL)	TONGUE-TEETH (LINGUA-DENTAL)	TONGUE TIP ALVEOLAR RIDGE (LINGUA-ALVEOLAR)	TONGUE AND HARD PALATE (LINGUA-PALATAL)	TONGUE AND SOFT PALATE (VELAR)	GLOTTIS (GLOTTAL)
Voiceless stops	p			t		k	
Voiced stops	b			d		g	
Voiceless fricatives	ʍ	f	θ	s*	ʃ†	ʍ¶	h
Voiced fricatives		v	ð	z*	ʒ†		
Nasals	m			n		ŋ	
Lateral semivowel				l			
Glides	w				r‡ j	w¶	
Voiceless affricate					tʃ		
Voiced affricate					dʒ		

* In [s] and [z], the channel is narrow.
† In [ʃ] and [ʒ], the channel is broad.
‡ The tongue tip in many instances is curled away from the gum ridge to the center of the palate.
¶ In [ʍ] and [w], both the lips and the back of the tongue are involved.

Distinctive Features of Consonants

If we apply the term *distinctive features* to the system just described, we base our distinctions on the differences in consonants on manner of production, place of articulation, and the vocal component. For example, let us contrast [p], [b], and [m]. The feature distinguishing [p] and [b] is the vocal component. On the other hand, [m] has three features to distinguish it from [p]: it possesses voice, is made with nasal resonance, and is a continuant whereas [p] does not possess these three characteristics.

The term *distinctive features* as applied in the literature refers to features presented as binary contrasts. The feature is present [+] or absent [−]. If we put the distinguishing features of [p], [b], and [m] as just discussed in this form it would appear as:

Distinctive Features of /p/, /b/, and /m/

	Voice/Lack of it	*Nasal/Non-nasal*	*Continuant/Non-continuant*	*Labial/Non-labial*
[p]	−	−	−	+
[b]	+	−	−	+
[m]	+	+	+	+

Distinctive features as used in most of the current literature is based on acoustic terms; the distinctive features are nine: vocalic/nonvocalic, consonantal/non-consonantal, compact/diffuse, grave/acute, flat/plain, nasal/oral, tense/lax, continuant/interrupted, strident/mellow. Those appearing in the literature about articulation problems usually are: grave/acute, strident/mellow, compact/diffuse. If you wish to read further concerning distinctive features as they relate to articulation problems, consult the H. Winitz book on articulation cited in the bibliography in Chapter 10. If you wish to read further concerning the distinctiveness criteria, read Harms cited at the end of this chapter.

The following definitions are included so that you may read the literature on articulation problems more easily. They are defined acoustically except for grave/acute which is also defined genetically.

Grave/Acute
    Acoustically, grave—Energy concentrated on lower frequencies of the spectrum. Large front cavity.

- Examples: [m], [f], [p], [v], and [b].
- Genetically, grave—Made at the periphery of the articulatory mechanism.
- Examples: [p], [b], [m], [k], and [g].
- Acoustically, acute—Energy concentrated on upper frequencies of spectrum. Large back cavity.
- Examples: [n], [s], [ɵ], [t], [z], [ð], [d].
- Genetically, acute—Made at the mid section of the articulatory mechanism.
- Examples: [s], [ʃ].

Strident/Mellow
- A high degree of noise (interference is high) versus a low degree of noise.
- Examples: Strident: [dʒ], [tʃ], [s], [t]
  Mellow: [g], [k], [z].

Compact/Diffuse
- Compact—A predominantly central formant with increase in total amount of energy and its spread in time.
- Examples: [r], [ŋ], [ʃ], [tʃ], [k], [ʒ], [dʒ], [g].
- Diffuse—No one central formant with decrease in total amount of energy and its spread in time.
- Examples: [m], [f], [p], [v], [b], [n], [s], [θ], [t], [z], [ð], [d].

The spectrogram shows us these sounds by indicating their resonance frequencies from which we can learn to identify them. The bands correspond to the basic frequencies of the vibrations in the vocal tract. The formants are the comparatively larger, darker regions that indicate the most intense frequencies.

From your newly acquired knowledge of the presence or lack of voice, the articulatory agents involved and the manner of production of consonants, examine the following changes and indicate what happens. For example, *tense* often becomes [tɛnts]. The insertion of [t], which is made with approximately the same articulatory agents as [s] and [n], takes place because the morpheme becomes easier to utter with the [t] inserted. Why, then, does *something* become ['sʌmp͵θɪŋ], *tenth* [tɛntθ] and *dance* [dænts]?

1. As you say *tackle* and *gargle*, the [k] and [g] are exploded laterally. Explain why.
2. As you utter *at the store* and *add the numbers*, the [t] and [d] are made with the tongue on the teeth rather than on the alveolar ridge. Why?
3. In *let out the dog, little, city mouse, cutting the grass*, [t] takes on some of the voiced characteristic of [d]. Why?

4. In *grandmother* and *handsome*, speakers frequently omit [d]. What characteristic of the [n] influences the omission of [d]?

5. In *campfire* and *obviate*, the [f] and [v] are made by some speakers with both lips, causing the sounds to become labial fricatives. Why does this happen?

6. In rapid speech, you are likely to omit [θ] in *fifth* and *seventh*. Explain in terms of the place of articulation.

7. Why in the speech of one individual do two pronunciations of *with* occur—*with Dan* [wɪð dæn] and *with Tom* [wɪθ tɑm]?

8. Why, in terms of the articulatory agents involved, does *Captain* become [kæpm]?

Vowels

Whereas consonants are important because they help bring intelligibility to the message, vowels through their variables of quality, pitch, time, and loudness bring emotion and feeling to the message. The word *no* printed singly carries some meaning as a written symbol, but *no* spoken singly carries more meaning and feeling. Spoken with loudness and a downward inflection, it conveys one kind of meaning and feeling; spoken softly with a rising inflection, it carries another kind of meaning and feeling.

Vowels are more variable than consonants; neighboring sounds influence vowels more than consonants. And the effect of the continuing movement of the vocal articulators during the utterance of a vowel in a word or phrase makes for differences both in acoustic results and articulatory movements. Although we describe vowels according to the previous discussion, you must remember that these characteristics are based on norms and that many individual variations exist.

Vowel sounds share the following characteristics in their manner of production: (1) All vowels are voiced, unless for special purposes the entire speech content is intentionally whispered; (2) all vowels are continuant sounds in that they are produced without interruption or restriction of the breath stream; (3) changes in tongue and jaw position are primarily responsible for the distinctive differences in vowel phonemes. To a lesser degree, lip activity accounts for some of the difference in articulatory activity and in acoustic end result.

PLACE OF PRODUCTION

All vowel sounds require activity of the tongue as a whole. It will be noticed, however, that each of the American-English vowels is produced with one part of the tongue more actively involved than the remainder of the tongue. For example, in the production of the vowel of the word *me*, the tip of the tongue remains relatively inactive behind the lower teeth, while the front of the tongue is tensed and raised toward the hard palate. In changing from *me* to *moo*, we may note that the front of the tongue is relatively relaxed, while the back is tensed and elevated toward the roof of the mouth. The vowel of *me*, because of its characteristic tongue activity, is considered to be a *front vowel*; similarly, the vowel of *moo*, because of the back of the tongue activity, is considered to be a *back vowel*.

HEIGHT OF TONGUE

Now, let us contrast the production of the vowels of *me* and *man*. Both of these are produced with front of the tongue activity, but the tongue is higher for the vowel of *me* than it is for the vowel of *man*. Similarly, the tongue is higher for the back vowel of *moon* than it is for the vowel of *mock*. In the words *mirth* and *mud*, where middle of the tongue activity is characteristic, we may also note that the vowel of *mirth* is produced with the tongue higher in position than it is in *mud*. The difference in height of tongue position, however, is not as great as for the other pairs of words.

Thus far, we have seen that vowels differ somewhat in individual production according to the part of the tongue that is most actively involved and the height of the tongue. We may also have noted that the change in the height of the tongue is likely to be accompanied by a change in the position of the lower jaw. That is, the jaw drops as the tongue drops, in going from a "high" to a "low" vowel. A third aspect of vowel production will now be considered.

MUSCLE TENSION

If we compare the vowels of *tea* and *tin*, we should be able to sense that the tongue is more tense for the vowel of *tea* than it is for the vowel of *tin*. Similarly, the vowel of *moot* is produced with more tongue tension than the vowel of *mock*. Further analysis will show that the differences in tension are not confined to the muscles of the tongue. The muscles of the chin also differ in degree of tension. A third muscle difference may be left by observing the changes in the position of the apex of the larynx—the "Adam's apple." When the tongue and under part of the chin are tense, the apex of the larynx is elevated and moves toward the front of the chin as it does in the act of swallowing. When the tongue and the under part of the chin are relatively relaxed, the larynx drops back to its normal position of rest as in quiet breathing.

On the basis of our discussion thus far, we may arrive at a threefold classification for vowel sounds.

1. Vowels differ as to place of production. They may be produced either in the front of the mouth, with the front or blade of the tongue most active; in the middle of the mouth, with the mid-tongue most active; or in the back of the mouth, with the back of the tongue most active.

Front Vowels		*Mid Vowels*		*Back Vowels*	
	PHONETIC SYMBOL		PHONETIC SYMBOL		PHONETIC SYMBOL
meet	[i]			boon	[u]
milk	[ɪ]			book	[ʊ]
may	[e]	Mirth	[ɜ] or [ɝ]	boat	[o]
men	[ɛ]	about	[ə]	ball	[ɔ]
mat	[æ]	upper	[ɚ]	bog	[ɒ]
ask*	[a]	mud	[ʌ]	balm	[ɑ]

* When the speaker compromises betmeen the vowels of *mat* and of *balm*.

2. Vowels differ as to height of tongue position.
3. Vowels differ as to degree of muscle tension.

LIP ROUNDING

A fourth feature which distinguishes some vowels from others, especially when the vowels are produced as isolated sounds, is lip-rounding. Back vowels, with the exception of the *a* of *calm*, are produced with the lips somewhat rounded. The vowel of the word *pool* is most rounded. There is lesser rounding for the vowels in *pull, boat, ball,* and *cot*. For persons who do not distinguish between the vowels of *cot* and *calm*, there will be no lip-rounding for either.

In the lists of words on this page, the first column contains front vowels, arranged in order of highest to lowest tongue position. The second column contains mid vowels, and the third back vowels, arranged in the same order.

The tongue position for the vowels of these words are shown in Figure 8. The dotted area represents the high points of the tongue.

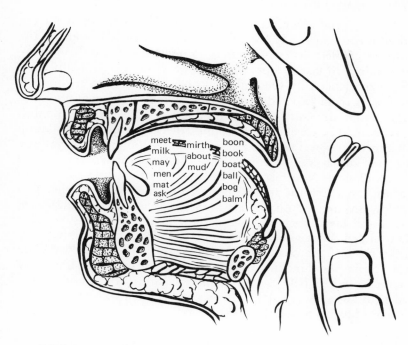

Figure 8. Representative tongue positions for American-English vowels. In actual speech there is considerable individual variation from these positions according to speech context.

DEGREE OF STRESSING

Vowels with greater stress tend to be longer than those with less stress; in fact, the stressed vowel often becomes diphthongized. Where [e] is stressed as uttered in the list of words, *vague, day, rain,* it is diphthongized. But when it is not stressed, as in the first syllable of *vacation* and in the last syllable of *mandate,* it is not diphthongized. Context is also important in the degree of stress. When you say, "Give me Kay's address," you are apt to use the monophthongal [e]. But when you say, "Are you meeting Kay?" you are apt to use the diphthongal [eɪ]. A second example involves [o]. When you say *obey,* the [o] not being stressed is usually [o], whereas in *row,* the [o] being stressed is usually [oʊ]. When you stress *throw* in "Throw it out," the [oʊ] is diphthongal. But when you do not stress *throw* in "Did Johnny throw away today's paper?" the [o] tends to be the monophthongal [o].

DEFECTIVE VOWEL PRODUCTION

Defects of vowel production do not occur as frequently as those for the production of consonants. The intensity of the vowels and possibly the visible aspects of their articulation help to make it comparatively easy for most children to learn to produce them accurately. Difficulties are sometimes experienced by the child who has hearing loss in the low-pitch ranges. A child exposed to foreign language influences may also experience some difficulty in the production of American-English vowels. We should be careful not to confuse defective vowel articulation with differences in vowel production on the basis of regional variations.

From our discussion of vowels, we can hypothesize that vowel phonemes will never contrast in voice but that they *will* contrast in such features as where the tongue is raised or bunched, whether it is high or low in the mouth, and whether the vowel is rounded or unrounded and lax or tense. Some of these features coexist. No front vowel is rounded. Back vowels tend to be rounded.

On the basis of the characteristics of vowels just discussed (height of tongue, raising or bunching of tongue) explain what has happened in the changes noted below. For example, *Patricia* is sometimes pronounced with an [i] not an [ɪ] in the second syllable. The [ɪ] used by most speakers has been raised to become [i].

1. Why does *keel* become [kɪəl]?
2. What happens as *milk* is pronounced [mʊlk]?
3. The final sound in *Monday, Tuesday, Wednesday* is usually pronounced [ɪ]. How in this different from the final sound being pronounced [e]?
4. Southerners sometimes pronounce *pen* and *pin* alike. In terms of the characteristics just discussed, what is happening?
5. What has occurred in these changes?
   [frʌm] for *from* in *from the farm.*
   [e haʊs] for *a house*
   [ði dɔg] for [ðə dɔg].
   [rʊf] for [ruf].
   [tʊrɪst] for [turɪst].
6. In *tomato salad* and *I bought a tomato*, what is the change in the last sound in *tomato*?
7. Some Southerners says [ra:t] for [raɪt]. What change has occurred?

Diphthongs

Diphthongs, like vowels, are produced as a result of modifications in the size and shape of the mouth and position of the tongue while vocalized breath is being emitted without obstruction of the breath stream. Diphthongs are voice glides uttered in a single breath impulse. Some diphthongs, such as the one in the word *how*, are blends of two vowels. Most diphthongs originally—as far as the history of the language is concerned—were produced as "pure" vowels but "broke down" to what is now a strong vowel gliding off weakly to another vowel lacking distinct individual character. The diphthongs in the words *name* and *row* are examples where the first element is emphasized and readily recognizable and the second element is "weak" and somewhat difficult to discern.

The following list of words includes the most frequently recognized diphthongs in American-English speech. Most phoneticians would limit the *distinctive* diphthongs to those in the words *aisle, plough, toil,* and *use.*

*ai*sle	b*ay*
pl*ou*gh	h*oe*
t*oi*l	d*ear*
f*air*	s*ure*
f*or*t	*u*se

References and Suggested Readings

Bronstein, A. J., *The Pronunciation of American English.* New York, Appleton-Century-Crofts, 1960.

Denes, P. B., and E. N. Pinson, *The Speech Chain.* New York, Bell Telephone Laboratories, 1963, Chap. 4. (Outlines anatomy and physiology of speech production.)

Harms, R. T., *Introduction to Phonological Theory.* Englewood Cliffs, N.J., Prentice-Hall, Inc., 1968. (Introduces the student to generative phonology.)

Liberman, A. M., K. S. Harris, H. S. Hoffman, and B. G. Griffith, "The Discrimination of Speech Sounds Within and Across Phonemic Boundaries," *Journal of Experimental Psychology,* LIV (November, 1957), 358–368.

Liberman, A., K. S. Harris, P. Einas, L. Lisker, and J. Bastian, "An Effect of Learning on Speech Perception: The Discrimination of Duration of Silence with and Without Phonemic Significance," *Language and Speech,* IV (October–December, 1961), 175–196.

Lloyd, D. J., and H. R. Warfel, *American English in Its Cultural Setting.* New York, Alfred A. Knopf, Inc., 1956.

Menyuk, P., "The Role of Distinctive Features in Children's Acquisition of Phonology," Journal of Speech and Hearing Research, XI (March, 1968), 138–146.

Thomas, C. K., *An Introduction to Phonetics of American English.* New York, The Ronald Press Company, 1958.

Problems

1. Distinguish spelling representation from sound representation:
   a. Pick out all words with the sound [ɪ] as in *hit* in *Women are undependable. Their so-called stability is but a myth.*
   b. List as many different spellings for these sounds as you can think of: [i] as in *tree*, [eɪ] as in *jail*, [aɪ] as *try*.
2. Note slight differences within these groups of phonemes:
   [k] *cool, key*
   [t] *stop, tape, rat*
   [p] *paid, spray, apt*
   [ʌ] *but, cut.*
3. Note the similarities and dissimilarities in terms of articulatory agents involved, manner of production, and vocal components in the final sounds of: *tank, tack; rat, race; lamb, can; taps, tabs; cough, five; truth, bathe; call, car.*
4. The following are pronunciations of other cultures as reported in various articles. What are the changes from a phonetic standpoint?
   duty [dʒutɪ]
   forget you [fəgɛtʃʊ]
   have [hæb]
   chicken [ʃɪkən]
   record [rɛkət]
   them [dɛm]
   man [men]
   set or sat [sɑt]
   ice [is]
   pig [piɪg]
   storm [tɔrm]
   lets [lɛs]
   lumber [lʌmɚ]
   children [tʃɪrən]
   On the whole do the above substitutions make more phonetic sense than the following:
   cat [tæk]
   squirrel [gɚdl]
   run [bʌn]
   look [lik]
   Sam [ræt]
   mule [mel]
   What substitutions would make sense in the above words?
5. Why, in teaching [s], would you use the phrases *can sing*, and *right song* rather than *bath soap*? The explanation is a phonetic one.
   Why, in correcting the substitution [f] for [θ], would you use the phrase *right through the door* rather than *come through the door*?

Why, in correcting the substitution of [w] for [l], would you use the phrase *the cat's long hair* rather than *blow long and hard*?

Why, in correcting the substitution of [w] for [r], would you use the phrase *turn red* rather than *barn door*?

Chapter 7

Development of Language

Speech—the capacity to learn an oral/aural code—we consider to be a specific function of the human species. The particular code acquired is, of course, a learned function. Almost all human beings acquire speech, or learn a given language code, because they are born with the capacities for this particular type of learning. Spoken language is a system of symbols, a code, which normally is produced by articulatory activity which associates sounds (utterances) and meaning in particular ways.

A child may be said to be speaking, to be using an oral/aural linguistic system* when he demonstrates by his productions that his utterances conform to the conventions of other speakers in his environment. These conventions include the acquisition of a phonemic or sound system, a morphemic system (the combination of sound elements into words), a semantic system (acquisition of vocabulary, and a syntactical system (the combining of words into "strings" or formulations that approximate the utterances of the mature members of his culture).

---

* Deaf children who learn to use a visible code or sign system are an exception in regard to the use of the oral/aural code. A visible code is, however, acceptable within our definition of speech.

Criteria for Language Acquisition

Sometime between the last quarter of the first year and the middle of the second year of life, the vast majority of children begin to speak. The acquisition of speech, the development of language,* is a continuous process throughout life. Normally, comprehension precedes production and exceeds production from the beginning to the end of life. We may, however, consider the following to be the criteria for the establishment of sufficient competence in comprehension and production to permit us to identify a child as one who has acquired language. A child may be said to be a speaker:

1. When he understands—derives meaning—from a conventionalized system of audible and/or visible symbols.
2. When, without specific and direct training, he can understand verbal formulations to which he has never before been specifically exposed. The child is then *listening creatively*. He understands what people say based on past understandings of what people have said.
3. When he can produce verbal formulations, new utterances that he has never before tried, and have them understood by others. The child is then *talking creatively*.

Criteria (2) and (3) reveal that the child is capable of generalizing from the specific words and utterances he has learned " directly " to the comprehension and production of an indefinite number of new utterances. In a very real and important sense, the child has become a linguistic generalizer and generator. He indicates that he has learned the rules of his language, and is applying these rules—the conventions of older and presumably proficient speakers—to what he hears and what he wants to say. He is likely to make many errors that are products either of overgeneralizing, or of correct generalizing where a linguistic system has exceptions—e.g., saying *sheeps* as a plural for *sheep*. He may

---

* We recognize that language is described by linguists according to hypotheses about competencies shared by a specific language community and that speech represents the performance of an individual user of the language. Speech, therefore, often provides the bases for linguistic research. We also recognize that a child may *know* the linguistic rules but may not be able to use them in speaking. In other words, that there may be a discrepancy between the actual speech output and the potential force for speech proficiency. In this chapter, describing the child's acquisition of linguistic proficiencies, we are not primarily concerned with abstract concepts of language but rather with the individual speaker's verbal output. We are therefore not making distinctions between the cognitive competence and the speech output.

make errors because he has not really caught on to the rules.* Such errors are good positive indicators that the child is " with it " linguistically and has become a verbal being and a member of a verbal culture.

Although the child begins to speak because he was born with the capacities for this achievement, his accomplishments as a verbal being will vary with a variety of innate and environmental factors. For the present we should like to emphasize that the *onset of speech* appears to be unrelated to the particular language a child will acquire, to his level of intelligence (unless the child is severely subnormal), or to the talkativeness of the members of his immediate environment, providing, of course, that they *do* talk. The child's proficiency as a speaker including his language development, is determined by a number of factors that we will consider later.

THE FUNCTIONS OF LANGUAGE

Primarily, the function of language is to permit the child to behave like a human being in the variety of ways in which human beings behave. More specifically, language is used for talking to and with others, to signal needs, intentions, feelings, and thoughts. Language is also used for self-talking (thinking), and for controlling and directing one's own behavior, as well as for controlling and directing the behavior of others. Language is used for deception and even for self-deception, for saying many nothings to avoid a vacuous existence and to becoming an accepted, socialized, and civilized human being. Language is used to disarm or delay nonverbal hostility, and for engaging and instigating hostility. In time, the maturing child will learn that not only does man have a way with language, but that language has a way with man. Not too long after the child acquires a command of language he begins to appreciate that language has a command of him.

In the discussion that follows we will consider the levels or stages of language development and some of the correlated maturational factors in these stages.

Language Developmental Stages

PRELINGUAL STAGES

Before a child speaks his first word—produces a verbal signal with an intended meaning—he normally goes through a series of stages in

---

* For an expanded exposition of this concept see N. Chomsky, " The Formal Nature of Language," in Lenneberg (1967, pp. 397–442).

vocalic and articulatory production that are characteristic and universal. That is, regardless of the linguistic code a child will begin to use during the second year of his life, he is likely to engage in some amount of vocal production characteristic of human infants. We assume, even though it is not clearly established,* that these stages are necessary precursors, at least of the modification of the child's sound (phonemic) productions. In our review of the stages we will speculate as to their implications for later language acquisition.†

UNDIFFERENTIATED CRYING

Babies cry, and parents, especially if they are new in this role, wonder why. Although we shall offer no philosophic speculation as to the reason for the early cries, we do know that babies enter the extrauterine world with a cry. Should a baby fail to do this, the attending physician is likely to give him a sharp slap on his tender backside to elicit such a cry. Perhaps the cry is a reflexive expression of the pain that comes initially with the baby's having to take care of his own breathing. If we cannot say positively that the child cries because of discomfort, we can certainly observe that the child cries when he is uncomfortable. In any event, the birth cry and the crying during the first few weeks of life are considered reflexive manifestations of discomfort. The cries are *undifferentiated*, in that the adult ear cannot distinguish or associate the nature of the discomfort with any features of the crying. The crying may be described as nasal, shrill wailing. It is essentially the same whether the child is hungry, thirsty, cold, in pain, or needs a change of linen.

We regard the first cry, and the subsequent undifferentiated crying, as reflexive expression of physiological (chemico-neuro-muscular) internal on-goings. The occurrence of crying indicates that for the time being the respiratory and laryngeal mechanisms are functioning normally. The child is responding as he should to internal changes. He can approximate his vocal bands, and they can be set into action as air on intake and breath on output are forced between them. If there are any identifiable sounds in reflexive crying, they are likely to be nasalized vowels.

Perhaps we should point that our observations about the child's

---

* Lenneberg (1967, pp. 140–141), a psychologist concerned with the development of language behavior, reports that some children have begun to speak without going through the prelingual stages normal to almost all children.

† Our discussion will be about children born after a normal, full-term pregnancy without any pre-, para-, or immediate post-natal factor to suggest any abnormality.

crying are based on assumptions relative to the changes that take place when an adult does something because the child is crying. Thus, we conclude that the child who stops crying after he is fed must have cried initially because he was hungry, or that the child who stops crying after he is given additional covering must have cried because he was cold. These may well be likely cause-and-effect changes in behavior. It is possible, nevertheless, that the child's cessation of crying may be the result of his being handled and receiving some direct human physical contact. The actual cause of the child's crying may not, however, have been alleviated. Perhaps that is why the child so quickly resumes crying when the adult leaves him.

COMFORT SOUNDS

A few children may vocalize during noncrying periods in states we consider comfortable, e.g., after a feeding and burping. Most infants are silent, awake or asleep, when not crying. Comfort sounds become considerably more evident during the second and third month. This is also the period of differentiated crying and more generally of differentiated vocalization.

DIFFERENTIATED VOCALIZATION

Beginning in the second month, most children become differentiated vocalizers, when crying or when otherwise engaged in sound production. In regard to crying, most mothers can tell when a child is hungry, not just because the child is crying when the mother thinks it is time for him to be hungry, but because his cry sounds characteristically different at such a time than when there is evidence that he needs his diaper changed, or when he is cold. There is a crescendo pattern to the child's hunger cry that is not present under other discomfort conditions.

The differences in crying constitute an early signal system for parents. Those who tune in are able to make associations between a kind of condition and a form of vocalization. We are not suggesting that the child has any intention or awareness about his vocalization. His productions are still reflexive. However, because his neuromuscular system has matured, his unwitting evocations become increasingly differentiated. The child is a reflexive producer, but those who attend may become interpreters of his status. Differentiated vocalization thus permits a one-way communication for the sensitive listener-respondent, usually the mother.

Cooing, gurgling, and "squealing," and sounds that approximate consonants are soon added to the vowel-like sounds in the child's inventory of sound production. Lenneberg (1967, p. 128) observes that beginning at 12 weeks of age, vowel-like (cooing) sounds may be sustained for 15–20 seconds. The infant is well on his way to becoming a proficient sound maker. He is, at this stage, an internationalist in his sound making. His products are by no means restricted to the language or languages of his home. We may, according to our prejudices, recognize front vowels in the child's squealings, and mid and back vowels, *ah*, *uh*, and *oo* in the child's cooing. We may also identify sounds that suggest *m*, *b*, and *g* and *k*.

By 16 weeks the child begins to make definite responses to human sounds and sound makers. The child, on hearing a speaker, turns toward him. His eyes begin to scan and search for the sound maker. If the child is himself engaged in vocalization, his initial response is likely to be an interruption of his effort. On making visual "contact" with the other speaker, the child may then respond by smiling or cooing. Vocal play may be maintained by an interchange of sound making between the child and another vocalizer. The evidence is strong that infant vocalization is reinforced by the presence and stimulation of an adult. Research on the sound making of children brought up in orphanages as well as on their early true speech development (Brodbeck and Irwin, (1946), Goldfarb, (1954), Lenneberg, (1967, p. 137) reveal that these children engage in less sound play than do those of peer age who are brought up in homes and receive parental attention.

It is possible to overwhelm the child by too much stimulation. Some children respond to adult efforts by ceasing their own vocalization. The wise adult can be guided by what needs to be done by observing the effects of what is done. If the child responds to adult sound play by more of his own, then the play should be continued. If the child stops his own vocalization, then the adult should cease too. We are not suggesting that the adult should refrain indefinitely from stimulating the child. The effort should certainly be resumed at a later time, and the results observed. A 16-week-old child may welcome stimulation that he rejected a week or two earlier. Few normal children will deprive adults of the enjoyment of vocal interchange.

The first three months take the infant from undifferentiated, reflexive crying to differentiated vocalization. Even the objective observer may conclude that the child's sound play, his cooing, gurgling, and more discernible oral products are fun. There are, however, some silent children who cry very little and with no suggestion of feeling or enthusiasm. Though some of these will ultimately become adequate if not loquacious speakers, a few will be among the small number who will grow up as nonverbal children. These, whom parents retrospectively recall as "very good" infants, whose cries were token whimpers, may later be identified as autistic children. Not only in their failure to respond to human speech, but in other aspects of their behavior, they are essentially silent and nonrelating children.

BABBLING

The period from three to six months is one characterized by a considerable increase in vocalization that includes identifiable sounds used in speaking. Some of these sounds, and combinations of sounds, are reduplicated. So we may hear "ga-ga" and "ug-ug" and "bah-bah." There is also a marked increase in the child's responses to the nonverbal behavior of members of his environment. The child may squeal with apparent pleasure at the sight of his mother, or when given a toy, or when picked up for play by a parent. He may respond with crying to loud sounds, or any suggestion of "No" or scolding in the voice of someone from whom he usually expects warmth and friendliness. By six months most children have reached the prelingual stage we designate as babbling.

We consider babbling an exceedingly important stage in speech development. Innate drives toward vocalization and sound play may be reinforced or discouraged. Environmental factors—the influence and effects of external stimulation—become determinants of what the child will be doing as a future sound maker. The child seems to be aware that sound making is pleasurable, both as an accomplishment in itself and as a technique for giving pleasure to others. We agree with Lewis (1959) that the primarily innate forces that bring the child to babbling will be enhanced and sustained by the nature of his environment. The child needs a favorable climate, with attentive but not overwhelming adults, to sustain him in his continued speech development.

By about the sixth month, differences in the vocalizations of deaf and hearing children may be discerned by a sophisticated listener. For the most part, these differences are more readily apparent in the deaf child's responses to the vocalization of others than in his own spontaneous efforts. The deaf child seems now to have a more limited repertoire of sounds than does his peer who can hear. Lenneberg (1964, p. 154) observes:

> . . . the total amount of a deaf child's vocalization may not be different from that of a hearing child, but the hearing child at this age will constantly run through a large repertoire of sounds whereas the deaf children will be making the same sounds sometimes for weeks on end

and then suddenly change to some other set of sounds and "specialize" in them for a while. There is no consistent preference among deaf children for specific sounds.

The voice of the deaf child in spontaneous utterance is no different from that of the hearing child. In response to inner drives the deaf child's voice is as true an indicator of his feelings as is the voice of the hearing child. The internal physiological mechanisms that create the neuromuscular state for vocalization are the same for the deaf child as for the one with normal hearing. So, too, the product is of the same variety. It is only when the deaf child's voice is part of a voluntary effort that differences appear, and the high-pitched, poorly modulated voice of the deaf begins to be heard.

LALLING

By eight months most children engage in a considerable amount of self-imitation in their sound making. We can begin to hear clear "ga-ga," "da-da," "ma-ma" utterances, often accompanied by intonation patterns that resemble those in the child's home. The child's voice will make it quite clear to his listener that he wants something *now*, or that he is pleased or displeased with what is going on around him. During this stage of development the child is not as random a sound maker as he was as a babbler. He makes fewer sounds, but has better control of his oral products. He is listening to himself, monitoring himself, and controlling his efforts. Sound reduplication is an expression of such control. Some of the sound combinations such as "da-da" and "ma-ma" resemble words. However, parental pride to the contrary, very few children who say "ma-ma" at eight months assign any meaning to their utterance. But some children do associate sound and meaning at eight months, and parental pride may not always be misplaced. Most children need a few months before they really mean what they utter. Part of this time is devoted to responding to what they hear with their own echolalic, imitative utterances.

ECHOLALIA

Echolalia is a normal stage in language development that occurs, as we have indicated, after the lalling stage. The echolalic child is an imitator, not of himself as he was and continues to be in part-time lalling, but of others. The imitative efforts begin to approximate what he hears. Thus he may imitate both the manual gesture and the syllables "bye-bye" without understanding the meaning of either. He may utter "ma-ma" or "da-da" or even "baby" without any intended meaning. Vocal intonations are also imitative, so that it is difficult for many parents to believe that the child's utterances are parrotlike and not true speech.

In another sense, however, the baby is developing speech. He is beginning to respond by differential behavior to utterances addressed to him. He may wave appropriately to the words "bye-bye" or reach in anticipation when asked, "Do you want your dolly?" When, perhaps between 10 and 12 months, he says "dolly" or "da" or "dada" on the presentation of his doll, the child has really begun to speak.

IDENTIFICATION LANGUAGE

By the beginning of the second year, many children have words to identify objects and persons in their environment. Because echolalic utterance continues, the one-year-old will seem to speak more words than he has meanings (appropriate behavior) for them. First words are likely to be reduplicated syllables, such as "dada" and "mama." The child may now be able to obey verbal "commands," such as pointing to his nose, ears, and so on, in response to the directions, "Show me your nose," "Where is baby's nose?" and so forth. The child may also play "Peek-a-boo," or bang his cup when he hears the word "cup." We should note that in these situations the child's utterances as well as his nonverbal actions are used to identify events. Unless he is somewhat on the precocious side, he is not likely to be using words to bring about an event, to get his doll, or his bottle of milk, or to call for his mother when any one of these is not in view.

TRUE SPEECH: ANTICIPATORY LANGUAGE

By the middle of the second year, most children are able to use language to bring about an event, to get something of someone not physically in view. We may observe that during this stage the child's utterance will be accompanied by a change in his "motor set" consistent with an appropriate reaction to what he expects to happen. Thus he not only says "up" but readies himself to be picked up. When he says "mama" he also looks to the door through which his mother is supposed to make her appearance. Words at this stage have a "magical" power for the child. They are a way of getting people to do his bidding, of satisfying his needs physically and psychosocially. Between 18 and 24 months most children have productive vocabularies of from three to 50 words, and much larger comprehension vocabularies. They are definitely "with it" linguistically, and ready for more complex verbal behavior.

The child's single-word utterances are, in effect, sentences. The meaning of the utterance is indicated by the manner of intonation. Thus "mama" depending on intonation, may mean an empiric "Mother, come here!" or "Where is mother?" or even, "Mother, I've had enough of you now." Similarly, "cup" may mean "Fill it up" or "I've had my fill of it." If we accept intonation as a form of syntax, then we may consider that the child's variously intoned words are complete sentences, which may have as many meanings as adults regularly give to the word forms "yes" or "no" or "uh-uh."

Children who will later be designated as severely intellectually retarded may not go beyond the stage of identification language, even though they may have a small vocabulary for naming (identifying) some objects and persons in their environment. A few retarded children may develop single-word or two-word utterances to bring about events, but growth of vocabulary is slow, both for comprehension and production of language. Retarded children have fewer words than their normal age peers, and fewer meanings for the words they know. Moderately intellectually retarded children will shadow the linguistic development of normal and bright children. Severely retarded children (those with intelligence quotients below low-grade idiocy) may be totally nonverbal or almost completely so.*

SYNTACTIC SPEECH

By two years of age the child is likely to have a vocabulary of between 50 and 100 words. Some children may be able to name all the familiar objects in their environment. The most distinctive achievement is the combination of words from their inventory into phrases which, though lacking in the conventional markers of syntax, nevertheless constitute sentences. The form of the words used may be two nouns—e.g., *cup* and *milk* to mean "Give me a cup of milk" or "I want milk" or, in the adult usage, an adverb+noun, e.g. "more milk" with the meaning apparent. Lenneberg (1967, p. 293) points out that it makes little sense to try to determine whether the child's vocabulary has a preponderance of nouns and some adjectives and a few conventional verbs that func-

---

* Here we may be dealing with circuitous thinking, with the effect as well as the cause of retarded onset of language. A child of three or more who has not begun to speak may get less stimulation than a normal child. If the severely retarded child is institutionalized, he may indeed never get around to speaking. Lenneberg (1967, p. 154–155) reports on a population of 54 mongoloid children who were raised at home (age range six months to 22 years). These children were observed over a period of from two to three years. At the end of the study period, 75 per cent of the children had reached a stage of at least identification language. The children had small vocabularies and could execute simple verbal commands. Lenneberg notes that progress in language development was noted only in the children who were below 14 years of age.

tion as sentences. Any of his words may be used contextually to indicate a variety of meanings. Frequently one word is used recurrently as a pivot [Braine (1963)], so that we get such phrases as "here cup," "here shoe," "here doll," as well as "doll here" and "kitty here." We may also have such phrase-sentences as "more milk" and "more up." The significance of this accomplishment is that the child is developing a sense of word combination, which in time will be modified by conventional word order and markers of syntax.

At two years of age an increasing number, perhaps 50 per cent, of the child's utterances are sufficiently intelligible to be comprehensible to persons who are not members of the child's family. Of great significance is the two-year-old child's ability to combine words that he has not been exposed to by older speakers. He is now speaking creatively, in that he is formulating sentences he has not heard, calling on his own lexical inventory. He has begun to reveal an ability to generalize, going from a phrase he may have heard, and so directly taught, to combinations he has not heard, but which conform in structure to those he has been taught. So from "baby up" he may go to "dolly up" or "mommy up," as well as "up baby." The ability of the child to alter the position of the pivot word, such as "up" in the examples just given, reveals that he is making functional distinctions in his phrase-utterances. We have a clear indication of sentence sense which, within another year, will conform both in word order and grammatical forms to the syntax of the older speakers to whom he is exposed.

COMMUNICATIVE INTENT

By two and a half years of age most children include functional words—prepositions, articles, and conjunctions—in their utterances. In other respects, too, their formulations approximate those of the older speakers to whom they are exposed. They begin to speak grammatically, or agrammatically, usually depending upon how those in their surroundings speak. Three- to four-word sentences are frequent. Between two and a half and three years, the child's increase in vocabulary is likely to be greater proportionately than for any other equal time period in his life. Between 24 and 30 months, the child's intention to communicate, to speak with the expectation that he will be both understood and responded to, becomes clear. If he is not understood, he manifests frustration. Fortunately, the normal three-year-old not only shows control of syntax, but control as well of most of the sounds of his language. So-called infantilisms, such as "wawa" for "water," decrease. The child's phonemic or articulatory proficiency is usually good enough for most of what he says to be readily intelligible.

Literally, the three-year-old speaks for himself, using "I" in contexts that a few months before contained "me." He understands and distinguishes between "I," "we," "me," and "you." The three-year-old can usually transform the "you" of a question addressed to him, e.g., "Do you want a cookie?" to "I want a cookie." Interestingly, autistic children, even when they begin to speak, are slow to make the distinction and transformation of "you" to "I" or "me." Characteristically, autistic children refer to themselves in the manner in which they are addressed. Thus, "Do you want a cookie?" is likely to be answered by "You want a cookie," or by a repetition of the entire sentence.

THREE TO FOUR—THE EMERGENCE OF AN INDIVIDUOLECT

We shall not attempt to discuss in any detail the language development of the child beyond age three. His progress is now so rapid, his ability to speak with conventional syntax so nearly complete, that little more than the niceties of complex sentences remain for him to master. By age four the child has improved considerably in his articulatory (phonemic) proficiency. Some children are in fact speaking much as they will as adults, except that they still, fortunately, vocalize as children. They intone correctly, and formulate sentences much in the manner of the older members of their environment,* and only few of them lisp and lall (substitute *w* for *l* or *r*). The four-year-old is a mature speaker who may begin to develop his own rhetorical style. He may have favorite words and even favorite ways of turning a phrase. The four-year-old not only speaks for himself, but begins to speak in a manner which *is* himself. We call this manner an *individuolect*.

Acquisition of Sounds; Phonemic Development

Thus far in our discussion we have emphasized the semantic (vocabulary) and syntactic aspects of language development. Neither, of course, can take place without the acquisition of the phonemic or sound system

---

* Syntactic proficiency is however by no means fully developed. As Chomsky (1969) reveals in her investigation, there are considerable differences in syntactic competence between five-year-olds and the adults in their environment. These differences tend to be reduced during the five to ten year period as children develop more semantic and generally more linguistic sophistication.

of the linguistic code. It is of interest to note that many children take longer to establish completely proficient control of the sounds of their language than to acquire the vocabulary and syntax of their system. To be sure, as infants engage in sound play, many sounds are produced that will not be voluntarily controlled, and intentionally articulated until the child is six or seven years of age. Children also show great variability in their phonemic proficiency. Some, especially girls, may arrive at an almost adult level of control by age four or five. Most children, however, need at least a year or two longer before they arrive at this level of proficiency.

Children's errors in phonemic production are not random. The child makes his words out of the sounds he is able to control. These, as we have noted, begin with vowels, nasals, and labials (lip sounds). The young child also engages in reduplication. So, with the few sounds he is able to control, he builds his first word inventory. Words such as *mama* present no problem. A *kitty* is, however, likely to be pronounced *kicky* because the child can usually produce a [k] before he can a [t]. So, he substitutes one stop-plosive sound for the other and, economically, uses the same sound twice. The production of *bummy* for *bunny* may be explained by the fact that [m] is a bilabial, as is [b]. The child beginning his word with one bilabial finds it easier to include a second [m] rather than to introduce a tip-tongue nasal [n].

As the child matures, both in his ability for auditory discrimination and articulatory control, he will make distinctions between sounds

Age at Which 75 Per Cent of Children First Uttered Various Types of Sounds Correctly

Chronological Age	Sounds
3	Initial, medial, and final nasals;* initial, medial plosives;* initial, medial semivowels; vowels; diphthongs
4	final plosives
5	final semivowels; final combinations; initial double consonant blends
6	initial, medial, final fricatives; final double consonant blends; reversed triple consonant blends; reversed double consonant blends†
7	initial, final, triple consonant blends

* These terms are explained in Chapter 6.

† Examples of blend: *pl* forms an initial consonant blend sound in *play*; *st* is a sound blend in *step*. Blend as used here is synonymous with the term " cluster."

that are acoustically similar. Usually, he establishes adult-level phonemic proficiency by age seven or eight. In general, we may note that the process of articulatory development is one of progressive differentiation. Children will almost always hear fine shades of differences before they can produce them. They will reject the adult's imitation of *wawipop* for *lollipop* or *bummy* for *bunny* before they can produce the word as the adult expects.

The table on p. 129, based on Templin's data (1957, p. 43) summarizes the phonemic development of children.

The list that follows gives the average age for the control of 24 consonants of English. (Templin, 1957, p. 53).

Sound	Age	Sound	Age
m	3	r	4
n	3	s	4.5
ng	3	sh	4.5
p	3	ch	4.5
f	3	t	6
h	3	th	6
w	3	v	6
y	3.5	l	6
k	4	th(voiced)	7
b	4	z	7
d	4	zh	7
g	4	j	7

In a more recent statement, Templin (1966) states that "Cross sectional normative studies have quite consistently shown that seven- to eight-year-old children can satisfactorily utter all the phonemes of English." Fry (1966) observes that "The rate of speech development varies greatly among individual children, but in the normally hearing child one can expect that by five to seven years of age the phonemic system will be completely and fairly well established."

SPEECH READINESS

If we review the semantic and syntactic acquisition (see the table that follows on Maturational Milestones), we will note that the child makes great spurts at particular periods in his life, e.g., the great (proportionate) increase in vocabulary at about 30 months of age; the development of syntax at about three years; the control of consonant clusters (blends) between five and six years. These may be considered periods of readiness in which basic skills are incorporated and the child then becomes ready for his next stage of development. Perhaps even more striking is the universal onset of speech, regardless of what language the child will speak, between 15 and 18 months of age. We indicated at the opening of this chapter that we consider speech to be a specific function of the human species. Children are born with the potential to speak if the opportunity is provided. The opportunity, so far as the onset of speech is concerned, is exposure to persons who speak. The rate at which children progress from their beginnings is determined by a combination of innate factors such as the integrity of the child's neurological system, his sensory system, his native intelligence, *and* cultural-environmental factors which, for the most part, are those that exist *within his own family*. We shall now consider some of these factors.

NEUROMUSCULAR SYSTEM

The child's nervous system must be capable of doing his bidding and of providing him with feedback as to what and how well he is doing. His nervous system must be adequate to make him sensitive to the sights and sounds in his environment, and to permit him to make differential responses to different conditions. He must not only be able to hear but to discriminate between speech sounds and other auditory events. It is possible, as we shall learn later in our discussion of brain-damaged children in Chapter 16, for a child to be able to discriminate, perceive, and make appropriate responses to nonspeech signals and yet not be able to perceive speech as a different form of sounds. Such a child may hear, and yet not learn to speak, for what he hears does not include the auditory perceptual capacities necessary for speech.

Cerebral-palsied children are, as a total special population, markedly retarded in speech development. Those cerebral-palsied children who are also mentally retarded by virtue of their brain damage are likely to be retarded in all aspects of speech development. In a study of the articulatory proficiency of cerebral-palsied children Irwin (1952, p. 269–279) found that these children at five and a half years of age are at a proficiency level equivalent to that of the 30-month-old child. The problems of some cerebral-palsied children are further complicated by hearing loss of both a peripheral and a central nature. Central hearing loss, as a consequence of damage to the auditory area of the brain, makes it difficult for the child to perceive speech differentially from other environmental noises.

Maturational Milestones: Motor Correlates and Language Development*

Age	Speech Stage	Motor Development
12–16 weeks	Coos and chuckles	Supports head in prone position; responds to human sounds by turning head in direction of sound source
20 weeks	Consonants modify vowel-like cooing; nasals and labial fricatives are frequently produced	Sits with support
6 months	Babbling, resembling one-syllable utterances; identifiable combinations include *ma, da, di, du*	Sits without props using hands for support
8 months	Lalling and some echolalia	Stands by holding on to object; grasps with thumb apposition
10 months	Distinct echolalia, which approximates sounds he hears; responds differentially to verbal sounds	Creeps efficiently; pulls to standing position; may take a side step while holding on to a fixed object
12 months	Reduplicated sounds in echolalia; possible first words for identification; responds appropriately to simple commands	Walks on hands and feet; may stand alone, may walk when held by one hand, or even take first steps alone
18 months	Has repertoire of words (between three and 50); some two-word phrases; vocalizations reveal intonational patterns; great increase in understanding of language	Walks with stiff gait; may build two-block tower; begins to show hand preference
24 months	Vocabulary of 50 or more words for naming and for bringing about events; two-word phrases of own formulation	Walks with ease; runs, can walk up or down stairs, planting both feet on each step
30 months	Vocabulary growth proportionately greater than at any other period in life; speaks with clear communicative intent; conventional sentences (syntax) of three, four, and five words; articulation still includes many infantalisms; good comprehension of speakers in his surroundings	Can jump; stand on one foot; good hand and finger coordination; can build six-block tower

Maturational Milestones—*Continued*

Age	Speech Stage	Motor Development
36 months	Vocabulary may exceed 1,000 words; syntax much like that of older persons in his surroundings; most of his utterances are intelligible to to older listeners	Runs proficiently; walks stairs with alternating feet; hand preference established
48 months	Except for articulation (phonemic production) the linguistic system is essentially that of the adults in his surroundings. He may begin to develop his own "rhetorical" style of favorite words and phrases	Can hop on one foot (usually right); can throw a ball to an intended receiver; can catch a ball in his arms; can walk on a line

* Adapted from E. H. Lenneberg. *Biological Foundations of Language* (New York, John Wiley & Sons, Inc., 1967), pp. 128–130.

THE AUDITORY SYSTEM

As we suggested above, the auditory system must permit the reception as well as the perception of speech events. That is, the speech signal must reach the brain (reception) and be processed differentially in the brain (perception). Children with a hearing loss, which impairs reception, are slower in speech development than hearing children. Deaf children are those whose receptive impairment is so severe that they cannot learn to speak through the auditory mode. However, some mildly or moderately hearing-impaired children, especially if their impairment is recognized early in life, may speak quite competently if given appropriate attention and training. The perceptually impaired (aphasic-dyslogic child) will be considered at some length in Chapter 16.

CEREBRAL DOMINANCE AND LATERALITY PREFERENCE

Human motor development is characterized by the preferential use of a paired organ, hand, foot, eye, or ear. This preference is an expression of laterality. Most of us are right-handed and right-footed *and* right-eyed. That is, given an opportunity to reach or grasp, to hop or stand on one foot, to view something with one eye, we are likely to use the same organ for the task—the one on the right side of the body—

with great consistency. About 7 to 10 per cent of us are left-sided. However, mixed preference, that is, the combination of right-handed-ness and left-eyedness, is quite common. A small percentage of us are ambilateral, that is, there is less consistency as to which hand will be used for reaching, or grasping, or executing some task that requires only one hand, or where one hand exercises a skill with the aid of the other hand. Among the ambilateral we have some who are also *ambi-dextrous*, who are equally skilled with either member of paired organs. Usually such skill is expressed in manual (hand) skills. Ambilaterality, we should note, does not imply ambidexterity. Among children who are intellectually and maturationally retarded we have a considerable amount of ambilaterality accompanied by ambi-nondexterity. The truly ambidextrous are a chosen few, most of whom are probably innately left-handed (sinistral) and who have developed more dexterity in the use of the right hand than innately right-handed persons are likely to develop in the use of the left.

The expression of laterality—let us use " hand preference " as an indicator of such expression—parallels critical stages in the development of speech. By 18 months, when most children have uttered their first true words, they have also begun to indicate hand preference. By three years, when syntax becomes acquired, hand preference, foot preference (standing or hopping on one foot), eye preference, *and* ear preference are also normally established. These laterality expressions mean that one hemisphere of the brain is dominant or controls a function.

Speech, however, employs paired organs for intake as well as output.* We listen with both ears, and take in visual events with both eyes. However, as we have seen, the perceptual appreciation of language events, the interpretation of what we hear or what we read, is normally processed in the left hemisphere for at least 95 per cent of right-handed persons and 60 per cent of left-handed persons. We may generalize therefore that *the vast majority of human beings have cerebral dominance for language behavior in the left hemisphere.* Such dominance is normally established by three years of age (Kimura, 1967). Cerebral dominance is delayed in the moderately and severely mentally retarded and in brain-damaged children. Nonspeech events, the noises of our environ-ment, and the perception of music are normally processed in the right hemsiphere. Thus, as we indicated earlier, it is possible for a child to respond appropriately to the barking of a dog, or the ringing of a bell, and even to listen to music, and yet not be able to make the discrimina-

---

* E.g. the tongue consists of two halves, which receive nervous innervations from both hemispheres of the brain.

tions and perceptions that are necessary to understand and acquire speech. This very special capacity—the processing of speech signals—is associated with cerebral dominance and the functioning of the temporal lobe of the left cerebral hemisphere.

INTELLIGENCE

The factor of intelligence is so intimately related to language development that we must be careful to avoid circuitous thinking. There is little doubt that intelligence is positively related to vocabulary growth and, perhaps to a lesser degree, also to syntactic competence (sentence length and complexity). Templin's study (1957, p. 117) is representative of most findings. She reports a correlation of .50 between intelligence and vocabulary growth in young children. Virtually all verbal intelligence tests for children, e.g., the Stanford Binet and the Wechsler Intelligence Scale for Children, include a vocabulary test as part of the scale because of the established relationship between language development, as measured by vocabulary, and intelligence.

One of the by-products of being born with good native intelligence is the likelihood that one's parents, and other members of the family, may also be intelligent, and provide an environment where proficient language usage will stimulate and encourage more of the same. Further, we have a likelihood that such a background will have books as well as parents for reading, for storytelling, and for the other social advantages that go along with good language development.

SEX

Though studies vary in their findings, we may accept as a general observation that up to age eight or nine, girls are somewhat more advanced than boys of like age in overall language development. McCarthy (1954, p. 492–630) reports such an advantage for girls over boys. Templin (1957), based on much the same procedures for collecting data as McCarthy, found smaller differences than those detected in earlier studies. Templin notes that while on overall language competence girls do tend to be somewhat superior to boys, the differences for specific language achievements are not consistent and are usually not great enough to be statistically significant. Girls do seem to be about a half year ahead of boys in articulatory proficiency. Boys, however, may exceed girls in word knowledge. Templin explains her findings of reduced differences between the sexes on the basis of changes in child rearing during the past few decades. We have changed from bringing up little girls as girls and little boys as boys to a single standard in child care and training (Templin, 1957, p. 147). This observation is supported by the findings of Winitz (1969) on a study of the language development of kindergarten children. Winitz found no significant differences between the sexes in regard to such language measures as length of response, the number of different words used, the structural (syntactic) complexity of the child's utterances, vocabulary skill, and articulatory proficiency.

ENVIRONMENTAL FACTORS

The most significant non-innate factor for the child's language development is his home. His potentialities for speech, from onset until the time when he begins to spend more time away from home than at home, are nurtured by members of his family, with his mother the primary influence. We assume, of course, that the child has a mother with normal maternal drives, one who enjoys and wishes to interact with her child. We assume that the mother enjoys talking to her child and is willing, when the child indicates readiness, to give him a proper opportunity for sound play. We assume that the mother will readily show delight at the child's vocalizations and babbling, lalling, and echolalia, enabling the child to derive pleasure from the delight he gives his mother and so be reinforced in his vocal efforts. All of these assumptions imply that the infant will be able to identify with a speaking adult and thus have a model for the shaping of his speech. We should note that what we say of the mother holds true equally for the father, or for a parent surrogate if, for some reason, a natural parent is not available to the child. Given such a home, a child may be expected to begin to speak by 15 months of age. Beyond this, other factors in the child's home environment and family constellation are important. Briefly, these include such factors as the number of children in his family, his place in order of birth, whether he is a singleton or a multiple-birth child, whether his home is monolingual or bilingual, and the educational level and socioeconomic status of his parents.

POSITION OF FAMILY

The first child with adult models is likely to have a somewhat earlier onset of speech than a second child. We may note, however, that a second child born four years or more after the first has the essential advantages of a first or only child. Twins, especially if they are born before a full-term pregnancy, are likely to have a later onset of speech and slower development than a single-born child. Davis (1937), who did a basic study comparing singletons with twins, found that twins were retarded in language development when compared with single-born children. The differences tend to decrease as the children mature and go on to school.

BILINGUALISM

If a child is born into a bilingual environment, his vocabulary may be below average for his age for either language or for a combination of both languages. M. E. Smith (1949), in a study of the vocabularies of 30 bilingual children (approximately three to six years of age) of Chinese ancestry in Hawaii, found, in both English and Chinese, that the children had below-average-sized vocabularies for children of their ages. Even when the vocabularies of the two languages were combined, only two fifths of the children exceeded the norm. When words of the same meaning were subtracted, only one sixth of the children exceeded the norm. On the basis of her study, Smith believes that it is probably wiser for young bilingual children to receive their two languages from separate sources. She therefore recommended that each adult in the home consistently use one language.

Research studies on bilingualism may not, in fact, be too meaningful for, as McCarthy (1954, p. 593) points out, most of these studies are based either on families from the upper social level who deem preserving language important because of cultural reasons or families from lower socioeconomic levels where parents may not be sufficiently intellectual or interested in learning to acquire the second language. The implications of bilingualism and the need for careful investigations of problems that are or may be related to exposure and the acquisition of more than one language may be appreciated by the following observation: "Americans in general and American academies in particular are so accustomed to a seeming monolingual environment that they are likely to be surprised by the extent of bilingualism. Indeed, few among them suspect that for the majority of those who speak it, English is a second language."*

SOCIOECONOMIC LEVEL

Children born of families in a higher socioeconomic status tend to develop language more rapidly than those born in lower socioeconomic families. Templin (1957, p. 147) points out that there are consistent

---

* Macnamara, J. (ed.), "Problems of Bilingualism," *The Journal of Social Issues*, XXIII, 2 (April, 1967). The student interested in or concerned with problems of bilingualism should study this monograph. It includes articles by authorities from a variety of disciplines dealing with important aspects and issues of bilingualism.

language differences in children from upper socioeconomic groups and lower socioeconomic groups. The children from the upper socioeconomic groups receive higher scores on all language measures at each level. These language measures include ability to articulate sounds, discriminate between sounds, recognize words, and utter longer and more complex sentences. A particular socioeconomic background is associated with many factors influential in language development; these may include intellectual level, amount of education of parents, cultural opportunities offered to children, and certain home attitudes. Furthermore, parents in upper socioeconomic classes tend to give their children more attention and to share more stimulating and interesting experiences with them.

Irwin (1952) did an interesting and provocative study on providing language stimulation to children. He had earlier found that children whose fathers were in the business and professional occupations acquired sounds more quickly than children born of fathers who were semiskilled or unskilled workers. Consequently, he wished to test the hypothesis that in the homes of working families the systematic reading of stories to infants during the year and a half period between 13 and 30 months would increase their phonetic production. Consequently mothers of 24 infants in the experimental group were instructed to spend 15 to 20 minutes each day reading stories to their children from illustrated children's books, talking about the books, making up original simple tales about them, and, in general, furnishing an enriched speech-sound environment. The results of the study suggest that systematically increasing speech-sound stimulation of children under two-and-a-half years in homes of lower educational status by reading and by talking about stories will lead to an increase in phonetic production over the level that might be expected without such stimulation.

STIMULATION TO SPEAK

As just indicated, stimulation to speak may come partly from the atmosphere of the home and partly from experiences that provoke linguistic activity. Some social environments provide more stimulation to speak and more good models to imitate than others. When a mother talks to her child frequently and simply and when her own speech is clear and intelligible, the child is likely to speak earlier. If, as he grows older, he lives with parents who share and enjoy interesting experiences with him, such as going on picnics and talking about books, he tends to speak more fully and with longer sentences than the child who has fewer experiences. Talk cannot thrive in a vacuum; it needs the stimulation of common experiences and adventures. An example of a child who had little stimulation to speak is that of a five-year-old boy who has a seven-year-old sister who is a chatterbox and who almost constantly interprets for him: "He doesn't like his cheese sandwich toasted; he likes it plain." When an adult suggested that he'd like to hear what the little boy thought of toasted sandwiches, the little sister replied, "He's too shy. He don't talk much." The poor lad never gets much chance to talk with a loquacious sister at his elbow.

Admittedly, some children are overstimulated. A seven-year-old boy lived with very verbal and alert parents, overly interested in bringing up their child with "broad horizons." From the time the child was two, they talked *at* him. As he grew older, they provided him with a wealth of sensory experiences such as listening to classical records and watching the ballet, but he never had time really to enjoy the experiences, for the parents accompanied each one with a barrage of words. Most of the words were polysyllabic. The overstimulation and the pattern of complex language were too much for him. The result was that he gave up trying to speak and appeared to be a child with "retarded language development." Though not truly retarded; he had become a reluctant speaker, at least in his home setting.

References and Suggested Readings

BRAINE, M. D. S., "The Ontogeny of English Phrase Structure," *Language*, XXXIX (January–March, 1963), 1–13.

BRODBECK, A. J. and O. C. IRWIN, "The Speech Behavior of Infants Without Families," *Child Development*, XVII (September, 1946), 145–156.

BROWN, R. and U. BELLUGI, "Three Processes in the Child's Acquisition of Syntax," *Harvard Educational Review*, XXXIV, 2 (Spring 1964), 133–151. (This article is an exposition of a study of two children, "Adam" and "Eve" who were selected because they were both very talkative and very intelligible.)

CARROLL, J. B., "Words, Meanings, and Concepts," *Harvard Educational Review*, XXXIV, 2, (Spring 1964) 178—202. (An exposition of how word meanings and concepts can be effectively taught by classroom teachers.)

CHOMSKY, C., *The Acquisition of Syntax in Children from Five to Ten.* Cambridge, M.I.T. Press, 1969. (This monograph describes the author's investigation of the acquisition of syntactic structures in children between five to ten years of age. Her findings indicate that the grammar of a five-year-old differs in a number of ways from adult grammar "and that the gradual disappearance of these discrepancies can be traced as children exhibit increased knowledge over the next four or five years of their development.")

DARLEY, F. L. and H. WINITZ, "Age of First Words: Review of Research," *Journal of Speech and Hearing Disorders*, XXVI, 3 (August, 1961), 272–290.

DAVIS, E. A., *The Development of Linguistic Skills in Twins, Singletons with Siblings and Only Children from Ages Five to Ten Years*. Minneapolis, University of Minnesota Press, 1937. (A classic and basic study of the language development of single and multiple-birth children.)

FRY, D. B., "The Development of the Phonological System in Normal and Deaf Child," in Smith, F. M. and Miller, G. A., *The Genesis of Language*, Cambridge, M.I.T. Press, 1966.

GOLDFARB, W., "Effects of Psychological Deprivation in Infancy and Subsequent Stimulation," *American Journal of Psychiatry*, XII (August 1954), 102–129.

IRWIN, O. C., "Speech Development in the Young Child," *Journal of Speech and Hearing Disorders*, XVII, 3 (September, 1952), 269–279.

KIMURA, D., "Functional Asymmetry of the Brain in Dichotic Listening," *Cortex*, III (1967), 163–178. (Dichotic listening, an approach to indicate ear preference, is explained in its relationship to cerebral dominance and language functions.)

LEE, L. L., "Developmental Sentence Types: A Method for Comparing Normal and Deviant Syntactic Development," *Journal of Speech and Hearing Disorders*, XXXI, 4 (November, 1966) 311–330. (An approach to the assessment of levels of syntactic development based on comparisons between a normally developing child and one with language delay.)

LENNEBERG, E. H., *Biological Foundations of Language*. New York, John Wiley & Sons, Inc., 1967.

LENNEBERG, E. H., "Language Disorders in Childhood," *Harvard Educational Review*, XXIV, (Spring, 1964), 152–177. (This issue is devoted to Language and Learning. It is highly recommended for teachers and language clinicians.)

LEWIS, M. M., *How Children Learn to Speak*. New York, Basic Books, 1959. (An English author's observations about speech development.)

McCARTHY, D., "Language Development in Children," in L. Carmichael (ed.) *Manual of Child Psychology* (Rev. ed.), New York, John Wiley & Sons, Inc., 1954, 492–630.

McNEILL, D., "The Development of Language," in Mussen, P. H. (ed.), *Carmichael's Manual of Child Psychology*, 3rd ed. New York, John Wiley & Sons, Inc., 1970, 1061–1161. (A survey of recent literature on language acquisition emphasizing the relationships among language development, intellect, and maturation in the child.)

MENYUK, P., *Sentences Children Use*. M.I.T. Research Monograph Series, Cambridge, Mass., 1969.

PIAGET, J. and B. INHELDER, *The Psychology of the Child*. New York, Basic Books, 1969. (Chapter 6 of this book is devoted to an exposition of the development (evolution) of language and thought in the child.)

SMITH, M. E., "Measurement of the Vocabularies of Young Bilingual Children in Both of the Languages Used," *Journal of Genetic Psychology*, XXIV (June, 1949), 305–310.

TEMPLIN, M. C., *Certain Language Skills in Children: Their Development and Interrelationships*. Minneapolis, University of Minnesota Press, 1957.

TEMPLIN, M. C., "The Study of Articulation and Language Development During the Early School Years," in Smith, F. M. and Miller, G. A., *The Genesis of Language*, Cambridge, M.I.T. Press, 1966.

WINITZ, H., "Sex Differences in Language of Kindergarten Children," *ASHA*, 1, (March 1959), 86.

WINITZ, H., *Articulatory Acquisition and Behavior*, New York, Appleton-Century-Crofts, 1969, Chapter 1. (An excellent review of the research literature on prelingual stages of language development and theories as about the onset of speech.)

Problems

1. What is meant by the statement: "Speech is a specific function of the human species?" Do you agree with this statement?
2. What are the criteria for true speech?
3. Listen to the free speech of a boy and a girl at each of the following age levels: two, four, and six years. Note differences in articulatory proficiency, vocabulary, and sentence length. Are there any consistent differences between the sexes?
4. Make the same observations as in (3) for a child whom you consider bright and one you consider of average intelligence.
5. Listen to children in the kindergarten and to children in the third grade. What language factors distinguish the two groups?
6. Ask a three-, a four-, and a five-year-old child to repeat the sentence: "Tomorrow Mommy, Daddy, and I will go on a picnic." Note the difference in their elicited imitations.
7. Read and report on two of the references from the list above.
8. Find a provocative picture in a magazine (one that is likely to induce a story). Ask a five-year-old and an eight-year-old to make up a story based on the picture. Note the differences in use of vocabulary, length, and complexity of each sentence, and in the total length of the story.

Chapter 8

Stimulating Language Development

Both the classroom teacher and the clinician are involved in the speech curricula of the elementary and high schools. These curricula implicitly pursue three aims for each child: (1) to correct any speech difficulty that calls attention to itself, causes the child undue concern, or detracts seriously from his communicative ability; (2) to help him eliminate minor articulation and voice difficulties and nonstandard pronunciations if he and the teacher elect this option; and (3) to assist him to become an effective speaker and listener. The first aim is usually achieved by speech and hearing clinicians or therapists. The program for it is ordinarily entitled "speech and hearing therapy." The last two aims are usually achieved by the classroom teacher under supervision. These two aims are incorporated in a program called "speech improvement," "language arts," or "speech arts."

Administration of Speech Improvement

The first aim is clear cut; the responsibility for achieving it lies clearly in the hands of those in charge of the remedial speech and hearing program. The second and third aims, which are aims of the speech improvement program, however, are not as specific, and the responsibility for achieving them may rest within several programs. In a

143

study (*ASHA*, 1961, pp. 81–82) conducted by a subcommittee of the Research Committee of the American Speech and Hearing Association (Geraldine Garrison, Chairman, Frederic Darley, Hilda Amidon, and Verna Breinholt), 70 per cent of the 98 supervisors consulted replied to a questionnaire concerning the administrative organization of the speech improvement program. Of the supervisors questioned, 35 per cent reported the program to be part of remedial speech and hearing services; 21 per cent, part of language arts; 5 per cent, separate programs; 6 per cent, part of both remedial services and language arts; and 3 per cent, part of other units. In the same study an analysis was made of nine outstanding speech improvement programs that had been in operation for some time. Of the nine, five were part of a remedial program in speech and hearing; one was a separate speech improvement program coordinated with remedial service; one was identified with the language arts program, but speech clinicians directed the speech work; and one was part of a two-year research study headed by remedial speech and hearing personnel.

Stimulation and Language Development

In the preceding chapter we talked about the functions of language: to signal needs, intentions, thoughts and feelings; to think; to control or direct one's own or others' behavior; to express one's own feelings or to encourage or distill aspects of feelings in others. The language arts program in the school deals with these very functions. For example, in expressing thought the child may compare, contrast, deduce, induce, make analogies, or point out relationships. In controlling others' behavior, he may present all his available evidence, may appeal to particular interests of his group, may role-play verbally or non-verbally a character with certain motivations, which portrayal may lead the receiver of the message to a value-judgment and eventually to a particular behavior. In expressing feeling or reacting to another's feeling, the child may give vent to his own hostile feelings or he may reduce these feelings in others.

The utterance of the child who uses language ably and purposefully tends to be fairly lengthy; his syntactical structure, complex; his vocabulary, sophisticated. He understands and responds to abstract thought. He is happy with and interested in many types of new experiences. There are probably two reasons for this facility with language: (1) a rich background of experience—trips, music, play activities, books, resulting in stimulating conversation, and (2) a positive, healthy self-concept. He is likely to have been brought up in a home and to have attended a school with many cultural advantages, a home and school where problems are "talked out" rather than "acted out." In talking about his experiences, the adults around him have enlarged upon what he has said, have developed the child's ideas and concepts rather than expanding the child's sentences, repeating the sentences with more adult syntax. In research at Harvard University (Courtney, 1965), two ways of talking to children were compared. In one group, the adults replied to the child by expanding his sentences; for example, the response to "Baby hungry" was "The baby is hungry." They supplied the missing bits of syntax. The other group who had the same number of daily conversations was responded to with comments that enlarged upon what the child said. For example, when the child said, "Baby hungry," the experimenter responded with, "Yes, he wants to eat." At the end of three months, both of these groups and a control group were given language ability tests. The expanded group showed a slight improvement over the control group but the enlarged group showed significantly greater improvement. The richness and variety of the responses in the enlarged group, even though the acceptable syntax was not stressed, brought greater language development. He feels secure. He respects himself and others. He perceives himself realistically and is aware of how others are receiving what he has to say.

From this discussion, we can deduce the ingredients of a successful language arts program.

First, it should involve a curriculum rich in experiences that will interest children. These experiences should be the basis for conversation wherein the teacher enlarges upon the ideas expressed and encourages other children to enlarge upon them. Loban notes the relationship of language, experience, and learning:

> Through experience and through language we learn. Experience needs language to give it form. Language needs experience to give it content (Loban, 1966, p. 73).

For young children, we believe in a variety of rich experiences: visiting farms, bus depots, fish markets, ice-cream plants, museums, airports, children's theater productions; taking short train or bus trips; discussing worthwhile, relevant problems where true interaction occurs, telling and listening to stories, painting, drawing, acting in a creative drama, putting on a puppet play.

We question, on present-day evidence, whether formal instruction in vocabulary or in grammar, transformational, structural, or traditional, is effective in appreciably improving expressive and receptive facilities of language. We do believe with Loban that "pupils need many opportunities to grapple with their own thought and express it in situations where they have someone to whom they wish to communicate successfully." (Loban, 1966, p. 71). In the account of speech activities in this chapter, we have attempted to suggest a variety of experiences that will stimulate language development.

Second, the teacher himself should feel basically adequate as a person and as a teacher as noted in Chapter 4 and should be able to help his children strengthen their self concepts. He must understand that the self concept is derived from what the child thinks of himself plus the appraisal of other meaningful persons in his realm. He should be able to create the kind of atmosphere where the child finds himself an adequate person and student; he should provide experiences that will assist the child in seeing himself positively and in discovering his worth as a person.* Furthermore, the teacher should be able to provide situations in which the reflected appraisal of others, namely the peer group, can play an important role in developing positive self concepts. Kaplan (1963), in improving the language skills of youngsters of other cultures, showed that growth in speech occurs in programs that attempt to improve the child's self image.

We believe that children's poor listening habits are related to a dearth of meaningful experiences and to an inability to communicate with others and with the teacher. As communication increases, as experiences are provided where the reward for listening is inherent and vital, children will listen more carefully, more thoughtfully, and more appreciatively.

Children must be able to communicate with each other and with their teacher. Sometimes the communication must involve the particular social dialect of the child. Loban, whom we quoted at some length in Chapter 3, emphasizes that children need to develop facility in speaking in their own social dialect first. We are inclined to agree with this assessment. In an experiment in Washington, D.C., financed by funds under Title III, special language arts teachers were first trained to communicate in the language of children's particular culture. The teachers then saturated their children with such vital experiences as drama, puppetry, play, and trips. These nonverbal children soon began to communicate with their teachers and made decided progress in language (Crow, 1966, p. 104).

That children learn about their own language is important. Consequently, the teacher's background in linguistics should be strong. In a recent issue of *Elementary English*, Keyser (Keyser, 1970) points out that linguistics is concerned with developing a theory to formally charac-

---

* See J. Strauss and R. Dufour, "Discovering Who I Am: A Humanities Course for Sixth Grade Students," *Elementary English*, XLVII (January 1970), 85–120.

terize the knowledge that a speaker of a natural language possesses, and that the questions the linguist asks are questions about formal properties of grammar based on the facts of a natural language. He goes on to say that this tells the linguist about the abstract principles of a language but it does not help him to write or speak better. He then explains how the teacher does make use of linguistic insights in the elementary and secondary curricula by looking at grammar as attempting to teach children how to make, critically examine, and reformulate hypotheses about language. Keyser follows this with four lesson plans, the first two of which will be briefly described. In the first, children list what objects the word *frighten* may take. The children finally deduce that the list contains "living things that move on their own." The teacher then goes on to encourage the children to find other verbs that can be classified according to the animacy of their subjects or objects. The goal of the second lesson is to point out differences between syntactic and semantic aspects of plurality of nouns in English. Similarly, in Chapter 3 we talked about encouraging children to compare the Scottish (or other) dialect with their own. For this exercise, the teacher must have some knowledge of comparative phonetics. Thus, although many of the linguistic principles may be utilized in teaching, to teach them to children as principles is probably not advisable.

That the teacher must possess a degree of linguistic sophistication is axiomatic. As a child ignores the [s] as in *he play*, the teacher may motivate him to change to *he plays* but frequently neglects to point out that *I play* and *you play* are representative forms in standard English. Consequently, some children will change *I play* and *you play* to *I plays* and *you plays*. To avoid such overcorrection, the teacher must understand that in the child's language system only one form exists in the three persons as exemplified by *he play, he have, he do*. Similarly a generation or two ago many teachers brought about overcorrection by insisting on [nju] for *new* and [stjudɪnt] for *student*; some apt pupils then turned blue into [blju] making themselves sound pretty ridiculous. The overcorrection was the result of lack of phonological sophistication that the teacher could have provided. Thus, the teacher utilizes many of the linguistic principles but rarely teaches the principles to the children directly.

Speaking activities that stimulate can take place in all kinds of environments—home, playground, speech clinic session, and classroom, and they range on a continuum from the very informal to the formal. The kindergartner may be telling a fellow kindergartner on the way to school what a fuss his family makes over a little bit of hot weather. Here the ideas are informally expressed by one person to another person. Organization is almost completely lacking. The kindergartner's only purpose is to express his feelings about one of the idiosyncrasies of adults. On the other hand, the president of an elementary-school student council may make an address to all the students of the school. This situation, the purpose of which is to welcome the students at the beginning of the school year, is a formal one involving hundreds of students. The president has planned his address carefully and has organized it according to a definite pattern. But the basic ingredients of these two speaking situations are the same. They include participants who are expressing ideas. They may be small or large in number, friendly or hostile, democratic or undemocratic, warm or cold, relaxed or rigid. These participants give forth a message—dull, mundane, or exciting, organized effectively or ineffectively, and which may or may not influence behavior. The other participants, in receiving this message, listen carefully or carelessly, critically or uncritically, graciously or ungraciously, in an atmosphere secure or insecure in a particular room, comfortable or uncomfortable, small or large, attractive or unattractive. In school or home situations, the teachers, the speech clinician, or the parents control these factors to some degree, regardless of the type of speaking situation, and regardless of where it occurs on the informal-formal continuum.

Factors in Speaking Situations

KINDS OF SPEECH SITUATIONS

Conversing, Talking, Discussing. One of the most frequent situations in speech is imparting ideas that inform or persuade. At the informal end of the continuum such talk is conversation. Conversation occurs both in the classroom and in the speech correction room. For instance, both the teacher and the clinician use the ingredients of "show and tell." Both strive to make "show and tell" a truly sharing time where students give and receive ideas. Both try to motivate children to express ideas that interest themselves but at the same time are exciting and vital to their listeners. The choice of ideas in this conversational speaking activity, as in other speaking activities, matures as the child grows older. Both the teacher and the clinician encourage this maturing process subtly and sensitively. For example, some first graders and many kindergartners are at the developmental level where they need the security of an actual object—like a small, furry make-believe kitten. The timid child manages only to show his treasure. Then he tells its story just to the teacher or to the clinician. With adult encouragement he tells it to the whole class or to a group.

In this sharing period, the clinician is not particularly concerned with organization, but the teacher is; he helps the children to organize their ideas. In the early part of the first grade, the teacher may, as the child talks, quietly and unobtrusively write on the blackboard the central idea of the sharing experience. As children mature, the teacher asks them to phrase their own central ideas as:

- We have a new blue and white rug.
- My daddy flew to California.
- My baby brother discovered his toes.

The teacher encourages the other youngsters to listen and then talk about the main idea and stay with it. With the flexible guidance of a good conversationalist, the teacher promotes an onward, somewhat organized flow of language. Consequently, as the child matures, he becomes more facile both with the expression and the organization of his ideas.

The informal end of the continuum of expressing ideas to inform or persuade is particularly important for the child with a speech defect. This child needs to feel that what he has to say is worthwhile and that others wish to listen to him. He needs to perceive himself as being adequate in a group speaking situation. Consequently, the teacher and the speech clinician often work together to give him the kind of stimulation to speak that will enhance his self-concept.

Mary Ann was a child with average intelligence, but with general marked language retardation, including many sound substitutions, use of short, very simple sentences, meager vocabulary, and little use of articles, prepositions, and conjunctions. Very few adults could understand her. The teacher and the clinician conferred on ways to stimulate Mary Ann to speak. Some were very ordinary; for instance, one day in the classroom the teacher asked Mary Ann to talk to Tommie's dog so that the dog wouldn't be lonesome. When Mary Ann became more sure of herself, the teacher encouraged her to read a poem she had dictated to the speech clinician to her classmates. At this time, Mary Ann was working on f and v:

> Fee, fie, fo, fum
> I come, I come, I come.
> Vee, vie, vo, vum
> The big, big, big bums
> They go, they go, they go.
> Fee, fie, fo, fum
> Vee, vie, vo, vum
> The five big bums
> They dive, dive, dive
> Like jive, jive, jive.

The first-grade children responding to her bit of nonsense laughed with her. In fact, one child said, "You ought to bring 'the wives' in now." Whereupon another remarked, "'Live' goes with it, too." Later on, when Mary Ann was ready, she talked to a stranger. The day the class went on a trip to a canning factory, the teacher asked its owner to respond to Mary Ann as Mary Ann thanked her for allowing the children to visit. The owner (fortunately a former speech clinician) graciously responded, understood Mary Ann's jargon, and provided another step forward in the child's language development.

At the high-school level, informal conversation exists both in the classroom and in the speech clinician's room. A speech class had attended a college play, *The Death of a Salesman*. The conversation that took place in the classroom as a result was spirited. One boy contributed considerable information about Arthur Miller's other plays. From here on, the teacher guided the conversation to include an analysis of the characters, the opposing forces in the play, and how the costuming and scenery helped to interpret it. The situation was informal; the ideas flowed onward with organization because of the teacher's skillful guidance. The classroom hour was an exciting one of good conversation, made possible because all the students had shared the same stimulating experience. If the speech clinician's student or students had attended the performance, the play might also have provided a topic of conversation for the therapy session.

Closer to the formal end of the continuum, four elementary higher grade students made Africa sound inviting. Two boys explained the tribal custom of telling stories around the fire. One of the boys told tales of animals who behaved like people and explained the tribal origin of each tale (from Edna Mason Kaula, *African Village Folktales*, New York, Harcourt, Brace and World, Inc., 1968). The second boy told how the frog lost his tail, why cats live with women, and dogs with men (from Eleanor B. Heady, *When the Stones Were Soft*, New York, Funk and Wagnalls Company, Inc., 1968). Another boy summarized the story of a boy driven by drought and his family's need for money to the dorp where he steers his course between the old and the new (from Fay Goldie, *Zulu Boy*, New York, St. Martin's Press, Inc., 1968). Still another boy illustrated the African racial cleavage by telling the story of Petrus and his brother, arrested by white authorities, who fled and made their way to Bechuanaland where they drew strength from the tribal life (from Naomi Mitchison, *Friends and Enemies*, New York, The John Day Company, Inc., 1968).

Books furnish the stimulation for much of this talk, both in the classroom and in the therapy session. They often make a special day or event significant. The first grader on St. Valentine's Day may enjoy Pamela Bianco's *The Valentine Party* (Philadelphia, J. B. Lippincott Company, 1955). The excitement of Pamela's finding that the party is for her rubs off on first graders. On Hallowe'en, the primary-school child may well delight in Nora Unwin's *Proud Pumpkin* (New York, Aladdin Press, 1953). Everyone admired the pumpkin, glowing on Hallowe'en. But then the pumpkin was lonely until a chipmunk made him his winter home. Or at Christmas the same child may well find pleasure in Will and Nicolas' *The Christmas Bunny* (New York: Harcourt, Brace and World, Inc., 1952), which tells of a young boy who, because of a rescue, is rewarded with a visit to the animals' Christmas in the woods. The beautiful illustrations of this book foster conversation in the classroom and in the therapy session.

Toys, visits, bulletin boards, and plants also promote talk. A farm run by high-school boys near a speech and hearing center is a truly exciting place for the center's children to visit. A visit furnishes plenty to talk about. On all levels in all classrooms and in the home, the more experiences the child has, the more he has to talk about and concomitantly the more to listen for.

Reading Aloud. A second effective activity is reading aloud. Here again both the classroom teacher and the clinician use oral reading to stimulate language development, and again the situation ranges from the informal to the formal with the formal situation occurring in the classroom. Sometimes the teacher or clinician reads a poem so that the children can talk about its ideas. Recently a teacher read to a group of nine-year-olds Rose Fyleman's poem about the rain coming down till the water was all over the town. It goes on to tell about cabs and buses floating, about everyone's living on the second floor. One nine-year-old responded with: "She'd have to row. I did once at Shawnee. I'd play in a boat—right in the middle—right out in the street—and pretend I was on the ocean. I'd like to take one of my friends with me. We'd talk, tell each other stories. Maybe I'd take my lunch in the boat, too. But if you'd open the door, the water would come in." Thus, the poem stimulated a flow of language. This same informal flow could take place in the clinician's room.

The same teacher read Rose Fyleman's poem that begins "Widdy-widdy wurkey is the name of my turkey." One of the children asked the teacher to read the poem a second time. After the second reading, the child remarked, "It's nonsense and silly but I like it. You know the names all rhyme. Remember? Wurkey, turkey, back again and hen, loose and goose." This child obviously had listened to the words and to their similarity in sound. Such stimulation to listen can occur in the classroom or in the therapy session.

One teacher motivated her youngsters first to think about the clouds in the sky and then to write about them. She asked a child to read to the class Rose Fyleman's poem about the bulls, wolves, and buffaloes in the sky—about their swimming, running, and flying. That afternoon and evening the children looked at the sky. When they returned to class next morning, they talked about what they had seen. Then they wrote about it. Finally they shared their selections with each other.

Another teacher uses sounds as a basis for original writing. Children listen to the sounds in wintertime. They hear tires screeching as they spin, doors banging, sleet hitting the windows, and wind whistling. Then they write about the noises and share their compositions with each other. Sometimes the teacher suggests that they use kitchen noises: the kettle whistling; the coffee pot going " ploppety, plop, plop, plop "; the toaster going " zing "; the dishes clattering; the pans banging; the stove bell saying " brrr "; the floor mop going " swish, swish." Such listening makes children in the classroom or therapy session more aware of sounds. The same group also uses the sounds of children's names as a basis for a poem like:

> Our little Jane likes sugar cane
> But chocolate ice cream to her is a pain.
> Now our big Jim likes to go to gym
> But drawing pictures is not for him.

A child comes to school prepared to like poetry, for he is intrigued with rhythm, the sounds of words, and the sensations of touch, taste, sound, and smell. His own rhythmic reactions are poetic in nature, as evidenced by his response to music. He is delighted with the way words sound. One six-year-old lovingly and caressingly used the word " delicious." The feeling of a fur piece was delicious. His stroking of fur, saying " delicious " at the same time, indicated his enjoyment and response to the sensation of touch. " Delicious " applied to ice cream showed his reaction to taste.

Just as vivid to the child of this age are sensations of sight, sound, and smell. He likes the sensuous quality of many of his experiences. Most teachers, by making use of this preparation to like poetry, enrich the child's school day by reading poetry aloud.

The teacher and the children read poetry aloud to bring out its melody, tones, movements, and quality. The teacher encourages children to select verse that meets their needs in terms of interest, emotion, and development. On the first day of a beautiful heavy snow, the teacher may read Frances Frost's *The Snow Man*, a poem about making the snow man, sticking the pipe in his mouth, tying a red scarf around his neck, and putting in his eyes. The children may do just that on their own initiative after school. Or why not provide an opportunity for them to build the snow man during school hours? Either the classroom teacher or the clinician may provide this opportunity. The day may be dull and need livening. On such a day a 10-year-old read Beatrice Brown's *Johnathon Bing*. Johnathon, going to Court to visit the King, discovered that he had forgotten his tie and his hat and finally that he was wearing pajamas. The children responded to this peculiar man Johnathon in this ludicrous situation. The dull day was brighter. Children also like lyric poetry that creates mood and calls forth pictures. One group of children again and again read and listened to Christina Rossetti's *Lullaby* with its pictures of the lambs sleeping, the stars up in the heavens, the moon peering, and with its mood of everyone quietly falling a-sleeping. Last, children like narrative poetry, such as Eugene Field's *Orphan Annie*, that tells of the adventures of an individual or a group of individuals. The good teacher and the perceptive clinician are alert to opportunities for sharing poetry suggested by the activities of the classroom and the school day.

At the more formal end of the reading aloud continuum one girl may be reading a particular poem or bit of prose to the entire class. Or the whole group may be speaking a poem together. The choral speakers may even perform in assembly. For example, choral speaking choirs may furnish the thread of the narrative for the story of important rivers. Or the choral speaking may be background for modern dance. Perhaps the poem tells the story of cities—like Sandburg's " Chicago "— while the modern dancers interpret it. At assemblies students frequently read selections from famous speakers. One vocational high school speech teacher said as a boy read, " He used to have trouble with his l's and r's. Now listen to him." The boy read well—with meaning and feeling.

Reading aloud both in the classroom and in the speech clinic room can be dreary. When the child is trying to read material that he does not quite understand, that he finds dull, and for which he feels no need, no stimulation is present. In a clinician's room when the only drill is reading loaded sentences over and over again, the result is equally dreary. Material to be read aloud should be material that in some way will stimulate the reader. It may have to do with the child's interests; it may be related to the occasion; it may be the kind of nonsense that appeals to him; it may express his particular feelings at a particular time. But it should prove stimulating. In each instance the children should have found out the meaning and feeling of the poem, and understood them clearly before they read aloud. The teacher then helps them to impart this meaning and feeling to the audience.

Dramatizing. Creative dramatics is almost universally successful with children of all ages and of all socioeconomic levels. In this activity where children get outside themselves, they feel free to express ideas. In addition they usually attend to the ideas expressed by their classmates with interest and thoughtfulness. Hayes reports that creative drama has been a powerful vehicle for developing thought and language, particularly in pidgin-speaking children. At Kalehi-Uka School in Honolulu, where many of the children are pidgin speakers, twelve teachers observed a year-long experimental creative drama program; they found that this medium supported independent and imaginative thinking, appreciation of ideas, and critical evaluation of the thinking of others. The children developed the ability to think and they displayed it in an ever-increasing use of language. Creative drama was especially helpful to the child who had very little language and to the pidgin speakers, who developed better speech patterns as a result of the experience (Hayes, 1970, p. 15).

Theater activities may range, as the others, from completely informal to the quite formal. From time immemorial children and parents have played a story, as evidenced in Robert Browning's poem "Development":

> My Father was a scholar and knew Greek.
> When I was five years old, I asked him once
> "What do you read about?"
> "The siege of Troy."
> "What is siege and what is Troy?"
> Whereat
> He piled up chairs and tables for a town,
> Set me a-top for Priam, called our cat
> —Helen, enticed away from home (he said)
> By wicked Paris who couched somewhere close
> Under the footstool, being coward
> But whom—since she was worth the pains, poor puss—
> Towzer and Tray,—our dogs, the Atreidai—sought
> By taking Troy to get possession of
> —Always when great Achilles ceased to sulk,
> (My pony in the stable)— forth would prance
> And put to flight Hector—our page boy's self.
> This taught me who was who and what was what:
> So far I rightly understood the case
> At five years old a huge delight it proved
> And still proves—thanks to that instructor sage
> My Father, who knew better than turn straight
> Learning's full flare on weak-eyed ignorance,
> Or, worse yet, leave weak eyes to grow sand-blind
> Content with darkness and vacuity.

Such playing stimulates language learning. For example, Robert Browning learned the meaning of *siege*, *Troy*, "who was who," and "what was what."

Teachers use this same kind of activity. One sixth-grade teacher wanted to prepare her children to view the television production of Shakespeare's *The Taming of the Shrew*. After she told the story, the children decided on what was to happen in each scene and who was to play Bianca, Katharina, Petruchio, and Hortensio. They then played *The Taming of the Shrew* in three scenes. As a result of this preparation, they watched the television production with understanding and interest. The discussion following their viewing was a lively one where the children began to learn some of the important elements of theater.

Teachers use not only stories as a basis for creative dramatics but also narrative poems, pairs of words like *ugly* and *beautiful*, sets of properties like an old bag, a scepter, and a blue teapot, and pictures that motivate but do not portray a story. Stories built from these sources stimulate children's language development. The degree of maturity makes a difference in the reaction to the stimulus. For example, two children, one aged seven and the other 13, were asked to make up stories that they could later play about the same picture. The picture was of a small girl looking rather wistful and dressed in a loose-fitting, white robe. The seven-year-old was mostly concerned with outward appearance and with descriptions, but the 13-year-old was interested in the relationship among persons. The seven-year-old saw just the present, but the 13-year-old viewed the past and looked to the future. The seven-year-old gave simple explanations and descriptions; the 13-year-old gave more complex ones. For example, she went into the motives of the child and her reasons for her actions. In addition, she saw the situation as a psychological problem of the child.

Speech clinicians, as well as classroom teachers, frequently use creative dramatics as material for teaching children to speak more clearly. A study by McIntyre (1959) evaluates the effect of a program of creative activities upon the consonant articulation skills of adolescent and preadolescent children with consonant articulation disorders. She selected 32 children from the speech therapy program of the Pittsburgh, Pennsylvania, public schools, who needed further therapy, and placed 16 in an experimental group and the remaining 16 in a control group. The experimental group participated in creative activities with 185 children for a six-week summer program of creative dramatics, creative music and dance, and arts and crafts. When the groups were retested, significant improvement in articulation was evidenced by a greater percentage of the children in the experimental group than was evidenced by children in the control group.

Many children's stories emphasize particular sounds, so that if the clinician is working on a sound, he can find a story that contains many words with the sound. For example, a first grader with a defective *k* and *g* might well play *Ask Mr. Bear* by Marjorie Flack (New York, The Macmillan Company, 1954). Danny tries to decide on a birthday gift for his mother. He meets a hen who suggests an egg, a goose who suggests a feather pillow, a goat who suggests cheese, and a cow who suggests cream. But finally Danny meets Mr. Bear who suggests a bear hug. All are happy. A second grader working with *k*'s might like to play Esphyr Slobodkina's *Caps for Sale* (New York, William Scott, 1947), which is the tale of a peddler and some monkeys and their monkey business. After going to sleep, the peddler looks up to see all of the monkeys wearing caps. A third grader who is working on *l* and *r* might enjoy playing Phyllis McGinley's *The Plain Princess* (Philadelphia, J. B. Lippincott Company, 1945), which involves a plan to make Esmeralda, the princess, beautiful. She goes to live with Dame's five beautiful daughters and learns not to be a spoiled princess but rather a person who is happy doing things for others. Thus, the princess becomes beautiful.

Adolescents, too, enjoy creative drama. A story such as Dorothy Canfield Fisher's *A New Pioneer* contains many *r* sounds and at the same time is the kind of material that interests adolescents. Magda is in bed crying, dreaming of all the horrible things that happened to her in Austria. Her grandfather comes to comfort her, telling her that everything will be all right now that they are in America. In school, some of the girls find her odd and different. As the students prepare for a Thanksgiving program, Magda writes and reads a prayer of Thanksgiving that she is now living in America. Her classmates are moved by her sensitive prayer.

All of the activities just mentioned are variants of dramatic activities on the informal end of the continuum. As the stories acquire more structure, as the "play" includes exposition, rising action, climax, falling action, and final outcome, as the teacher gives more direction, as the lines become set, as costumes and scenery are added, and as the size of the audience increases, the creative drama becomes less informal and approaches the more formal end of the continuum.

At the formal end of the continuum is the play where lines are learned, where the director gets exactly the results he wants, where the scenery and costumes are designed with care, and where the production is put on before an audience who pays to attend. But sometimes children learn lines and give plays to just another class. The direction is not as detailed. The costumes and scenery are improvised, and the result may be less formal than a carefully staged creative dramatic activity.

RELATIONSHIP OF SPEECH ACTIVITIES TO CURRICULUM

Speech education involving such stimulating speech activities is part and parcel of all school curricula. Teachers at both the elementary and high school levels frequently plan their work with their students. As the work of the unit progresses, many speech activities take place. Children give talks, report, discuss, debate, interview, read aloud, and dramatize.

For example, children in an eighth grade were studying the early history of New York State. While studying this era, one 12-year-old, reporting on his trip across New York State on the Thruway, compared the Thruway to the Erie Canal. The report of this trip motivated members of the class to study the building of the canal more thoroughly. The writer of their social studies text explained the reasons for the building of the canal and its values to the country, but the children wanted more information than their text contained. They discussed what more they would like to know about the Erie Canal. Specifically they wanted answers to:

- What were the factors that made a canal seem advisable?
- Who decided a canal was necessary?
- Why was Van Buren opposed to it?
- Why did Clinton approve the building of the Canal?
- What were the times like in the early 1800's?
- What kind of clothes did people wear then?
- What did they do for entertainment?
- How did they live?
- What did they do for a living?
- How was the building of the Canal planned?
- What was the route of the Canal?
- What were some of the difficulties encountered in building the Canal?
- Who built the Canal?
- What was its opening like?
- What were the effects of its opening?

After they had listed these questions on the blackboard, they broke into groups to decide how to do their research and how to report on their findings. The project demanded oral communication in its planning and in its execution.

Throughout this activity groups frequently gave progress reports. As the children read, they found other items that they thought should be included. Finally, individuals and groups of individuals reported on what they had read. One boy gave an account of the way people talked in the 1800's. This item was not included originally, but he and the members of his group felt it added to their understanding of the period. "Oh, go sandpaper your nose" became one of the favorite expressions of the group. Another panel of students gave a very interesting discussion of the songs sung during this era. Through such activities children learn to speak better and to participate in discussion more capably.

The teacher helped these children in a number of ways to prepare for and to give their talks. He reminded them of the necessity of gaining and holding the interest of their listeners. He suggested ways and means of collecting material and of organizing it. He stressed their having a thorough knowledge of their topic, a real interest in it themselves, and a desire to communicate this interest to their listeners.

The teacher also taught them to be more successful participants in a discussion group. He taught them how to state a problem, analyze it, and examine its solutions. The children learned that they must have a basis for the choice of a particular solution. Although these children had already learned to be fairly effective members of a discussion group, the teacher reinforced their learning. Frequently he stressed that they must have knowledge and background before speaking. Because the discussion sometimes went off on a tangent, he emphasized that they must keep it relevant. He helped the students to consider all points of view, participate well, and listen carefully. He encouraged each boy and girl to be a responsible member of the group.

In this work on the Erie Canal the students found it necessary to read aloud from various sources. One boy read the speech made by DeWitt Clinton at the opening of the Canal. The teacher helped him to prepare this speech for reading aloud by making sure he understood the material both intellectually and emotionally. As the boy mentioned bringing together the waters of the Hudson River and Lake Erie, his classmates felt pride in his voice. Because he knew the background so well, he needed almost no help in preparing his material to read aloud.

Finally, as a culminating activity, the class wrote and produced a play that depicted the struggle to build the canal. The play included a chorus of singers who sang about the Erie Canal and a choral-speaking group who, dressed in overalls, carrying shovels, and pushing wheelbarrows, spoke, "We are digging the ditch through the mire." The play, quite elaborately staged and executed, ran for three nights. It was the most formal of the speaking activities involved in this unit.

Such school activity also provides material for conversation for the speech clinic session.

SOCIAL CLIMATE

In all of the speaking activities the stimulation to speak is increased or decreased by the social and physical environment. In classrooms and in therapy sessions, where the social climate is warm, friendly, and wholly accepting and where the teacher or clinician listens graciously, carefully, and understandingly and where he places value on the contribution of each child, students are encouraged to talk, listen, and react. Such a climate cannot be created for speech situations alone; rather it must pervade every activity. It comes from a class framework that includes many opportunities for working together cooperatively in large and small groups at tasks or ideas that promote initiative. From such enterprise grows respect of group members for each other and for each other's contributions. Moreover, from such enterprise develops concern for the well-being of every member of the group. This setting provides the social climate conducive to a meaningful, gracious, and thoughtful interchange of ideas. Such a climate should prevail both in the classroom and in the speech clinician's room.

PHYSICAL ENVIRONMENT

Last, the teacher and the clinician do what they can to encourage a favorable physical environment. When the classroom has tables and chairs, the teacher's task is easier than when it has permanently installed seats. A group at one table may be talking about last night's baseball game; another, at a different table, about feeding dogs; another, about a visit to Disneyland; and still another, about an astronaut's latest trip. Similarly, the clinician's room should be comfortable, give the students a chance to walk around, and invite members of a group to talk with one another. Both the clinician and the teacher bring to the environment materials that stimulate children. Books, magazines, toys, pictures, valentines, masks and jack o'lanterns on Hallowe'en, and puppets that induce the children to handle them and to talk for them. A good-looking, comfortable room with materials that stimulate but do not distract invites talk. Both the classroom teacher and the clinician should provide such material.

INFLUENCE OF VARIOUS CULTURES ON LANGUAGE

Earlier we stressed two aspects of the linguistically advantaged: (1) rich experiential home and school background, and (2) positive self-concept. In the homes of people of middle and higher socioeconomic status the verbal environments in some ways tend to be richer than they are in families of lower socioeconomic status. From her research, John has concluded that the home environment of children of low socioeconomic status hampers the acquisition of abstract and integrative language (John, 1963, p. 14ff.). Deutsch notes that conversation in so-called disadvantaged homes consists largely of brief sentences and commands, that there is little labeling of actions and objects, that there are few books and magazines (Deutsch, 1967, p. 149). Bernstein maintains that early experience with "elaborated codes" (specific messages in terms of situation, topic, and person) allows for the expression of complex thought and tends to discriminate between cognitive and affective communication. On the other hand, "restricted codes" (nonspecific messages, clichés, generalized statements, or observations), although readily understood, are not conducive to careful, critical thought. Bernstein points out that the two codes do not necessarily develop as a result of the speaker's innate intelligence. The level at which the child operates a particular code is related to his innate ability, but the orientation is related to the sociological restraints upon the speaker (Bernstein, 1966, p. 430).

We also indicated that a positive self-concept helps language to develop. The communication that takes place in school may foster a negative self-concept for the child of a different culture. Deutsch (1965) talks about the cumulative language deficit wherein as the so-called disadvantaged child progresses in school, his language abilities fall further and further behind the advantaged. Unless the verbal environment of the school is within the capabilities of its participants, the school loses its socializing force. Frost has recognized that the continued lack of success in communication between the teacher and the child of a different culture can lead to confusion, resentment, and a negative self-image; the negative self-image results because the child cannot relate verbally to the teacher and in some instances is made to feel that his language is inferior (Frost, 1966, p. xv).

In the chapter on standards we noted that some writers believe that in regard to morphology and syntax, the Negro dialect has its own systematic structure and set of rules. Baratz (1969) points out certain of these rules:

1. The morpheme for the plural is not added with a numerical quantifier, as *fifty cent, two foot.*
2. The contiguous relation of *John* and *cousin* may mark the possessive, as *John cousin.*
3. Word order expresses the conditional, as "I aks did he want to go."

4. The third person singular lacks the third-person morphological ending as, "She work here."
5. Verb agreement differs from standard American, as "She have a bike," or "They was going."
6. The copula may be omitted, as in "I going" or "He a bad boy."
7. The double negative is used, as "I don't got none."
8. *Ain't* is used in expressing the past, as "He ain't go."
9. *Be* expresses habitual action, as "He be working every day." This is in contrast with "He working right now" (Baratz, 1969, p. 89).

We should like to note here as we did in the Chapter 3, "Standards of Speech," that some writers emphasize that the language of the child of the inner city, although a different one, is not one wherein a language deficit exists. They question whether some environments are more successful than others in stimulating language development (Baratz, 1968), whether if the language of the child in the inner city were equated with the language of the child in the suburbs, the measurements of cognitive differences might not be more nearly equal. They also point out (Baratz and Povich, 1968) that whereas language of Negro children contains structures that can be considered "restricted forms" when compared with standard English, in reality they indicate a level of syntactic development where transformations are used appropriately in terms of lower-class dialect. The lower class negro child is using the same forms as the lower class negro adult and has thus acquired the forms of his particular linguistic environment.

The writers believe that by using the child's own social dialect and by providing vital, stimulating experiences, the child's interest and desire for success in communication can be aroused. Research shows that inner city children express themselves best in unstructured situations, and because they do well in the land of make-believe, creative, dramatic, and puppetry activities seem to work. Because they understand more language than they use, pantomime can be utilized, for they will be able to understand situations that are described and then will be able to portray them. This nonverbal kind of communication can lead to verbal communication. After the child feels success in communication, the teacher can begin to teach the prestigious dialect. The child becomes aware that he substitutes [t], [f], or [s] for [θ], that he omits weakly stressed syllables, as *surance* for *insurance*, that he shifts the primary stress frontward as in *police* or *guitar*, and that he gives heavy stress to final weakly stressed syllables as in *accident* or *evidence*. He becomes aware of morphological differences—that he says *hisn, hern, those here dogs, them there cats, more prettier.*

As noted in Chapter 3, this process of teaching a second mode of communication is not begun in the early grades but in the later ones. Changes take place gradually, until the child is writing and speaking the prestigious dialect. On certain occasions and in some environments, he will continue to use his own social dialect—the first language he acquired.

Relationship of Speech Improvement to Speech Correction

Several studies that have investigated the effect of speech improvement upon articulation have been completed. One such study (Byrne, 1960) is reported in the October, 1960, issue of *ASHA*. Teachers, after an in-service training period that emphasized ear training (identification of the sound, listening for it, and discrimination between sounds), provided kindergarten and first-grade children with speech improvement lessons daily for 21 weeks. The experimental kindergartners achieved scores on two of the three articulatory measures and the one auditory discrimination test that were significantly different from those of the control group. The experimental first graders had scores on one articulation test that differentiated them from the control group; on word recognition the experimental first graders did significantly better than the controls.

Van Hattum (1959) reports similar results in a study published in *Exceptional Child*. He instituted a speech improvement program in Rochester, which provided ear training for part of the first-grade population. After the training period, he checked the number of students who needed speech work in the third grade. Of the 1,503 pupils who did not receive speech improvement, 20.1 per cent had speech defects. Of the 467 students who did receive speech improvement, 12.9 per cent had speech defects. Concomitant with the speech improvement program, the dismissals from clinic climbed from 19 per cent to 41 per cent.

A study done by Sommers and others (1961) explores the effects of speech improvement and speech therapy on the articulation and reading of first-grade children. The results of this study were interesting. Speech improvement was found to affect reading skills, as expressed in reading factor scores in a significant way. Speech clinic procedures did not significantly change reading comprehension scores for children with misarticulation or for children with normal articulation, but they did improve scores for a matched group of 25 children with severe articulation problems. Speech therapy did not affect reading factor scores in any significant way but it did improve articulation significantly more than did speech improvement. In fact, three months of speech therapy appeared about as effective in reducing articulation errors as nine months of speech improvement. Children receiving speech improvement improved significantly more in articulation than those who did not receive it. Children with severe articulation problems improved significantly when they received both speech therapy and speech improvement, as compared with a matched group who received speech improvement only (Sommers, 1961, p. 37). This study was followed by one designed to test the effectiveness of speech improvement on reading and articulation of school children beyond the first grade. The data support these conclusions about articulation:

a. Speech improvement conducted by clinicians who used analytical ear-training procedures was significantly better in improving articulation of first-grade children when it was provided for nine months rather than 16 weeks beginning at the middle of the school year.

b. Speech improvement for eight weeks in second grade was ineffective in providing further improvement in articulation for children who received nine months of it in first grade.

c. The consonant sounds which were most easily corrected under a program of nine months of speech improvement in first grade and eight weeks in second grade were studied. They were found in order of highest to lowest percentage of correction to be: [v], 50 per cent; [f], 41 per cent; [r], 38 per cent; [g], 37 per cent; [k], 36 per cent; [θ], 33 per cent; [s], 26 per cent; [ʃ], 22 per cent; [tʃ], 20 per cent, and [l], 18 per cent. Additional investigation was given to the [s] sound. Misarticulations of [s] were analyzed in terms of interdental and lateral sigmatisms. Twelve per cent of children with lateral sigmatisms were corrected; 32 per cent of the children with interdental sigmatisms were corrected (Sommers, 1962, p. 58).

The data support these conclusions about reading:

a. Subjects who were provided with speech improvement both in first and second grades made significantly higher reading factor scores at the end of the second grade than did subjects who were not provided with speech improvement.

b. Higher reading factor scores for subjects who experienced speech improvement in first and second grades did not result in higher reading comprehension scores at the end of the second grade, compared with those who never received this treatment.

c. No significant difference was found in the improvement of reading factor scores for first-grade subjects who received 16 weeks of speech improvement compared with those who received nine months of this treatment (Sommers, 1962, p. 59).

The very important study referred to earlier, made by a committee of the American Speech and Hearing Association, also points to the need for a speech improvement program. To be clear as to what this committee means by speech improvement, we include its definition of speech improvement and its statement of purposes of the program:

> For the purposes of this study speech improvement takes place in the classroom. It consists of systematic instruction in oral communication which has as its purpose the development of articulation, voice, and language abilities that enable all children to communicate their ideas effectively. Speech improvement is not concerned with the work of the speech clinician with speech -and hearing-handicapped children outside of the regular classroom (*ASHA*, 1961, p. 78).

The committee describes the purposes of the program:

> Similarities in curriculum development and instructional practices in speech improvement are more common than are differences and contrasts. There appears to be general agreement on the purposes of instruction in speech improvement. Teachers indicate that curriculum experiences should be provided in the classroom to permit all children to develop the best speech, voice, and language patterns of which they are capable, correct minor speech and voice difficulties, and express their ideas clearly and effectively. There also seems to be general agreement that ability to hear and to discriminate between speech sounds is of first importance in speech and language development and in the correction of minor speech difficulties (*ASHA*, 1961, p. 84).

The activities that accomplish these purposes include exercises in discriminating between similar sounds, in articulating and pronouncing clearly, in use of stress, and in use of voice. Seven speaking actitivities used as procedures in teaching speech improvement are auditory training drills, voice and articulation practice, discussion and conversations, dramatic presentations, oral reading, parliamentary procedure, and talks and reports (*ASHA*, 1961, pp. 84–85). These seven activities fall into the categories mentioned earlier in this chapter.

The committee says about measuring the effectiveness of speech improvement:

> The principal means of measuring the effectiveness of speech improvement is judgment—the judgment of supervisors, teachers, parents, and children. However, 29 per cent of the speech improvement teachers use articulation tests and 16 per cent use voice ratings. While 67 per cent of the teachers depend upon their judgment together with that of their supervisors, 31 per cent use the judgment of parents and 45 per cent use the judgment of children in evaluating speech improvement.

Teachers of speech improvement are strongly convinced that speech improvement helps children not only to develop good speech, voice, and language patterns but also to correct minor speech and voice problems. They also believe that children are helped to organize their thoughts and to express them clearly and effectively (*ASHA*, 1961, p. 87).

Supervisors are not convinced that speech improvement decreases the number of students requiring speech therapy. Only 23 per cent believe it does.

Except for those on the West Coast, speech and hearing clinicians throughout the nation, however, are more certain than their supervisors that speech improvement has decreased the number of children requiring therapy. Of the clinicians, 61 per cent believe that speech improvement reduces the number needing therapy. The same committee makes suggestions for a model program in speech improvement, noting that all classroom teachers are teachers of speech improvement and that speech improvement programs should provide the kinds of assistance classroom teachers need to help all children learn to organize their thoughts and express them effectively in the best speech, voice, and language of which they are capable. They base their plan in part upon the description of ongoing programs of speech improvement. The following are the committee's recommendations:

All children are carefully screened by speech and hearing personnel and records are kept on each child. Those children who indicate that they can respond to speech improvement techniques are not referred for remedial speech, although they may be later if they do not make expected progress.

When a program is being started, all elementary teachers are given in-service training covering a period of two to three years; the length of training is dependent upon the previous preparation and experience of the classroom teachers and the amount of time clinicians can devote to programs in the classroom. After the program is begun, in-service training is limited to teachers new to the system. In-service includes a planned series of workshops and demonstrations held during the year either by the supervisor of speech improvement or by persons recognized for their leadership in the work. When possible, college courses in speech improvement are offered locally. Provision is made for teachers' attendance at regional and state conferences.

Speech improvement is not taught as a separate subject in any classroom from kindergarten through grade 12. Instead, it is part of the regular curriculum in that it is integrated with subject-matter areas and with school activities.

In the classroom during the in-service training period the clinician does demonstrations of speech improvement at least once a week to set a pattern for the classroom teacher to follow between demonstrations. Major emphasis is placed upon developmental and preventive aspects of speech, voice, and language, but attention is given to correction of minor speech and voice problems. Through conferences the clinician helps the teacher to integrate speech improvement with class and school activities, and she assists the teacher to conduct speaking activities as part of instruction. The clinician makes specific suggestions for helping children receiving remedial services to participate in speech improvement and to use newly acquired skills. The clinician assists the teacher to use standardized evaluative criteria as well as judgment in measuring the effectiveness of the work. With the period of in-service training completed, the classroom teacher assumes responsibility for speech improvement and the clinician serves as consultant.

Since parents can do much to help their young children develop speech, voice, and language abilities, an able clinician is assigned to work with parents of children in kindergarten and in grades one and two. Conferences begin with the initial visit of parent and child at school in preparation for the child's entering school. In larger school systems this clinician devotes full time to work with parents individually and in groups.

At the senior high school level speech improvement is integrated with work in fundamentals of speech, public speaking and debating, and dramatics and is correlated with academic subjects and with activities such as student government, class organizations, assembly programs, and clubs. In-service training and assistance are provided by the supervisor of speech improvement (*ASHA*, 1961, pp. 90—91).

From these studies it seems obvious that schools need both speech clinic and speech improvement programs. Speech clinical services help the handicapped to overcome their difficulties. Speech improvement services help all children to speak and listen better and reinforce the teaching given in speech therapy sessions. Stimulation to speak through speaking activities and through a democratic, friendly classroom atmosphere is important in both speech improvement and speech therapy.

References and Suggested Readings

ABERNATHY, R. L., "The Role of Storytelling," *The Speech Teacher*, IX (November, 1960), 283–286. (Gives a preliminary report on the role of storytelling in the United States.)

ALLEN, P. D., "An Elementary Teacher's-Eye View of the Disadvantaged," *Elementary English*, XLIV (January, 1967), 53–56. (Gives the characteristics of the disadvantaged child in terms of his feelings, of his lack of experiences in some areas and wealth of them in others, and of the disparity between the language spoken at home and at school.)

ARBUTHNOT, M. H., *Children and Books*. Chicago. Scott, Foresman & Co., 1947. (Considers how to select books for children and how to guide their reading. Contains excellent sections on storytelling and choral speaking.)

ASHA Subcommittee of Research Committee, "Speech Improvement," Chapter 7 in "Public School Speech and Hearing Services," *Journal of Speech and Hearing Disorders*, Monograph Supplement 8 (July, 1961).

BIRCH, J. W., and J. MATTHEWS, *Improving Children's Speech*. Cincinnati, Public School Publishing Company, 1958. (Presents goals in speech improvement for various grades and means of achieving these goals.)

Board of Education of the City of New York, *Puppetry in the Curriculum*. Curriculum Bulletin I, 1947–48 Series.

————, *Toward Better Speech*. Curriculum Bulletin V, 1952–53 Series.

BOWDEN, F. B., "Conversation and Discussion in the Elementary School," *Elementary English Review*, XXIV (May, 1947), 293–302.

BRETT, S. M., "A New Measure of Language Maturity," *Elementary English*, XLII (October, 1965), 666–668. (Notes the length of the T-unit, the minimal sentence as a valid indicator of maturity.)

BROWN, H., and H. HELTMAN, *Let's-Read-Together*. New York, Harper & Row, Publishers, 1950. (One of the most comprehensive and usable collections of poetry for choral speaking.)

BROWN, K. L., "Speech and Listening in Language Arts Textbooks: Part I," *Elementary English*, XLIV (April, 1967), 336–341. (Reports on the kind and quantity of speech and listening content in textbooks in language arts in the elementary schools.)

BYRNE, M. C., *The Child Speaks: A Speech Improvement Program for Kindergarten and First Grade*. New York, Harper & Row, Publishers, 1965. (Contains a speech and language development program which is sound-oriented.)

————, "Results of a Speech Improvement Program for Kindergarten and First-Grade Children," *ASHA*, II (October, 1960), 360—361. (Studies the effect of a daily speech improvement program on articulation ability of kindergarten and first-grade children.)

CARLTON, L., and R. H. MOORE, "The Effects of Self-Directive Dramatization on Reading Achievement and Self-Concept of Culturally Disadvantaged Children," *The Reading Teacher*, XX (November, 1966), 125–130. (Reports that significantly greater gains in reading can be achieved with groups of culturally disadvantaged elementary school children through the use of classroom self-directive dramatization of stories than through methods involving traditional use of basal readers.)

CARROW, SISTER M. A., "The Development of Auditory Comprehension of Language Structure in Children," *Journal of Speech and Hearing Disorders*, LII (May, 1968), 99–111. (Tells how to evaluate comprehension of linguistic structure of children.)

CAZDEN, C. B., *Environmental Assistance to the Child's Acquisition of Grammar*. Ph.D. Dissertation. Harvard University, 1965.

Contest Committee of the Speech Association of America, "A Program of Speech Education," *Quarterly Journal of Speech*, XXXVII (October, 1951), 347–358. (Shows the place of speech in society.)

CORBIN, R., and M. CROSBY, *Language Programs for the Disadvantaged.* Champaign, Ill., National Council of Teachers of English, 1965. (Defines the problem, tells about various programs of teaching the disadvantaged, gives some of the linguistic and philosophical background.)

DIZNEY, H. F. and R. W. ROSKINS, "An Investigation of Certain Qualitative Aspects of Verbalization," *American Educational Research Journal,* III (May, 1966), 179–180. (Reviews certain qualitative aspects of verbalization of 15 bright fourth-grade children. Measures used include average words per response, type-token ratio (unique words used), adjective-noun ratios, adverb-noun ratios, average number of words per second.)

EISENSTADT, A. A., "Who Teaches Speech?" *American Childhood,* XLIII (May, 1958), 26–27. (Stresses the importance of the classroom teacher in developing acceptable patterns of speech in the child.)

EMERICK, L. "Speech Improvement in the Kindergarten," *Education,* LXXXIV (May, 1964), 565–568. (Shows that articulation errors of those children receiving speech improvement decrease significantly more than do the errors in those who do not receive this training.)

ERWIN, J. C., "Speech Improvement in the Elementary School," *The Speech Teacher,* VII (September, 1958), 185–190. (Reviews activities of classroom teachers in speech improvement.)

EVERTTS, E. L., ed., *Dimensions of Dialect.* Champaign, Ill.: National Council of Teachers of English, 1967. (Contains a series of articles on language deprivation, dialectal barriers, and means of teaching language to children).

FROSTIG, M. and P. MASLOW, "Language Training: A Form of Ability Training," *Journal of Learning Disabilities,* I (February, 1968), 105–115. (Discusses developmental functions of language.)

GLAUS, M., *From Thoughts to Words.* Champaign, Ill., National Council of Teachers of English, 1965. (Shows how to help children interpret their individual thoughts into spoken and written words.)

HAHN, E., "An Analysis of the Content and Form of the Speech of First Grade Children," *Quarterly Journal of Speech,* XXXIV (October, 1948), 361–366. (Shows that where speaking is fun, speaking skills are high. Explains that the length of response, sentence structure, and completeness of structure depend on the immediate situation more than the topic.)

HAYES, E., "Drama Big News in English," *Elementary English,* XLVII (January, 1970), 13–16. (Cites the advantages of creative drama.)

HUNT, K. W., *Grammatical Structure Written at Three Grade Levels.* Champaign, Ill., National Council of Teachers of English, 1965. (Shows the consistency of patterns of change from one grade level to the next.)

HUNT, K. W., "Recent Measures in Syntactic Development," *Elementary English,* XLIII (November, 1966), 732–739. (Suggests that clause length is a better index of language maturity than sentence length or number of subordinate clauses.)

HUNTER, M. A., "Lessons in Articulation," *The Speech Teacher,* IX (November, 1960), 290–292. (Tells how classroom teachers can teach discrimination and production of sounds.)

IRWIN, R. B., "The Role of the Speech Therapist in the Speech Improvement Program," *The Speech Teacher*, IX (November, 1960), 278–282. (Shows relationship of speech improvement to speech therapy. Suggests a limited role of speech therapist in speech improvement services.)

KAPLAN, B. A., "Issues in Educating the Culturally Disadvantaged," *Phi Delta Kappan*, XLV (November, 1963), 71–76.

KEYSER, S. J., "The Role of Linguistics in the Elementary-School Curriculum," *Elementary English*, XLVII (January, 1970), 39–45.

KRIPPNER, S., "Reading Improvement and Scores on the Holtzman Inkblot Technique," *The Reading Teacher*, XIX (April, 1968), 519–522. (Suggests that children with disordered thought processes, bizarre perceptions, and emotionally disturbing fantasies may not be expected to do well in remedial reading until a personality change has been effected.)

LEASE, R., and G. B. SIKS, *Creative Dramatics in Home, School, and Community*. Harper & Row, Publishers, 1952.

LEWIS, C., "Language and Literature in Childhood," *Elementary English*, XLIV (May, 1967), 518–522. (Tells about dramatizing scenes from *The Iliad*.)

LOBAN, W., *Problems in Oral English*. Champaign, Ill., National Council of Teachers of English, 1966. (Reports the first phase of his longitudinal study of language development.)

McDAVID, R. I., ed., *An Examination of the Attitudes of the NCTE Toward Language*. Champaign, Ill., National Council of Teachers of English, 1965. (Shows historically changing attitudes toward language.)

MacDONALD, J. B., *Language and Meaning*. Washington, D.C., Association for Supervision and Curriculum Developments, NEA, 1966. (Discusses language, meaning, and motivation, curricular language as related to classroom meanings, what language reveals, and the relationship of meaning and thinking.)

McINTYRE, B., "The Effect of Creative Activities on the Articulation of Children with Speech Disorders," *ASHA*, I (November, 1959), 80.

MARGE, M., "The Influence of Selected Home Background Variables on the Development of Oral Communication Skills in Children," *Journal of Speech and Hearing Research*, VIII (September, 1965), 291–309. (Studies the effects of permissiveness of mothers, parental demands, techniques of speech training at home, differences between the ratings of speech teachers and other teachers in evaluating the speaking abilities of youngsters.)

MARTIN, B., Jr., "Helping Children Claim Language Through Literature," *Elementary English*, XLV (May, 1968), 583–591. (Talks of three general levels of language: the "in-group" language of the home, the public language of society, the life-lifting language of literature. Stresses the use of language as a communicative tool—that we must help the child use language to create and solidify his personal world and to bridge from his world into the lives of other people. Many examples.)

MIEL, A., ed., *Practical Suggestions for Improving Teaching*. New York, Bureau of Publications, Teachers' College, Columbia University, 1958. (Contains A. Bingham, "Improving Children's Facility in Problem Solving.")

MUKERJI, R., and H. F. Robison, "A Head Start in Language," *Elementary*

English, XLIII (May, 1966), 460–463. (Gives examples of language deficits. Explains the types of structured experiences and teacher-child language activities that will stimulate language growth.)

MUNKERS, A., *Helping Children in Oral Communication*. New York, Bureau of Publications, Teachers' College, Columbia University, 1959. (Presents an example, an explanation of the teaching efforts which led up to the product, and comments and questions concerning the decisions made by the teacher involved.)

NURK, M., "Motivating Speech Improvement in the Upper Grades," *The Speech Teacher*, IX (November, 1960), 301–303. (Tells how to use records of *My Fair Lady* and the story of *Pygmalion* to motivate speech improvement with upper elementary and junior high school students.)

OBERLE, M., "A Contemporary View of Elementary Speech Education," *The Speech Teacher*, IX (November, 1960), 267–270. (Explains the importance of speech training to the elementary school child.)

O'DONNELL, R. C., *Syntax of Kindergarten and Elementary School Children: A Transformational Analysis*. Champaign, Ill., National Council of Teachers of English, 1967. (Analyzes the language of white middle-class families' children in grades 1, 2, 3, 5, and 7.)

OGILVIE, M., "Creative Speech Experiences in the Elementary School," *The Speech Tracher*, VII (January, 1958), 5–10.

———, "Oral Communication in Elementary School Living," *The Speech Teacher*, VII (January, 1957), 43–47.

———, *Speech in the Elementary School*. New York, McGraw-Hill, Inc., 1954.

———, and M. N. SEARLES, "The Important Place of 'Sharing Ideas,'" *The Speech Teacher*, IX (November, 1960), 287–289. (Suggests how the teacher may guide the show-and-tell period.)

OLSEN, J., "When Children Are Silent," *Elementary English*, XLIII (December, 1966), 877—879. (Looks for an explanation of the reticent child.)

PETTY, W. T., and R. J. STARKEY, "Oral Language and Personal and Social Development," *Elementary English*, XLIII (April, 1966), 386–393. (Cites research evidence to show the interrelatedness of language ability, environmental, physical, and interpersonal factors, and several behavioral tendencies such as the expression of fright.)

POSSIEN, W. M., *They All Need to Talk*. New York, Appleton-Century-Crofts, 1969. (Covers the areas of creative drama, discussing, reporting, using children's literature, poetry, and choral speaking.)

POTTS, M., "The Effect of Second-Language Instruction on the Reading Proficiency and General School Achievement of Primary-Grade Children," *American Educational Research Journal*, IV (November, 1967), 367–373.

PRONOVOST, W., with L. KINGMAN, *The Teaching of Speaking and Listening in the Elementary School*. New York, Longmans, Green and Co., Inc., 1959. (Includes guides for teaching speech activities in the elementary school program. Shows very clearly the integration of speech education with various elementary-school academic areas. Contains many examples.)

RASMUSSEN, C., *Speech Methods in the Elementary School*. New York, The Ronald Press Company, 1947.

ROBINSON, HELEN, ed., *Oral Aspects of Reading*. Chicago, University of Chicago Press, 1955.

RUDDELL, R. B., "The Effect of the Similarity of Oral and Written Patterns of Language Structure on Reading Comprehension," *Elementary English*, XLII (April, 1965), 403–410. (Indicates that reading comprehension is a function of the similarity of patterns of language structure in the reading materials to oral patterns of language structure used by children.)

――――, "Oral Language and the Development of Other Language Skills," *Elementary English*, XL (May, 1963), 489–498. (Discusses various relationships: vocabulary and syntactical language development; oral language development and reading achievement; listening development and reading achievement; oral language development and writing. Shows the interrelationships of language skills.)

SCHELLENBERG, J. A., "Group Size as a Factor in Success of Academic Discussion Groups," *Journal of Educational Sociology*, XXXIII (October, 1959), 73–79. (Found that students who were placed in discussion groups of four experienced greater freedom of expression than those placed in groups of six, eight, or 10.)

SCOTT, L. B., "What Values, Puppetry?" *Elementary English*, XXX (April, 1953), 210–213. (Explains the use of puppetry in helping the speech-defective child.)

SHRINER, T. H., "A Comparison of Selected Measures with Psychological Values of Language Development," *Journal of Speech and Hearing Research*, X (December, 1967), 828–835. (Develops composite scale value of language development from two to 12 years.)

SHRINER, T. H., and D. SHERMAN, "An Equation for Assessing Language Development," *Journal of Speech and Hearing Research*, X (March, 1967), 41–48. (Develops an equation based on: mean of five longest responses, number of different words, structural complexity score. Based on a language sample consisting of 50 responses to pictures.)

SIKS, G. B., *Creative Dramatics*. New York, Harper & Row, Publishers, 1958. (Tells how to guide and find material for creative drama.)

SIMMERMAN, A. J., "Lessons in Creativity," *The Speech Teacher*, IX (November, 1960), 293–295. (Describes a creative experience involving poetry.)

SLADE, P., *Child Drama*. New York, Philosophical Library, 1955. (Gives directions to the teacher doing creative drama.)

SOMMERS, R. K., et al., "Effects of Speech Therapy and Speech Improvement upon Articulation and Reading," *Journal of Speech and Hearing Disorders*, XXVI (February, 1961), 27–37. (Explores the effects of speech improvement and speech therapy upon the articulation and reading of first-grade children.)

――――, "Effects of Various Durations of Speech Improvement upon Articulation and Reading," *Journal of Speech and Hearing Disorders*, XXVII (February, 1962), 54–61. (A continuation of the preceding study.)

STRANG, R., and M. E. HOCKER, "First-Grade Children's Language Patterns," *Elementary English*, LXII (January, 1965), 38–41. (Describes oral language used by a heterogeneous group of first-grade children.)

STRICKLAND, R., "Needed Research in Oral Language, Part I," *Elementary English*, XLIV (March, 1967), 257–259. (Reviews the need for children to attain the standard of speech that will be an asset and not a liability in achieving the objectives in their lives.)

VAN HATTUM, R. J., "Evaluating Elementary-School Speech Therapy," *Exceptional Child*, XXV (May, 1959), 411–414. (Gives the effect of training in speech improvement upon a number of cases of speech defects.)

VAN RIPER, C., "They Too Need Speech," *Journal of Exceptional Children*, XII (February, 1946), 134–136. (Stresses the importance of communication for the handicapped. Shows the relationship of mental hygiene and speech.)

————, and K. G. BUTLER, *Speech in the Elementary Classroom*. New York, Harper & Row, Publishers, 1955. (Contains many suggestions for improving speech in the classroom. Particularly good for teaching sounds and for work on discrimination of sounds.)

WELLS, C., "Speech in the Full School Program," *Elementary English*, XXVIII (April, 1951), 201–204. (Stresses the idea that every class is a speech class and every teacher a speech teacher. Describes a good climate for speech.)

VOLC, J., "Storytelling in the Language Arts Program," *Elementary English*, XLV (November, 1968), 958–965. (Includes a bibliography of stories that tell well, filmstrips, movies, records, and books on storytelling. Sound advice.)

WILSON, R. M., "Oral Reading Is Fun," *The Reading Teacher*, XIX (October, 1965), 42–43. (Shows gains in oral reading with twelve one-hour sessions.)

WILT, M., "Talk, Talk, Talk," *The Reading Teacher*, XXI (April, 1968), 611–617. (Surveys problems of the development of language.)

ZIMBARDO, P. G., and J. S. BARNARD, "The Role of Anxiety and Defensiveness in Children's Verbal Behavior," *Journal of Personality*, XXXI (March, 1963), 79–96. (Shows how anxiety interacts with types of interview conditions to influence both comprehensibility of speech and intrusions of affect in children's speech.)

Suggested Readings in Language of Children from a Different Culture

ALLEN, P., "An Elementary Teacher's-Eye View of the Disadvantaged," *Elementary English*, XLIV (January, 1967), 53–67.

BARATZ, J. C., "Language and Cognitive Assessment of Negro Children," *ASHA*, III (March, 1969), 87–91.

————, "Language and Cognitive Assessment of Negro Children: Assumptions and Research Needs." Washington, D.C., ERIC. Ed. 020 518, 1968.

————, and E. Povich, "Grammatical Construction in the Language of the Negro Preschool Child," Washington, D.C. ERIC. Ed. 022 157, 1968.

BERNSTEIN, B., "Elaborated and Restricted Codes; Their Social Origins and Some Consequences," in A. G. Smith, ed., *Communication and Culture*. New York, Holt, Rinehart and Winston, Inc., 1966, pp. 427–441.

BLOOM, B., A. DAVIS and R. HESS, *Compensatory Education for Cultural Deprivation*. New York, Holt, Rinehart and Winston, Inc., 1966.

BLACK, M. H., "Characteristics of the Culturally Deprived Child," *The Reading Teacher*, XIX (March, 1965), 465–470.

CAZDEN, C. B., "Subcultural Differences in Child Language: An Inter-Disciplinary Review," *Merrill Palmer Quarterly*, XII (April, 1966), 185–219.

CROW, L., W. MURRAY and R. SMYTHE, *Educating the Culturally Disadvantaged Child*. New York, David McKay Company, 1966.

DEUTSCH, M., *The Disadvantaged Child*. New York, Basic Books, 1967.

——, "The Role of Social Class in Language Development and Cognition," *American Journal of Orthopsychiatry*, XXV (January, 1965), 78–88.

FROST, J., and G. HAWKES, eds., *The Disadvantaged Child: Issues and Innovations*. Boston, Houghton Mifflin Company, 1966.

GERBER, S., and C. HERTEL, "Language Deficiency of Disadvantaged Children," *Journal of Speech & Hearing Research*, XII (June, 1969), 270–280.

GLADNEY, M., and L. LEAVORTON, "A Model for Teaching English to Non-Standard English Speakers," *Elementary English*, XLV (October, 1965), 20–25.

HAMLIN, R., R. MUKERJI and M. YONEMURA, *Schools for Young Disadvantaged Children*. New York, Teachers' College, Columbia University, 1967.

HERTZLER, J. *A Sociology of Learning*. New York, Random House, Inc., 1965.

HUNT, J. M., "The Psychological Basis for Using Pre-School Enrichment as an Antidote for Cultural Deprivation," *Merrill Palmer Quarterly*, X (July, 1964), 209–248.

JOHN, V., and L. GOLDSTEIN, "The Social Context of Language Acquisition." *Merrill Palmer Quarterly*, X (July 1964), 265–275.

KRUGMAN, M., "The Culturally Deprived Child in School," *National Education Association Journal*, C (April, 1961), 23–25.

LOBAN, W., "Language Proficiency and School Learning," in J. D. Krunholtz, ed., *Learning and the Education Process*. Chicago, Rand McNally & Company, 1965, pp. 113–131.

LORETAN, J. O., and S. UMANS, *Teaching the Disadvantaged*. New York, Teachers' College, Columbia University, 1966.

POSSOW, H., ed., *Education in Depressed Areas*. New York, Teachers' College, Columbia University, 1967.

REISSMAN, F., *Helping the Disadvantaged Pupil to Learn More Easily*. Englewood Cliffs, N.J., Prentice-Hall, Inc., 1966.

STOFFEL, F. "Once Upon a Time," *American Education*, IV (September, 1968), 53–55.

WILLIAMS, F., and R. C. NAREMORE, "On the Functional Analysis of Social Class Differences in Modes of Speech," *Speech Monographs*, XXXVI (June, 1969), 77–102.

Suggested Readings in General Teaching Methods in Language

ANDERSON, V. D., et al., eds., *Readings in the Language Arts*. New York, The Macmillan Company, 1964.

BAKER, S. W., *The Language Arts, the Child and the Teacher*. San Francisco, Fearon Publishers, 1955.

BROGAN, P., and L. FOX, *Helping Children Learn*. Yonkers, New York, World Book Company, 1955.

DAWSON, M. A., *Guiding Language Learning*. New York, Harcourt, Brace & World, Inc., 1963.

GRAY, W., and H. and P. GREEN, *Developing Language Skills in the Elementary School*. Boston, Allyn and Bacon, Inc., 1963.

HERRICK, V. E. and L. B. JACOBS, eds., *Children and the Language Arts*. Englewood Cliffs, N.J., Prentice-Hall, Inc., 1955.

National Council of Teachers of English, *Language Arts for Today's Children*. New York, Appleton-Century-Crofts, 1952.

National Society for the Study of Education, *Teaching Language in the Elementary School*, 43rd Yearbook, Part II. Chicago, University of Chicago Press, 1964.

SHANE, H. G., et al., *Improving Language Arts Instruction in the Elementary School*. Columbus, Ohio, Charles E. Merrill Books, Inc., 1962.

STRICKLAND, R. G., *Language Arts in the Elementary School*, 2nd ed. Boston, D.C. Heath and Company, 1957.

WOLFE, D. M., *Language Arts and Life Patterns, Grades 2–8*. New York, The Odyssey Press, Inc., 1961.

Problems

1. Visit a classroom and list the different speech activities that went on while you were there. Did anything happen that could not be considered a speech activity?

2. Visit an elementary or high school classroom and analyze the effect of the seating arrangement, the social climate of the room, and the interests of the children on their motivation to speak in the classroom.

3. Indicate in some detail specific classroom activities that may promote conversation, group discussion, creative dramatics, reading aloud, and speaking before the class.

4. Show how three pieces of children's literature could be used as a basis for speaking situations.

5. Find a story and three poems that the children of the level you intend to teach might well enjoy.

6. Visit a classroom. List the experiences that stimulated the development of language. Indicate why they seemed to be effective.

7. Indicate how a speech clinician might make use of creative drama in a therapy session.

8. Visit a classroom. Give examples of teacher responses that enlarged upon what the child said and those that expanded upon what the teacher said.

Chapter 9

Delayed or Retarded Language Acquisition and Development

Delayed Development

The child who is severely delayed in language development is not likely to be found in the "normal" classroom. Even if the severe delay is not associated with mental retardation, the child's admission to graded classes may be postponed. In some instances, a child with moderate language retardation may be enrolled in a class for exceptional or educationally handicapped children. Occasionally he may be found in a class with normal children of a younger age group. For the most part, however, the classroom teacher is more likely to have children with mild language delay, children whose history may include slower onset of speech and somewhat slower development in articulatory, vocabulary, and syntactic (grammatical) proficiency.

The term *delayed language development* may be applied among school-age children to a range of problems, from cases in which there is a complete failure to use oral language* to those where the child's vocabulary

---

* Complete failure to develop language in children with hearing, as we noted earlier, is likely only for those who are in the low-grade idiot range of intelligence.

and sentence control seem adequate, but his speech is not readily intelligible. However, as we will consider later, children who persevere in infantilisms are also likely to be retarded in their syntactic development. We should note at this time that exceptions of all kinds are to be found. There are some late starters who catch up quickly once they get going, and who by school age are on a par with their age peers. There are some children whose speech is faulty for one or two sounds, who may lisp or lall, but who are nevertheless completely intelligible with good or better than average vocabularies and with comparable syntactical proficiency. At the other extreme we may find some children who employ gestures as substitutes for oral language as well as those who use single words or phrases accompanied by gestures at age four or five. A few, after making a slow start with a vocabulary of a dozen or so single-word utterances, may give up the effort and withdraw to become almost silent children by age four or five.

Many children who enter school with delayed language development are likely to present articulatory problems by the time they reach the second or third grade. These children do not suddenly develop their articulatory difficulties. For the most part, their articulatory proficiency was delayed as one aspect of their language development. By the time the children begin to manage language, the articulatory aspect of their overall development becomes more apparent.

Menyuk (1964) compared 10 children diagnosed as using infantile speech with 10 matched children, ages 3.0 years to 5.10 years. The I.Q.s of the two groups were approximately 126, based on the Ammons Full-Range Picture Vocabulary Test. Menyuk concluded from her data that the term "infantile," in regard to articulation, appears to be an incorrect designation because "at no age level did the grammatical production of a child with deviant speech match or closely match the grammatical production of a child with normal speech from two years on." Our own observations support those of Menyuk, with even greater differences found for children who are within the normal or below-average range of intelligence.

Children with serious delay in the language (oral words) per se are not likely to be advanced beyond the early primary grades. There are, of course, occasional and important exceptions. We sometimes find children with severe oral linguistic impairments who nevertheless learn to read and to write and so evidence their educational achievement. More often, however, children with serious delays in language development also have difficulties in learning to read and to write and are generally retarded in educational achievement.

For the most part, the classroom teacher of the nonexceptional child may have one or two children who have the residuals of delayed language. These children often need the help of the speech clinician to improve their articulatory proficiency. They are likely also to need help with other aspects of language development.

MENTAL RETARDATION

The chief cause of seriously prolonged language (speech) delay is mental retardation. The most severely mentally retarded may never acquire functional speech. Moderately retarded children usually do acquire speech, but often with numerous defects in articulation, impoverished vocabularies, and very limited syntax. Mildly retarded children may acquire speech, but are likely to have limited vocabularies and use relatively simple sentence constructions.

Lillywhite and Bradley (1969, p. 11) report that in a survey of communication impairment among the educably mentally retarded in the Portland, Oregon, public schools, 12 per cent were found to have speech and/or language defects, as compared with 4.5 per cent among the nonretarded. Generally, in their survey, Lillywhite and Bradley observed that the most severely retarded, those with I.Q.s ranging from 40 to 70, presented a variety of defects, including articulatory, functional, and organic voice quality disturbances such as excessive nasality, huskiness, and language delay. "All of the children showed speech and language functioning in one way or another significantly inferior to expectation based upon mental age." They were, of course, considerably more inferior based upon actual age expectations. Contributing causes of speech defects are hearing loss, found in greater incidence among retardates than among nonretardates, as well as sluggish control of palatal and pharyngeal structures.

If we accept Newland's (1960) use of the term "mentally retarded" to denote "those children whose competently ascertained learning aptitudes are approximately one half to three fourths those of their chronological peers and whose limitations in this regard are believed to be attributable to biologic rather than psychologic or environmental factors," we would find a positive relationship between the degree of mental retardation and the amount of language delay as well as the quality of the language when it is acquired. We sometimes find children with moderate mental retardation who seem to have as many words as their age peers. A discerning listener may be able to note, however, that these children use the words less meaningfully and that the words lack depth and richness of concept. It is our observation that some mentally retarded children who are well trained and well taught are able to acquire appropriate words on a low level of meaning for many situations and events. We agree with Newland that even if the mentally retarded child "is able to acquire as many lower-level tidbits of learning as the average . . . he would presumably integrate them less well, less meaningfully, less fully . . . to such an extent that the results of his integrations are discernibly different from those of his nonretarded brothers" (Newland, 1960, p. 81). Some mentally retarded children who "know the words but not too many of the meanings" may manage to get through the primary grades without too much trouble. These children, by virtue of the "halo effect" of their apparent linguistic ability, may not seem to be mentally retarded until they reach a level in school where the teacher begins to note their difficulty in dealing with concepts or ideas that cannot be readily objectified.

It is also important to recognize that there are some children whose difficulty with oral language makes them appear to be mentally retarded when they are not. Some children who are suspected of being mentally retarded because of their delayed development may, upon examination with nonlanguage tests of intelligence, turn out to be normal, or even above average, in intelligence. Other causes, such as slow general physiologic development, emotional disturbances, or hearing loss, may account for the language delay. The possibility of error in arriving at a causal diagnosis of mental retardation for language delay points to the need for a competent clinical psychologist or school psychologist to examine the suspected child and make an evaluation. If this cannot be done, the classroom teacher may entertain hypotheses about the concerned child, but judgments should be withheld until justified. The teacher should be especially careful to reserve judgment about possible mental retardation for the child with uneven school achievement. If the child does average or better work when oral language is not required, but does poorly in areas that require speech competency, we should seek the cause for the disparity rather than conclude that we are dealing with a "nontypical" but nevertheless mentally retarded child. The Illinois Test of Psycholinguistic Abilities (ITPA, Kirk and McCarthy) may be used for the assessment of language competencies.

THERAPEUTIC APPROACHES: THE MENTALLY RETARDED

Treatment for the mentally retarded child—for the one who, by our definition, is so for biological rather than pathological reasons—should take the form of education and training geared to the capacities of the individual child. Stimulation and improvement of the home environment, if this is possible, should help to bring the retardate to a level where his potential for language usage and articulatory proficiency become highly and positively correlated. Specific training for the correction of specific articulatory and vocal defects is indicated for the higher grade retardates. Such children may be members of slow progress or "special" classes. For most children a reasonable achievement objective is to strive for the proficiency level of a normal child whose chronological age is equal to that of the mental age of the retardate. In the absence of sensory, motor, or personality involvements, this level of achievements may be reached for most higher level retardates. Little progress, however, may be expected beyond age 14 (Goda and Griffith, 1962).

Figure 9, taken from Lenneberg (1967, p. 169) presents a graphic comparison of the language development of retardates and normal children in relationship to milestones for sitting and walking.

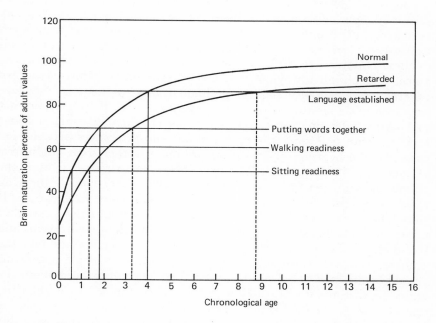

Figure 9. On the ordinate, Lenneberg combined all the parameters of brain maturation into a single factor. "Retarded children presumably attain the maturational values later in life than normal children. Attainment of brain maturation is correlated with behavioral achievements shown here as 'horizons.' A comparison of the growth curves of normal and retarded children explains why the relative distances among the various milestones become greater with advancing age. Normally, a child begins to join words together about 15 months after he is ready to sit up; in a retarded child it may take 24 months to achieve this. It takes about two years to acquire the general basis for language establishment once a normal child has begun to put words together. In a retarded child it may take five years or more to acquire the same facility in language."*

---

* From E. H. Lenneberg, *Biological Foundations of Language*, New York, John Wiley & Sons, Inc., 1967, p. 169.

We should like to emphasize that although, as we have noted, voice and articulatory defects occur in a higher incidence in retardates than in children of normal intelligence, the chief factor in the mentally retarded child's communicative difficulties are to be found in his inadequate language. This, as Wood (1964, p. 39) points out, may have either organic or nonorganic associated causes.

HEARING LOSS: THE DEAF*

A deaf child is one whose hearing was insufficient, at the time when speech normally is learned, to enable him to acquire oral language ability through the sense of hearing. Children with a hearing loss severe enough for them to be diagnosed as deaf do not learn to speak unless specially trained to do so through the use of devices and techniques that are not necessary for children with normal hearing. Virtually all of these children are likely to have significant defects of articulation, voice, and almost always of language development. However, as we observed in our discussion of the prelingual stages in language development, up to six months of age the vocalizations of deaf children are not ordinarily different from those of hearing children. Between six and eight months, deficiencies in vocalizations and utterances between the deaf and the hearing tend to be quantitative rather than qualitative (Lenneberg, 1964, p. 153). The deaf infant has a reduced inventory of sounds, and spends less time in sound play than does the hearing child. This observation has an important therapeutic implication. If the child is recognized early as one with a severe hearing loss, every effort should be made by his parents to encourage his vocalizations and sound play. The parents should, for example, make certain that the child sees the parent who is talking to him. Simple repeated statements should be directed to the child. A mirror, strategically placed above the child, may stimulate his talking to his mirror image. Such activities will encourage the deaf child not to become a silent child. He may be responsive to the low-pitched vocalization of the adult, that is, to the voice per se, and then learn to look and see, and perhaps begin to face-read some of the speech of the adult. Appropriate gestures accompanying the speech of the adult may well enhance the deaf child's understanding of the adult's speech.

The problems of the deaf child for language learning are sometimes complicated by some degree of associated mental retardation or by slower mental maturation. However, Lenneberg (1964, p. 156), after

---

* The problems of the deaf and hard-of-hearing children are considered in some detail in Chapter 14.

reviewing the literature on cognitive, nonverbal investigations of deaf children, observes: "On strictly cognitive tasks it has been experimentally shown that even pre-school and thus 'pre-language' deaf children perform no worse than hearing children."

The extent of delay in language development for many, if not for most deaf children, may be appreciated when we realize that the normal hearing child has a *speaking* vocabulary of 2,000 or more words—and several times that number for comprehension—by the time he is of school age. In sharp contrast, the deaf child who enters a school for the deaf at age five may have no working vocabulary at all. If, in addition, he has not developed a gesture (sign) system, he has in effect no functional communication.

This is the basis of the position taken by Furth (1966, pp. 226–228) on the need to establish an early visual language (gesture) system for congenitally deaf children. Learning to talk, and so to think, without recourse to oral language enhances the deaf child's cognitive and intellectual development. Waiting to establish an oral language system may impair such development. So, Furth argues, "as a direct result of linguistic incompetence, the deaf fail or are poor in all tasks which are specifically verbal or on a few non-verbal tasks in which linguistic habits afford a direct advantage." As an indirect result, the deaf lack information and exhibit a minimal amount of intellectual curiosity. Moreover, "they have less opportunity and training to think." Based on these observations, Furth proposes that the deficiencies associated with the linguistic incompetence of the deaf "would be avoidable if non-verbal methods of instruction and communication were encouraged both at home in the earliest years and in formal school education." He suggests that at home "parents must have recourse to distinguishable signs and use these together with speech. Practically all deaf children, instead of the present 10 per cent, could then be expected to reach a basic competence in English, just as all hearing children in any society learn the language to which they are exposed."

Furth may be overoptimistic in his projection of the training of deaf children through nonverbal (we believe he means non-oral) means. However, we accept his position that the intellectual potentials of most deaf children, as well as their linguistic limitations, could be improved if the implications of his suggestions were followed.

There are some exceptions among deaf children in regard to language development. Most of the exceptions are found among bright deaf children, especially among those whose parents were aware of the hearing impairment and initiated early training along the lines suggested above. Other exceptions may be found among deaf children with sufficient residual hearing who are able to make use of their limited hearing, those who have learned to attend to speakers and to read their faces and their articulatory and accompanying manual gestures. Some children, though deaf, may have their residual hearing enhanced by a properly fitted hearing aid and so learn considerably more about speech and speakers than if they relied on vision alone. Still other exceptions are found among children who became deaf (adventitious deafness) after they had acquired speech. In general, however, the incidence of speech defects and of language retardation is almost universal among preschool deaf children.

Most deaf children of school age have a slower rate of academic achievement than do their hearing peers. However, unless mental retardation is an associated problem, most deaf children learn to read and to write, and to progress in other school subjects. Myerson (1955, p. 148) sums up the situation in regard to language development with this observation: "For the present and past generations of the deaf upon whom the test results were obtained, language and communication skills have lagged far behind intelligence, chronological age, and interests." The implication in this observation is that deaf children are not being taught as they need to be taught to take full advantage of their intellectual potential.

Deaf-Aphasic Children. Before leaving the subject of the deaf, we will briefly discuss a small subgroup of congenitally (developmentally) aphasic-deaf.* Such children, who are also referred to as having central deafness, are not able to perceive and assign meanings even to sounds which, when reinforced by amplification, are physically received. We assume that such children, in addition to peripheral hearing loss, also have incurred damage or have severe maturational delay of an area, or areas, of the cerebral cortex that normally serves for the analysis of speech sounds. If a child is both peripherally and centrally deaf (aphasic), he is likely to ignore and reject even very loud speech, and may be disturbed by and refuse to use hearing aids. He is probably wise in doing so, because if he is unable to make sense out of any received human speech sounds, confusion and frustration may result from mere reception without perception. Such a child should be trained through a straight visual approach, with gesture and finger spelling and later through graphic media alone for reading and writing. We need to emphasize, however, that the deaf-aphasic child constitutes a very small subgroup of the deaf. Nondeaf congenitally aphasic children, also a small group, will be considered in Chapter 16.

---

* See Chapter 16 for a discussion of the aphasic (dyslogic) child.

THE HARD-OF-HEARING

Language retardation and voice and articulation defects are prevalent in children who have sufficient hearing to learn to speak through the auditory modality, but whose hearing is sufficiently impaired to create problems in the easy and comfortable reception of speech signals. O'Neill (1964, p. 4) considers the term "hard-of-hearing" to designate "a person who experiences difficulty in auditory reception but not complete loss of auditory reception (as exists in the deaf). Auditory reception can be improved by amplification or training."

With important exceptions, the incidence of speech (voice and articulation) and language defects are positively related to the severity of hearing loss and to the time in the child's life at which the loss began. The child who develops a hearing loss at age three or four, when his speech is well established, is likely to have much less impairment for language, and possibly also for voice and articulation, than is the congenitally hard-of-hearing child, or one whose hearing loss was acquired before he spoke in sentences. Some children whose pure-tone audiometric results might lead us to expect severe speech difficulties may do better than those whose hearing impairment might be considered relatively mild judging by their audiograms. "Just as there are gradations in the usefulness of hearing, so there are gradations in the quality and intelligibility of the speech of the hard-of-hearing" (Silverman, 1961, p. 451). We need to appreciate that both the quality and the quantity of the language of the hard-of-hearing child depend on many individual factors. These include the intelligence of the child, the early recognition of the hearing loss, and the motivation of both parents and child toward speech learning. A bright child, well motivated and with well-informed parents may achieve normal speech through combining lip (speech) reading and the maximum use of hearing. Amplified sound and the use of a hearing aid, if possible and appropriate, may be of considerable help.

Speech Defects Associated with Hearing Loss. Almost all children who are more than mildly hard of hearing have some degree of difficulty in articulation and appropriate vocalization. Depending in part on the type and degree of hearing loss, distortions and omissions of consonants, and especially fricative sounds, are common. There is also likely to be some difficulty in distinguishing between voiced and voiceless cognates such as *b* and *p*, *d* and *t*, *v* and *f*, and the *th* sounds. Vowels and diphthongs may be distorted.

The improvement of the speech of the child with a recognized and appreciable hearing loss is the task of the professional speech clinician rather than the classroom teacher.

Intermittent or Occasional Hearing Difficulty. Many teachers have had children who on occasion seem to have some difficulty in hearing. It is possible that some of these children have relatively slight though chronic difficulty with hearing, but are usually able to make up for the loss by good attentive effort. However, if such a child has a head cold, or suffers from enlarged adenoids because of a temporary inflammation, his hearing problem may be temporarily increased. Fatigue or ill-health may produce comparable results. There are, of course, other children who, for reasons related to their emotional problems in or out of the classroom, on occasion seem not to be able to hear. Perhaps these children block out human speech sounds because of difficulties that arise when they hear, understand, and respond to speech. If the teacher suspects the latter to be the case, an understanding of what may be the basis for the nonhearing rather than a scolding is in order.

Whenever hearing loss is suspected, an audiological evaluation, which should by all means include speech perception, is recommended. If hearing loss is found, its cause and possible treatment should be determined by a physician. Fortunately, in some instances medical treatment can minimize or entirely clear up temporary difficulty in hearing, resulting from pathology.

*The Hard-of-Hearing Child in the Classroom.** The teacher can be of appreciable help in the classroom for a child believed to have a hearing loss. Among the things he can do to be of direct help to the particular child are:

1. Make certain that he is looking in the direction of the child when giving the class instruction or direction.

2. Seat or reseat the child so that he will be both close to the teacher and readily able to see his face when he is speaking. This means that if the teacher is to stand in any part of the room for any length of time, the child suspected of hearing loss should be permitted to change his seat.

3. Speak louder and somewhat more slowly, when an activity is anticipated that will involve a specific response from the child suspected of having a hearing loss.

EMOTIONAL PROBLEMS

The history of many children with language delay includes an item indicating that they began to speak at an age within normal limits but

---

* See Chapter 14 for a more detailed discussion of the teacher's role.

then seemed to give up speaking. On questioning, one or both parents may reveal that the cessation of speaking seemed to be associated with an unhappy familial situation. In some instances it becomes apparent that the parents were disturbed about their own relationship, and frequently spoke harshly to each other in the presence of the young child. Occasionally, an admission is obtained that when the parents spoke to each other at all, it was in emotional outbursts. The young child, we would gather, became afraid of the consequences of speech and retired into the relative safety and security of not speaking at least to his parents or in his own home. Such a child may, after he resumes speaking, continue to be fearful about its consequencees when he enters school. If he meets with any penalty resulting from speech behavior during his early school experiences, his original fears may be reconfirmed. This is the type of child who may prefer to be thought uninformed, or prefer to be given a talking-to for his apparent inattention, rather than risk the assumed greater penalty of saying the wrong thing. He may well decide that it is better to be the "quiet one" than the one who gets involved in difficulties by freely verbalizing his thoughts.

Another situation associated with regression or cessation of speech and occurring frequently enough to be worthy of note is the birth of a new child. The two- or three-year-old may look upon the crying, non-speaking infant as a usurper of attention and affection. With what seems fair logic, the older sibling may decide that he may be able to regain his original position in the family if he imitates some of the behavior of the newcomer, and so gives up speech.

Responses to Parental Attitudes. Several investigators (Peckarasky, 1952, and Wood, 1946) have found that parents of delayed-speech children are frequently unrealistic in their expectations about them. Sometimes both parents, but mothers perhaps more so than fathers, expected their children to develop and learn more than the Gessell Developmental Scales (1957) present as norms for "average" children. Individual case studies revealed that some children who had not gone beyond single-word utterances at age three had toilet training initiated, usually with failure, before one year of age. Some children were expected to feed themselves after their first attempt to pick up a spoon. To be sure, occasionally a child not only achieves this, but insists on trying. Most one-year-old children, however, enjoy being helped to food and the incidental interchange with the feeder.

Other findings reveal that the parents of delayed-speech children are often inclined to be rigid and restrictive in their demands upon their children, as well as upon one another. Possibly as a result of the frustration experienced by the parents, there is an air of excessive tension in the conduct of the home. Many of the parents admit to being "perfectionists" but use the term with pride rather than insight. It is possible that children brought up in such homes unconsciously feel rejected. It is possible also that the parents, consciously or unconsciously, are rejecting their children. Certainly these parents are rejecting the efforts and accomplishments of their children, and the children respond to this attitude as if they were entirely rejected. If a child's early speech attempts are ignored as being unworthy of notice, or criticized for not being readily understandable, he may well hesitate to talk in order to avoid an unfavorable parental response.

Some of the feeling of apprehension continues to characterize the behavior of children who once were delayed in speech. The classroom teacher in the first or second grade would do well to be permissive in attitude and to avoid correcting the articulation or pronunciation of children who have a delayed-speech history. These children need the security of acceptance of themselves as they are so that speech efforts will not be conducive to disapproval or fear. Remedial speech work of specific speech faults may well wait until the third or fourth grade for these children. Of course, indirect efforts at correction take place whenever the child is exposed to a kind and permissive environment that stimulates good but not perfectionistic speech. An attitude of permissiveness, incidentally, should be consistent and should not vary from day to day according to the whims of the adult.

Faulty Motivation. A child is likely not to develop many new skills, language acquisition included, unless such skills provide him with a sense of satisfaction and accomplishment not otherwise obtainable. Though we believe that almost every child is born to speak, and will have a normal age for onset of speech, the members of his family may nurture or retard such development. The child whose wants are regularly anticipated may be denied the opportunity for expressing his wants, and have his need to do so frustrated in consequence. The magic of speech is the right of each child who is capable of exercising such potency. Parents who are overprotective, because of past or present injuries or illnesses of their child, and who hover over him when he first stands alone, or when he attempts to walk, who cannot wait until the child completes even a gesture before he is overwhelmed with a number of things he might possibly mean by that gesture, deny their child the need to learn to do things for himself, speaking included. Such a child, unless he is able to identify himself with others in his environment who are less anxiety-ridden and less anxiously protective, may be delayed in language development and may be slow in developing language skills even though he may have begun to speak at about the expected age. Among the immediate improvements sought for the child and parents are the following:

1. An understanding on the part of parents, and any other over-anxious, overzealous members of the child's environment, that he is deserving of the right to entertain a want or a need, even if he has to cry about it.

2. When an attempt at speech is made, the attempt is to be heard out before the adults jump to do something about it.

3. A repeated vocalization, especially if it accompanies a repeated gesture in association with a given situation, may be the beginning of word usage. The adult should imitate the vocalization in the recurring situation, before responding to the act of gesture and vocalization. In this way attention is directed to the oral activity rather than to the pantomime.

4. Once repeated vocalization is established, the parent should take the initiative and give a simple monosyllabic name to a toy or object frequently used and desired by the child. This name should include sounds the child has successfully made and repeated in his sound-play activity. For example, if "da" is frequently uttered by the child, the name "da" can be given to a doll or some other plaything enjoyed by the child. The sound should be spoken by the parent each time the object is given to the child, and each time the adult, when present, observes the child reaching for the object. After one or two days of this practice, the object should be withheld until the child makes some attempt to utter the sound-name for it. If the child is reasonably successful in making a sound that closely resembles, if not directly reproduces, the sound-name he should be given quick approval for his effort. This, however, *does not mean* that he is to be rewarded by another toy or overwhelmed with a flow of words too numerous and too rapid for assimilation or understanding.

BILINGUAL ENVIRONMENT

As indicated in our discussion on language development, children who come from a multilingual environment may be seriously delayed in the onset and growth of their own language abilities. Many children are without question able to acquire two or more languages that they are exposed to from infancy. Research data strongly suggest, however, that for an appreciable number of children the effect of multilingual (usually bilingual) exposure beginning at an age before a single language is established is to cause some degree of impairment in overall language proficiency. As we indicated earlier, Smith (1949), who studied the effects of bilingualism (Chinese and English) among children in the

Hawaiian Islands, found that as a group the children had vocabularies of below-average size in both Chinese and English. Beyond this, Smith found that even when the vocabularies of the two languages were combined, only two fifths of the children exceeded the expected norms for monolingual children. On the strength of her data Smith concluded that "only the superior bilingual child is capable of attaining the vocabulary norms of monoglots. . . ."

Occasionally, we find that the single significant factor in a delayed-speech child is multiple language exposure. On the whole, it would seem much safer for a child to have one language well established before he is exposed to a second. If multiple language exposure cannot be avoided, as is the case in many homes and many cultures, it would seem that the use of a given language be identified consistently with a person or a situation. Some children seem to find it necessary to fit themselves and the speaking situation into a linguistic "groove" and to maintain that groove in a consistent manner. For example, if the parents spoke only English, and the grandparents, nurse, or housekeeper spoke a second language, the child would learn to associate a language pattern —a way of speaking—with a person and so have less conflict than if his own parents spoke English on some occasions and a second language on others. When the other times are unpredictable, or when the other times are reserved for admonishments, difficulty with the second language may intensify. So also, unfortunately, may the child's attitude toward language behavior in general.

The observations we have made in regard to bilingual exposure hold true also for children who appear to have difficulty in language development. Many children present no such difficulty. Such children are often found in middle and upper socioeconomic-class homes. Penfield (1959, pp. 221–255) in fact recommends that children who live in bilingual environments, as, for instance, in Montreal, Canada, should intentionally be taught two languages by the direct method—that is, by having the child exposed to both languages in his home, but each in a systematic way—during the early, preschool years. The argument for this natural and direct approach is that the child's brain before he is of school age has a maximum of plasticity and capacity for acquiring more than one language. A young child may respond "reflexively" to the language in which he is addressed. He will not, of course, realize that he may be speaking French on one occasion and to one person, and English to another person or on *different* occasions.

If, however, a child who has been exposed to more than one language appears to have difficulty in learning to speak, we strongly recommend that the parents decide which language is to be essential for the child and that he be exposed to only that one until his speech behaviour has become established. This frequently calls for control and modification of the home environment as well as aspects of the environment outside of the home. Though this is not always easy to achieve, it is important that it be done.

Bilingualism may present a variety of problems relative to language proficiency, and psychological and social development. These are discussed in a monograph edited by Macnamara (1967).

TWINS

As indicated in our discussion in Chapter 7, the incidence of delayed speech and slow language development is greater among twins than among single children. Day (1932), for example, found that preschool-age twins had age-interval increments approximately half of those of single-born children. Language retardation among twins may be attributed to both organic and atypical environmental causes. Both will be briefly considered.

According to Nelson (1959, p. 305) most twins are prematurely born. Prematurity of birth is associated in many instances with vascular defects and with brain damage. Even when there is no clear evidence of damage to the brain, there is considerable evidence of a lag in overall physical maturation, which continues at least until the time the child is of age to enter school. Lags in psychological and social development parallel those for physical development. These disadvantages, we should emphasize, are associated with the combination of twinning and premature birth. Though there is evidence that some prematurely born children "may never catch up" (Silvern, 1961), we are more inclined to accept the point of view of the geneticist Newman (1940), who maintains that if twins survive the hazards of being born and the consequences of prematurity, by the time they are well along in school they are as capable as their single-born peers.

Twins provide an atypical environment for one another. As they grow up they seem to be satisfied with their mutual social situation and so are less demanding of the attentions of older persons. Even if attention is demanded, it must be divided. Unfortunately, twins are not well qualified as language stimulators. The result is that they are exposed less to adults than are single children, and more to poor language stimulation. An interesting linguistic phenomenon among twins is their development of a special code for expression and communication—an idioglossia—which seems to serve the twins adequately but baffles all other members of the family. Because of the evident satisfaction twins derive from their idioglossia, they may not be motivated to learn the language of their homes or their more extended environment.

If twins arrive at school age still using their special language, we recommend that, if at all possible, they be put in separate classes. If this is not possible, they should be put in separate groups so that they may associate with children using more conventional language.

The Role of the Classroom Teacher with Delayed-Language Children

As indicated at the beginning of this chapter, the classroom teacher is not likely to have many children with seriously retarded language development among his pupils. By the time children of normal intellect who began by being delayed in language reach school age, they are likely to be speaking well enough to be accepted in the regular class. However, some of the residuals of the problems may remain. Some of the children formerly delayed in speech may still be apprehensive about speaking and show anxiety when responsibility for communication is fixed upon them. These children are likely to be freer when responding as members of a group than when they are required to recite alone or to speak with, rather than in front of, their classmates. Others may have limited vocabularies or more than a normal number of speech faults. If the teacher can determine which of the causes of retarded language development were present for any of the children, he can be of great help in controlling or preventing the pressures associated with the original cause for language retardation. These children need to learn that speech is enjoyable before they become aware that with the acquisition of speech there is an assumption of communicative responsibility. When pleasure replaces apprehension, goals for increased speech proficiency can be set. The child should be gently directed toward these goals and not goaded toward their attainment. Incidentally, we strongly urge that the child who has just started his school career be given no cause to become self-conscious about his lack of speech proficiency. The teacher must provide motivation, stimulation, and good and attainable models, as well as reinforcement for improvement. However, the teacher should avoid any negative indications that might lead the child to hold back on talking, or worse still, cause self-interruptions of what the child, however improficiently, might be trying to say.

References and Recommended Readings

BROWN, S. F., "Retarded Speech Development," in W. Johnson et al., *Speech-Handicapped School Children*. New York, Harper & Row, Publishers, 1967, Chap. 6. (A survey of major causes and therapy for children who are retarded in speech development.)

DAVIS, H., and S. R. SILVERMAN, *Hearing and Deafness*, Rev. ed. New York, Holt, Rinehart and Winston, Inc., 1961.

DAY, E. J., "The Development of Language in Twins," *Child Development*, III (September, 1932), 179–199.

FURTH, H. G., *Thinking Without Language*. New York, The Free Press, 1966.

GESSELL, A. I., and C. S. AMATRUDA, *Developmental Diagnosis*. New York, Paul B. Hoeber, 1957.

GODA, S., and B. C. GRIFFITH, "Spoken Language of Adolescent Retardates and Its Relation to Intelligence, Age, and Anxiety," *Child Development*, XXXIII (September, 1962), 489–498.

KEASTER, J., "Impaired Hearing," in W. Johnson et al., *Speech-Handicapped School Children*. New York, Harper & Row, Publishers, 1967, Chap. 8.

LENNEBERG, E. H., *Biological Foundations of Language*. New York, John Wiley & Sons, Inc., 1967.

LENNEBERG, E. H., "Language Disorders in Childhood," *Harvard Educational Review*, XXXIV, 4 (Spring, 1964), 152–177. (A review of causes, prognoses, and therapeutic procedures for children with moderate and severe language disorders.)

LILLYWHITE, H. S., and D. P. BRADLEY, *Communication Problems in Mental Retardation*. New York, Harper & Row, Publishers, 1969. (Includes discussions of background, causes, and management of communication problems of mentally retarded children.)

MACNAMARA, J. (ed.), "Problems of Bilingualism," *The Journal of Social Issues*, XXIII, 2 (April, 1967).

MENYUK, P., "Comparison of Grammar of Children with Functionally Deviant Articulation," *Journal of Speech and Hearing Research*, VII, 2 (June, 1964), 109–121.

MYERSON, L. "A Psychology of Impaired Hearing," in W. M. Cruickshank, ed., *Psychology of Exceptional Children and Youth*. Englewood Cliffs, N.J., Prentice-Hall, Inc., 1955.

NELSON, W. E., *Textbook of Pediatrics*, 7th ed. Philadelphia, W. B. Saunders Company, 1959.

NEWLAND, T. E., "Language Development of the Mentally Retarded," *Monographs of the Society for Research in Child Development*, XXV, 3 (May, 1960), 71–87.

NEWMAN, H. H., *Multiple Human Births*. New York, Doubleday Doran & Company, Inc., 1940.

O'NEILL, J. J., *The Hard of Hearing*. Englewood Cliffs, N.J., Prentice-Hall, Inc., 1964.

PECKARASKY, A., *Maternal Attitudes Toward Children with Psychogenically Delayed Speech.* Doctoral dissertation (unpublished), New York University, School of Education, 1952.

PENFIELD, W., and L., ROBERTS, *Speech and Brain Mechanisms.* Princeton University Press, 1959, pp. 251–255.

SILVERN, W. A., *Dunham's Premature Infants,* 3rd ed. New York, Paul B. Hoeber, 1961, pp. 76–83.

SMITH, M. E., " Measurement of Vocabularies of Young Bilingual Children in Both of the Languages Used," *Journal of Genetic Psychology,* LXXIV (June, 1949), 305–310.

VAN RIPER, C., *Speech Correction,* 4th ed. Englewood Cliffs, N.J., Prentice-Hall, Inc., 1963, Chaps. 5 and 6. (The chapters survey the causes and treatment of delayed speech and contain suggestions for stimulating language in reluctant speakers.)

WOOD, K. S., " Parental Maladjustment and Functional Articulatory Defects in Children," *Journal of Speech Disorders,* XI (December, 1946), 255–275.

WOOD, N. E., *Delayed Speech and Language Development.* Englewood Cliffs, N.J., Prentice-Hall, Inc., 1964. (A concise monograph on language development, causes of delayed speech, and therapeutic procedures; includes many pertinent annotated references on delayed speech.)

Problems

1. What are the chief causes of delayed speech? What is *the chief* cause?
2. What is the relationship between emotional upheavals in the family and possible speech delay? Can you recall such a case?
3. Check with the parents of some children as to the ages when their children began to speak. Average the ages for the boys and for the girls. Which group had an older average age?
4. Twins have been found to begin to speak at a later age than single children. How do you account for this?
5. Read the article by Ruth W. Metraux, " Speech Profiles for the Child 18 to 24 Months," *Journal of Speech and Hearing Disorders,* XV (March, 1950), pages 37–53. Check the language development of a child you know between the ages of 18 and 54 months with the Metraux profiles. If there are any differences, can you account for them?
6. There is considerable evidence that children who have difficulty in learning to read include more than a " normal " number of children with delayed-speech onset. Can you account for this?
7. Compare a three-year-old child's motor and speech development with the motor and language milestones of the table adapted from Lenneberg. (See Chapter 8 on language development.) Make the same comparisons for a three- or four-year-old child who has been designated as being delayed in speech.

Chapter 10

Defects of Articulation (I)

Of all speech disorders, teachers encounter articulatory defects most frequently. The studies cited in Chapter 1 show that from 3 to 6 per cent of schoolchildren have articulatory defects. The number is more than all the other speech difficulties combined; in fact, in the school-age population, about three fourths of all speech defects are of an articulatory nature.

Definition of Articulatory Defects

Articulatory defects fall, in general, into three categories: (1) the substitution of one sound for another; (2) the omission of sounds; and (3) the distortion of sounds.

This categorization is based on the way the listener perceives the sounds. Since clinicians today generally diagnose articulatory defects in this way, the categorization based on listener perception is used. On the other hand, we might have looked at the problem of articulatory difficulties from the viewpoint of the child-speaker who may be applying a deviant but consistent set of phonological rules.

193

SUBSTITUTION OF ONE SOUND FOR ANOTHER

The substitution of one sound for another is the type of articulatory error that children in the primary grades make most frequently (Patton, 1942). In a detailed study, Snow (1963) reports on the sounds most frequently substituted for other sounds. She found these substitutions most frequent: /ʃ/, /ts/ and /s/ for /tʃ/; /ɵ/ and /f/ for /s/; /f/, /s/, /t/ for /ɵ/; /s/ and /tʃ/ for /ʃ/; /d/ and /v/ for /ð/; /dz/ and /tʃ/ for /dʒ/; /dz/ and /s/ for /z/; /z/, /dʒ/, /dz/ for /ʒ/; /w/ for /r/; /w/ for /l/; /w/ for /ʍ/, and /l/ for /j/. An examination of these data reveals that the substitutions have many of the same phonetic features as does the incorrect sound. For example, in comparing /ɵ/ and /s/, both are fricatives and both are unvoiced; the difference lies in the parts of the articulatory mechanism involved. /ɵ/ involves the tip of the tongue and the cutting edges of the teeth, whereas /s/ involves the tip of the tongue and the alveolar ridge or the ridge behind the lower teeth. In comparing the sounds in the substitution /w/ for /r/, both are glides and both are voiced. The difference again lies in the involvement of particular articulatory agents. In /d/ for /ð/, both are voiced but the manner of articulation is different, for /d/ is a stop whereas /ð/ is a fricative. Furthermore, the articulatory agents involved are different, for /d/ is made with the tip of the tongue on the teeth ridge and /ð/ is made with the tip of the tongue against the cutting edges of the teeth. All in all, the phonetic features of the substitutions and the correct sounds share many characteristics; despite their differences, there are many basic similarities.

The following are substitutions made by a seven-year-old boy and those made by a six-year-old girl. Indicate the substitutions and indicate in what way each substitution is different from the correct sound.

Substitutions made by Mary, a six-year-old girl in a large school system:

[sʌm]	for *thumb*
[tusbrʌʃ]	for *toothbrush*
[tæt]	for *cat*
[stos]	for *stove*
[naɪs]	for *knife*
[tɪkɪ]	for *chicken*

Substitutions made by Jimmy, a seven-year-old boy:

[stɝəl]	for *squirrel*
[prʌʃ]	for *brush*

[trʌm]	for *drum*
[lɛlo]	for *yellow*
[fɜdɚ]	for *feather*

Most children are seemingly not consistent in their substitutions. They may substitute [f] for [θ] in one word and not in another. They may substitute [f] for [θ] but substitute [θ] for [s]. Consistent patterns of substitution may seem to occur infrequently. But when the substitutions are analyzed carefully, a pattern usually emerges. In general, children are more likely to make errors when the sound occurs in the middle or at the end of a word, rather than when it occurs at the beginning of a word.

THE ROLE OF DISTINCTIVE FEATURES IN SUBSTITUTIONS

In Chapter 6, on the production of speech sounds, we indicated certain similarities and differences in sounds. We noted that sounds differ in place of articulation, presence or absence of voice, and manner of production. In terms of these three attributes, you were asked to analyze children's frequent substitution of sounds. Recent research by Menyuk (1969) points to the importance of the distinctive features of consonants. She studied the mastery of consonantal sounds in terms of gravity and diffuseness (aspects of place of articulation); stridency, nasality, and continuancy (aspects of manner of articulation); and the vocal component (presence or absence of voice) for two groups: (a) children with normal speech development for whom data were obtained by transcribing phonetically the substitutions made as the children were spontaneously generating sentences, and (b) children with articulatory difficulties, for whom data were obtained by giving the Templin-Darley Articulation Test and analyzing the results.

The data for the group with normal speech development were analyzed by determining the percentage of sounds containing a feature that was used correctly at various ages in the developmental period of two and a half to five years of age. The rank order of use of features in correctly uttered phonemes was: (1) nasal, (2) grave, (3) voice, (4) diffuse, (5) continuant, (6) strident. In other words, the feature first mastered in terms of percentage of correct usage was nasality (the presence of nasal resonance as in /m/ and /n/); the second, grave (being produced at the periphery of the speech mechanism as /p/, /b/, /k/, and /g/); the third, the voicing or unvoicing feature; the fourth, the diffuse feature (involved in anterior sounds such as /t/, /d/, and /ө/); the fifth, the continuant feature; and the sixth, the strident feature, where interference is high as in the /tʃ/ and /s/. Interestingly enough, as Menyuk analyzed phonological developmental data, she found the rank order for Japanese children to be identical with that for American children. From this, one can hypothesize that the ability of children to perceive and then to produce distinctive linguistic features of sounds is universal. The features dominating the acquisition of phonemes in the early stages of morphemic structure are two aspects of manner of production—use of nasality and use of voice—and one aspect of place of articulation, grave—placement in periphery of the mechanism.

In her analysis of distinctive features of phonology of children with articulatory defects, Menyuk makes the point that children in learning to utter a phoneme must perceive several features. She notes that distinction between sounds which differ in the feature of place of articulation causes the greatest difficulty. In *tate* for *cake*, /t/ and /d/ are alike except that /t/ is an alveolar sound and /k/ is a palatal sound. The other feature she mentions is continuancy in manner of production, as *tink* for *think*. She observes that when two features are disturbed, as *date* for *cake*, where the substitution involves both the place of articulation and voicing, the speech becomes less intelligible. The need for more research and more analysis of phonological data is evident.*

OMISSION OF SOUNDS

A sound may be omitted. The following are examples of omissions of sounds by David, a 10-year-old boy:

[bɛd]	for *bread*
[dɛs]	for *dress*
[taɪ]	for *try*
[ten]	for *train*

Most youngsters will not be as consistent as this child in omitting sounds. Their omissions may be more like those of Susie, a five-year-old, whose examples follow:

Air you dowin? [er jʊ doɪn]	for *Where are you going?*
Me ante o too. [mi ɑntɔ o tu]	for *I want to go too.*
I or? [aɪ or]	for *Why for?*

Omissions occur much more frequently in the young child's speech than they do in the older child's speech. Children omit final consonants more often than the initial or medial consonant. They commonly

---

* For an analysis of this research, see H. Winitz, *Articulatory Acquisition and Behavior*, New York, Appleton-Century-Crofts, 1969, page 61.

omit one of the sounds in clusters of two consonants, such as *tr*[tr], *pr*[pr], *st*[st], or *sl*[sl].

Omissions are not common. According to Templin (Templin, 1957) they comprise about 13 per cent of all errors from ages three through eight.

DISTORTION OF SOUNDS

A sound may be distorted. The listener recognizes the sound for what it is, but is distracted by it. The way the sound is made calls attention to it. Laymen, in describing a distorted *s*, make such remarks as: "Her *s* whistles" or "Her *s* has a slushy *sh* sound." In the whistling *s*, too much air is escaping, and in the slushy *s*, air is escaping over the sides of the tongue.

Degree of Severity of Articulatory Difficulty

The severity of an articulatory difficulty depends on how greatly it reduces the intelligibility of the speech of its owner and the concern it gives him. The degree of intelligibility is related to the number of sounds omitted and the number of substitutions; the distortion of sounds is of least importance in intelligibility. When the child omits many sounds and when he substitutes many sounds for others, his speech becomes almost unintelligible. Children judge the severity of the articulatory defects in accordance with the number of errors. Kleffner (1952) notes that fourth-grade children react unfavorably to a consistent error on a frequently occurring sound and even more unfavorably when many errors are present. When a sound that occurs frequently in our language, like [t] or [s], is defective, it has more effect on intelligibility than a sound, like [ʃ] or [ʒ], that occurs infrequently. The simplest way for a classroom teacher to evaluate the severity of a defect is to count the number of sounds that are omitted, substituted, and distorted. Many quite complex systems of evaluation of degree of severity have been devised. Most of these still need refinement and are used only by speech clinicians.

The child may either accept and acknowledge his difficulty, reject it and insist that it does not exist, or be overly concerned with it. A teacher is of inestimable worth in fostering the attitude of acceptance and in motivating the student to do what he can to correct the difficulty. Both the teacher and the clinician may have to help the child who believes his inadequate speech is adequate. They must assist him in isolating the error and in perceiving it. In some cases, parents help insulate the child against therapy because they believe that a particular error is attractive. On the other hand, overperfectionist, nagging parents may cause the child to be unduly anxious about his difficulty. In one instance the deviation or difference is approved; in the other it is penalized. The teacher must be aware of how the child perceives his own difficulty.

Related Difficulties

Other difficulties are closely related to articulatory difficulties. For example, the child with a denasal voice has three defective sounds: *m*[m], *n*[n], and *ng*[ŋ]. The child with the muffled voice keeps his mouth almost clenched shut; the quality is due in part to the lack of clear-cut articulation of sounds. These two difficulties are labeled voice disorders. The term "retarded speech development" includes many articulatory defects—omissions, substitutions, and distortions; in fact, some writers include their discussion of the articulatory defects of the primary-grade children under retarded speech development. Retarded speech development, however, does connote, in addition to articulatory difficulties, small vocabulary, overly simple sentence structure, and, in general, retarded language development. Cleft-palate speech and defective speech due to impaired hearing are also characterized by articulatory difficulties. Even in cluttering, because of its rapid rate, the child noticeably slurs over and distorts the consonantal sounds. Thus, defective articulation may be a single problem to a child or it may be a symptom of a more complex syndrome.

Articulatory Disorders and Maturation

Because some parents show undue concern about their young children's ability to articulate, teachers must be particularly aware of the need for recognition of the maturing factor in diagnosing articulatory defects. One mother of a five-year-old boy in kindergarten came to a school to demand speech help for him. The only error he made with any consistency was to substitute [t] and [d] for the two *th's*[θ], [ð]. But at times even these sounds were correct. Occasionally he said a [w] for [l]. The mother insisted his speech was not "normal," explaining that his sister had spoken better at the same age, that his cousins of the same age spoke very well, and that the neighborhood youngsters who were even younger spoke more clearly. The little boy was a verbal child who expressed himself unusually well with very few articulatory errors. The teacher explained the part maturity plays in the development of articulation. Because the mother remained unconvinced, the teacher called in the clinician to reassure the mother. The teacher also suggested that the mother remain in the kindergarten room to listen to how other kindergartners spoke.

Studies made where no speech correction was available show that maturation alone takes care of many articulatory errors in the first four grades, but that it does not have any appreciable effect in the higher grades. Roe and Milisen (1942) indicate that the percentage of children making articulatory errors decreases from grades one through six, and that the average number of errors decreases as the grade level increases from grades one through five. A statistically significant difference between grades one and two, two and three, and three and four reveals that growth and maturation eliminate many articulatory errors in these grades. But the lack of a significant difference between grades four and five and five and six tends to prove that maturation does not effect any noticeable improvement in the speech sounds of higher grades. Sayler (1949) notes that there was a slight decrease in the average number of articulatory errors from grades seven through 10. Landers (1959) did a study with 22 matched pairs of kindergarten children, including children with incorrect productions of between five and nine sounds in one or more positions. To one group he gave speech therapy; to the control group he did not. It appeared that the children improved their speech as much by maturation and the regular kindergarten curriculum as by both of these factors and speech therapy.

Some studies, however, show that speech therapy brings an increased rate of decline in articulatory errors in kindergarten and in very young children. Reid (1947) found that speech therapy produced a greater decline of articulatory errors than could be attributed to maturation alone. Ventura, Ingebo, and Wolmut (1960) showed that speech therapy in the kindergarten classroom, with the whole class participating, achieved the greatest change in articulatory ability and that speech therapy outside the classroom achieved the greatest change in the articulation of certain consonants. Both methods, however, achieved significantly greater change than maturation alone. A study by Carter and Buck (1958) determined the feasibility of including first-grade children in a speech therapy program. Their control group received two 30-minute speech therapy periods weekly for nine months; of these 72.2 per cent made 100 per cent final correction while only 9.1 per cent made no correction. Of the 26 children in the experimental group who received no therapy, eight made 100 per cent correction, while about one half made no correction of their defective sounds.

From a study by Sommers and others (1967) involving 288 public school subjects with articulatory difficulties, the following conclusions concerning the advisability of work with children with articulatory problems in kindergarten, first and second grades were drawn:

1. Second grade children with poor stimulability scores require speech therapy if they are to make significant improvement.
2. Children in kindergarten, first and second grades with poor stimulability scores will benefit more from speech correction than those children with good stimulability scores.
3. Exclusion of kindergarten, first and second grade children from therapy classes is unwarranted because they seem to make significant improvements in articulation as a result of their experiences.
4. Speech therapy is effective for children in kindergarten, first and second grades regardless of the severity of the articulation problem.

NORMS FOR ACQUISITION OF SOUNDS

A table on page 130 shows the age at which most children are able to articulate certain sounds. Templin notes that by eight years essentially mature articulation of speech sounds is attained. At this age about 95 per cent of correct articulation, as measured on a 176-item test, has been reached. Only 14 sound elements are not articulated correctly by 90 per cent of the children, and, with the exception of *wh*[ʍ], most of the sound elements approach this level of accuracy (Templin, 1957, p. 144). Using terminal status scores in the articulation of consonant sounds, the boys took one test interval (.5 year) longer than the girls to reach a comparatively mature level of articulation (Templin, 1957, p. 147).

PROGNOSIS FOR IMPROVEMENT THROUGH MATURATION

Since maturation may take care of some of the articulatory difficulties in the primary grades and not of others, guidance is needed in the selection of children for therapy. Such guidance has been provided by three studies. The results of a study by Carter and Buck (1958) suggest that therapy be given to those children who cannot correct their articulation when given a nonsense syllable test. From their study it appears that the higher the percentage of correction on the nonsense syllable test, the more accurate is the prediction of achieving accurate articulation without therapy. A study by Steer and Drexler (1960) indicates that certain measures at the kindergarten level can predict later articulatory ability. The most effective and reliable predictive variables appear to be: (1) the total number of errors in all positions within words; (2) errors in the final position; (3) errors of omission in the final position; and (4) errors on the *f*, *l* consonant group. The amount of improvement in articulatory ability, independent of the number of errors, at the kindergarten level also appears to be significant. Farquhar (1961) reported that the child's ability to imitate the clinician's correct production of his misarticulated sounds seemed to be predictive of subsequent improvement.

Recently, however, a test (The Predictive Screening Test of Articulation, Van Riper, 1969) has been devised to help the clinician identify those children who will overcome their articulatory difficulties without professional assistance. The authors of the PSTA indicate that it should be regarded as a first step in the development of prognostic articulation testing. They observe that both lateral emission of sibilants and /r/ distortions are seldom overcome without professional help and that new tests of oral motor and sensory characteristics and of phonemic synthesis, analysis, and discrimination may contribute to the ability to identify children who persist in articulatory errors.

More generalized predictive factors are reported by Irwin (1966). In a study to identify factors or measures predicting improvement in speech, language, and auditory skills, she found that improvement in articulation can be predicted by mental age, scores in articulation, and stimulability. The more severe the articulatory defect, the more improvement appears to occur. Good stimulability scores at the beginning of therapy will predict probable success.

Testing for Errors

When a child's articulation does call attention to itself or when the child himself is disturbed about his difficulty, the teacher should determine what errors the child is making. The teacher can get a general impression of the child's speech through conversation. For younger children, pictures cut from magazines motivate conversation. Pictures that tell a story, such as children having a good time at a birthday party, a small child crying as he looks at a broken doll, a farmer feeding his cows, or children playing in the sand and building castles, are particularly effective in motivating conversation. Certain picture books promote talk. For example, Mrs. Newberry's *Percy, Polly and Pete* (Harper and Row, Publishers, 1952) contains pictures that induce children to comment about the activities of the three cats. With older children, the teacher may talk about common interests, hobbies, vacation plans, or some other interesting topic. From such conversation, the teacher gains a picture of the child's speech.

Often times, however, a teacher wants a more accurate analysis and wishes to test each sound. Jordan (1960) shows that such an analysis does give valid information on how the child says the sounds, even in connected speech. He studied the relationship between measures of articulation from phonetic analysis and measures of articulation obtained from listener ratings of connected speech. He found that the articulation test responses provided valid information on articulatory behavior in connected speech. In addition, he discovered that listeners' reactions to defective articulation are dependent on (1) the frequency with which articulatory defects occur and (2) the degree of the defect. To the listener, omissions are more deviant than substitutions, and substitutions are more deviant than distortions. The number of defective sounds is highly related to the measure of articulation derived from listener response to connected speech.

Frequently, the teacher is asked to refer students to the speech clinician. A Subcommittee on Diagnosis and Measurement of the Research Committee of the American Speech and Hearing Association (ASHA, 1959, p. 52) indicates that for speech screening, surveys and referrals by teachers are used most frequently. Because the teacher does often make the referral, he should make the referral for articulatory defects on some organized basis—preferably an articulatory test which tests all the consonantal sounds. His purpose is not to evaluate the precise articulatory abilities of the children but rather to decide whether their abilities lie within the normal ranges of the group. The speech clinician to whom the child is referred will take care of the more detailed therapeutic examination.

A study by Siegel (1962) suggests that classroom teachers can be trained to test articulation. The experiment consisted of three articulation-testing occasions. On the first occasion two experienced and two inexperienced examiners each tested 26 mentally retarded children with the Templin-Darley Screening Articulation Test and with the criterion measure being the number of correct responses. The inexperienced examiners were then given about four hours of training and experience in articulation testing. After this training, all the examiners retested 22 of the children. The next week, all the examiners tested a new group of 21 children. The results indicated that inexperienced examiners could be trained to be quite reliable with a minimum of training. Reliability, however, did not guarantee examiner equivalence since, in spite of high reliability, examiners tended to differ significantly in absolute scores assigned to children.

Testing, whether done by the clinician or by the teacher is influenced by many factors: The subject being tested is not the same today as he was a week ago. A study by Winitz (1963) suggests that articulatory testing may not always be temporally reliable. He tested 100 youngsters with a mean age of 65.3 months and then retested them after an interval of 6–12 days. An examination of the data revealed that for some sounds considerable intrasubject variability was introduced in the two testing times. The rapport the child feels with the examiner may make considerable difference; psychological studies show that reinforcement with nothing but an appreciatively uttered "m-m-m-m" makes a difference in psychological scores. The distractions within the environment play a role. To test a child in a teacher's room with teachers constantly entering is bound to modify the child's performance. The amount of noise can affect scores. Nichols (1967) indicates that noise in the testing environment and the intensity of the responses of the testee affect articulation scores. Finally, the instrument itself can be a variant.

Testing is either done auditorily ("Say after me"), in which case the child is imitating the tester, or visually ("Look. Tell me the name of ———"), in which case the child is spontaneously giving the name of the object; or in a combination of the two. Studies seem to indicate that the spontaneous method elicits more errors. A study by Lencione and Trent (1965) reported in *ASHA* indicates that, in testing 80 children between the ages of six and 11 years with both spontaneous and imitative test procedures, a significant difference between the two methods for testing consonants in the three positions and for substitutions and omissions exists, but that for testing distortions and double and triple consonants, no significant differences occur.

Somewhat similar findings are reported by Siegel, Winitz, and Conkey (1963) who compared the imitative and spontaneous methods of presenting word stimuli during articulation testing. The tester's face was screened while he uttered the words in the imitative procedure. In the spontaneous procedure, children looked at pictures of objects likely to be familiar to kindergarten children and gave the name of each object. The results indicated that eight out of 40 sounds were produced correctly by significantly more children on the imitative than on the spontaneous condition. These results suggest that the imitative mode may result in better articulation performance than the spontaneous mode.

A study by Smith and Ainsworth (1967) support the findings of the Siegel, Winitz, and Conkey study. The purpose of this study was to determine whether children with defective articulation produced the same number of articulatory errors when their speech was stimulated by three different methods: picture stimulus, auditory stimulus ("Say after me") and auditory-visual stimulus ("I want you to watch my mouth as I say the word"). The subjects were first graders with articulatory errors, who had had no speech therapy. The sounds selected were /r/, /l/, /θ/, /ð/, /s/, /z/, /dʒ/, /k/, /g/, and /b/. The results indicated that the picture stimulus mode was more effective in eliciting articulation errors than the other two modes, and that the auditory stimulus was more effective in eliciting articulation errors than the auditory-visual mode.

Sounds are usually tested in three positions: initial, where the sound begins the word, medial, where it is in the middle of the word, and final, where it ends the word.* For the young child the teacher may test with pictures.

Irwin and Musselman (1962) have devised a picture articulation test that checks more than one sound in a word and that includes all of the consonants in the initial and final positions, all of the vowels, and all of the diphthongs. The 61 phonetic elements are incorporated in the 27 words shown in the table on the facing page; in the study these words were represented by original India-ink drawings.

The study shows that this test may be used to evaluate more than one error in a word with reliability by both experienced and inexperienced judges. This test takes half as much time to administer as the conventional test. The study also showed that there was no significant difference between the experienced and inexperienced judges.

Fristoe and Goldman (1968) support the feasibility of testing more than one sound in a single word. They compared testers' ability to listen for and evaluate two or three sounds in a word with their ability to evaluate a single sound in a word. That there was little difference in the testers' performance suggests that speech clinicians can effectively evaluate more than one sound per word and that articulation tests can thereby be condensed.

---

* Authorities now debate whether the medial position should be legitimately included, because a sound in a medial position usually begins or ends a syllable. If one considers position in relation to syllables, only initial or final sounds would be included. Curtis and Hardy note that Stetson's analysis of articulatory dynamics, supported by considerable experimental data, appears to indicate that a consonant's function as either an initiating or terminating element of a syllable may be more significant than its position in a word (1959, p. 245). They note that classifying a sound as medial denotes the possible difference in functions, since a consonant in the medial position may be either initiating or terminating with respect to the syllable. Hence they use the classification as to whether the sound occurs before a vowel (prevocalic) or after a vowel (postvocalic) within a syllable. Keenan (1961) also suggests that the medial concept be discarded and that the classification be based, as Curtis recommends, on whether the consonant begins a syllable and precedes a vowel, whether it ends a syllable and follows the vowel, or whether it is part of a cluster (as the *l* in *pl*). Certain writers also express concern about the effect of neighboring sounds on the sound to be tested. Most current tests take these factors into consideration.

Word	Sound		
	INITIAL	MEDIAL	FINAL
pig	p		g
boy	b		ɔɪ
teeth	t		θ
door	d		r
cage	k		dʒ
book		ʊ	k
garage	g	ɑ	ʒ
fish	f		ʃ
valentine	v	æ	n
glove		ʌ	v
thumb	θ		m
this or that	ð		
smooth		u	ð
saucer	s	ɔ	ɚ
mouse		aʊ	s
zebra	z		ə
ship	ʃ		p
hand	h		d
church	tʃ	ɝ	tʃ
jail	dʒ	eɪ	l
music	m	ju	
nose	n	oʊ	z
leaf	l	i	f
web	w	ɛ	b
white	ʍ	aɪ	t
yellow	j		o
ring	r		ŋ

Avant and Hutton (1962) have devised a measuring tool that: (1) permits examination of articulation in connected speech with reliability and validity; (2) permits evaluation of such other facts as rate, voice quality, pitch, loudness, and breathing; (3) uses a stimulus that produces a consistent response; and (4) can be administered quickly and easily. The tool is a short reading passage for upper elementary school children. In constructing the test, they emphasized: (a) inclusion of a wide variety of speech sounds, with emphasis on those occurring most frequently and those most often defective; (b) readability (simple structure, and vocabulary from first 1,000 words of the Rinsland list); (c) rapidity in administration. The tester may use phonetic transcriptions. Instructions on a scoring procedure for articulatory errors include: (a) an omission, by marking a diagonal line through the symbol for the omitted sound; (b) a substitution, by writing the phonetic symbol; (c) a distortion, by a question mark above the symbol; and

(d) an added sound, by an insertion of the phonetic symbol representing the sound.

The selection follows:

One day Jim was looking out the kitchen window. "Mary," he called, "Father is coming in the front door with a big white box."
"I have something to show you," said Mr. Jones.
"Is the box for us?" they both cried.
When he took the paper off, they saw it was a red doll house.
Jim said, "There are some people in it. The man is reading and the woman is washing a baby."
"She looks like Mrs. Green," Mary said.
"Do you see the girl in the play room?"
Mary saw the girl was sitting on a large ball.
Just then Mother came in. Mary and Jim said, "Look at the pretty toys Father gave us. Thank you very much for them" (Avant and Hutton, 1962, p. 41).

Goldman and Fristoe (1967) have devised a filmstrip articulation test that examines all the necessary phonemes, and obtains an adequate and accurate sample of a child's behavior. This test consists of 35 pictures depicting objects familiar to young children. The tester obtains a total of 44 responses by asking the child questions about the pictures, in addition to the names of the 35 objects. All words except one are in Thorndike's list of 10,000 most commonly used words.

The Arizona Articulation Proficiency Test (Barker and England, 1962) includes each phoneme of American English and /l/, /r/, and /s/ blends, with the norm age of the acquisition of each sound. All articulation errors are recorded and when a sound is defective in one position, one numerical value is recorded; when it is defective in two positions, the value is doubled. The total value is entered if the sound is defective in all three positions. The total of the error value of the consonants and vowel columns are totaled and substracted from 100 to give the Arizona Articulation Proficiency Score.

One of the most widely used articulatory screening tests is the Templin-Darley Screening Test (1960). This test consists of 50 items selected on the basis of which best discriminates between good and poor articulators. A cutoff score is available for each age level.

Most of the tests just mentioned fall into the category of screening tests, which are used to assess the adequacy of the child's articulatory performance. They are used in school surveys to determine which students need the help of the speech clinician. A second type of test, much more detailed, determines the ability of the child to use sounds in various phonetic contexts. In consequence, it provides the clinician with information on the child's ability to produce sounds in various positions and phonetic contexts. In addition, it can be used to compare therapy, to evaluate progress, to select case loads, to determine consistency of misarticulations, and to identify factors related to misarticulations—such as distinctive features related to sound substitutions. For this purpose Templin and Darley (1960) use a 176-item test as a diagnostic articulation test.

Another diagnostic test is McDonald's Deep Test of Articulation: Picture and Sentence Forms (1964). This test offers a different approach to the assessment and treatment of functional articulatory problems, for it is based on constructs derived from motor and acoustic phonetics, control theory, developmental psychology, and linguistics. It disavows the traditional concept of initial, medial, and final consonants, and tests instead simple and abutting consonants in a representative sampling of phonetic contexts.

Factors Associated with Articulatory Difficulties

LANGUAGE DEFICITS

Many authorities believe that most children with deficiencies in articulatory development also have deficiencies in other aspects of language development. Ferrier's (1966) study, reported in some detail in Chapter 1, indicates that children with articulatory difficulties do not do as well in language as measured by all nine tests of the Illinois Test of Psycholinguistic Abilities (First Edition) as do children with normal speech. For the children with articulatory defects, the scores on four tests were substantially lower, indicating that these children do not do as well as normal-speaking children in expressing ideas verbally, using grammatical structures automatically, recalling a series of digits presented to them orally, and recalling a series of geometric forms presented to them visually. Smith (1967) supports the finding on recalling digits, both in immediate and delayed recall.

Schneiderman (1955) studied the relationship of defective articulation to language ability. She included in language ability spoken vocabulary, sentence length, and a rating by the classroom teachers on the children's ability to express themselves verbally. She found that children with the lowest level of language ability were also the children with the largest mean number of defective speech sounds, whereas the children with the highest language ability had the lowest mean number of defective speech sounds. She states that this relationship is due in large part to other factors, such as mental age.

Still other studies indicate deficits in language development. Three of the studies point to the ability of normal-speaking children to use more sophisticated syntactical structures than do children with functional articulatory difficulties. Menyuk (1964) reports that in comparing children with infantile speech* with children with normal speech (ages 3–5.10), the normal-speaking children used significantly more transformations than the defective-speech group, and the group with infantile speech used more restricted forms and used them much more frequently than the normal-speaking group. The child with normal speech rapidly acquired structures that required increasingly complex rules for their generation over the two to three-year period, and exceeded in acquisition of structures even the oldest infantile-speech child. There was no significant difference in the mean number of sentences used.

The results seem to indicate that the most meaningful factor is the difference in the two groups' ability to determine the complete set of rules used to generate and differentiate structures at any level of grammar. Examples of transformation types are:

Negation—*He isn't a good boy.*
Question—*Are you nice?*
Contraction—*He'll be good.*
Auxiliary *be* placement—*He is not going.*
Relative clause—*I don't know what he is doing.*
Iteration—*You have to drink milk to be strong.*

Examples of restricted forms are:

Verb phrase omission—*This green.*
Noun phrase redundancy—*I want it the paint.*
Preposition substitution—*He took me at the circus.*
Pronoun subject substitution—*Me like that.*

Similarly Vandemark and Mann (1965) found that the significant difference between a group of 50 normal-speaking children and 50 children with defective articulation was in the syntactical complexity, which involved grammatical completeness and complexity of response. According to this study, children with defective articulation are not

---

* This category would seem to be comprised of the more severe articulatory cases. According to Menyuk (1964, p. 119) the most frequent sound errors were omissions and substitutions. Furthermore, 50 per cent of the infantile-speech children omitted initial /s/ and final /t/, and more than 50 per cent of the children used these substitutions: /w/ for /r/ and /l/, /t/ for /k/ and /θ/, /d/ for /g/ and /ð/.

inhibited in terms of amount of verbal output but are deficient in areas of grammatical completeness and complexity of response.

Shriner, Halloway, and Daniloff (1969) in a study of 30 children with normal articulation and 30 with defective articulation found that the mean number of words per response was significantly lower for the speech-defective group than for the normal-speaking group. They agree with Vandermark and Mann that the children with defective articulation do not use as developed a syntactical structure as the normal-speaking children. This study used a method of evaluating the complexity of sentences that differed from the Vandermark and Mann study in that these researchers counted the number of noun phrases and verb phrases.

Lee (1966) compared the syntactical development of two boys— one normal, the other deviant in articulatory development. She found marked differences between them. Not only was the speech deviant slower in following a normal pattern of behavior but he failed to produce certain types of syntactic structures.

The lack of syntactical development may be related to the lack of articulatory development. Perhaps a neurological impairment, or a defective auditory and/or proprioceptive feedback which causes the defective articulation, may bring about syntactical lags. Or the child who misarticulates, having been made aware of his inadequacy, may speak infrequently and thus have less of an opportunity to experiment with syntactical forms. More research is needed before the significance of the coexistence of deficits in syntactical and articulatory development can be explained.

LOW INTELLIGENCE

Any number of studies show a high incidence of articulatory defects among children who are definitely feeble-minded. Many organic conditions, such as brain injury, contribute to both deficient articulatory and mental ability. Speech defects are more frequent among children of low than of high intelligence. Gladys Reid (1947), however, points out that articulatory ability is not related to and cannot be predicted from intelligence when the intelligence is above that indicated by an I.Q. of 70. Yedinack (1949) also indicates that there is no significant relationship between articulatory defects and intelligence. Similarly, a study by Steer and Drexler (1960) predicting later articulatory ability of kindergartners, notes that intelligence as measured at the kindergarten level appears to be unrelated to articulatory ability five years later.

When the comparison is refined so that the type of articulatory defect is considered, a difference does seem to exist. Prins (1962b) in a comparison of speech-handicapped and normal children found that children with defective articulation errors of the omission type were lower in intelligence as measured by a receptive vocabulary test than were the normal-speaking children. But when the articulatory errors consisted chiefly of interdentalization of /s/ or /z/, or the use of phonemic sound substitutions in which only one articulatory feature is altered, there was no significant difference in intellectual ability as measured by a receptive vocabulary test.

In a study, representative of others, of the articulatory development of 415 mental retardates, Wilson (1966) found that 53.4 per cent had defective articulation, while 46.6 per cent had normal speech. As the mental age increases, the total number of deviant sounds decreases but the articulatory pattern is not orderly. Several sibilant, affricative, and fricative sounds are never produced by 90 per cent of the children through the nine-year mental age level. The articulatory development of mentally retarded does not parallel the development of normal children even when the mental age of the retardate is matched against the chronological age of the normal child.

SOCIOECONOMIC STATUS

Prins (1962) also did correlations between a variety of articulatory variables and socioeconomic status. He found that subjects with a high proportion of interdental lisping (where /s/ is produced with the tongue visible between the teeth) tend to come from high socioeconomic levels whereas subjects with a high proportion of omission-type errors come from low socioeconomic levels.

HEARING LOSS

We have already stressed the relationship between adequate hearing and the ability to learn to speak. Although the child's hearing may be sufficient for understanding conversation and what goes on around him, it may be insufficient for learning to make all the sounds. Some sounds the child may not hear at all. His own speech, therefore, reflects his inability to hear. When D. J. Mase (1946) was selecting his subjects for a study of the etiology of articulatory defects, he discovered five boys with pronounced hearing loss. No teacher or principal was aware of a hearing loss in any one of these five boys even though the symptoms of total monotony and inarticulate speech were clearly evident. Peripherally deaf children almost always have defective articulation, for they are unable to imitate sounds. They cannot compare the sounds they utter with those produced by others. In fact, they cannot hear the sounds of any model. Their abilities to see and to feel cannot make up for their inability to hear. We will discuss the problem of the child with a hearing loss more fully in Chapter 14.

EMOTIONAL OR PERSONALITY DIFFICULTY

A child learns to speak to help him adjust to his environment. A large part of man's social adjustment to his surroundings is verbal. Hs environment and surroundings influence his ability to adjust through verbal means. Some children's environment is so difficult that they cannot learn to adjust to it. An articulatory defect may be a symptom of this inability to adjust. Solomon (1960) notes that the child with the functional articulatory difficulty tends to be passive and to internalize his responses. He indicates that this child is characterized by submissiveness, timidity, and a need for approval. He interprets the findings to indicate that speech and behavior problems are found together and may both represent refusals to acquire socially acceptable functions because of unfavorable stress or environmental pressures.

Wood (1946) did a study on the adjustment of parents who had children with articulatory defects. He found, by administering personality tests, that the mothers of children with articulatory defects as a group were more neurotic in tendency, more submissive, and more self-conscious than average mothers as measured by test norms. Furthermore, the scores of the mothers of children with articulatory defects were lower than the test norms in self-adjustment, social adjustment, and total adjustment. The scores of the fathers on one test did not differ significantly from test norms; on another they showed that the fathers rated lower on self-adjustment than the norms. Wood concludes that articulatory defects are definitely and significantly associated with maladjustment and undesirable traits of the parents and that such factors are usually centered in the mother. As mentioned in Chapter 7, his study also indicated that when the mothers of children with articulatory defects were treated clinically to help them secure better adjustment, their children improved more quickly with speech correction help than did children whose parents were not treated. Moll and Darley (1960) studied the attitudes of mothers of children who had articulatory impairments. They found that mothers of such children have higher standards and are more critical of their children's functioning than are mothers of children whose speech is not impaired.

Dickson (1962) studied the differences in the emotional characteristics of parents of two groups: (1) those children who outgrew functional articulatory errors, and (2) those who did not. He found after an item analysis of the Minnesota Multiphasic Personality Test that there were some indications that the mothers of children who retain their errors tended toward "emotional immaturity and instability."

STRUCTURAL ABNORMALITIES

Anomalies of the tongue, lips, teeth, and palate have long been associated with articulatory difficulties. Recently, however, attitudes have changed on the responsibility of organic deviations of the articulatory mechanism for articulatory defects. For instance, the literature in the field of speech therapy presents opposing viewpoints on the responsibility of dental abnormalities for defective articulation. Undoubtedly, for some children, malocclusion of the teeth or an abnormally large tongue contribute to the child's lack of articulatory development. But some children with similar organic difficulties do not misarticulate the same sounds whereas other children with a normal mechanism do misarticulate them. Poor structures may, however, be a contributing factor in explaining poor articulation.

Teeth and Gum Ridge. The teeth and/or the gum ridge are involved in the sounds [f], [v], [θ], [ð], [s], [z], [ʂ], [ʃ], [ʐ], [ʒ], [tʃ], and [dʒ]. In [f] and [v] the upper teeth touch the lower lip. In [θ] and [ð] the tongue tip is placed against the biting edge of the upper teeth or between the two rows of teeth. In the sibilant sounds, the air is directed against the teeth in a variety of ways. In some cases the teeth have difficulty reaching the lower lip, the biting edge is badly located, or the teeth are so formed that it is difficult to find a surface of teeth against which to direct the air.

The condition where the upper front teeth protrude abnormally beyond the lower teeth is called an overbite. When the upper lip meets the lower one with difficulty, [p], [b], and [m] may be defective. The tongue lies forward in the mouth, sometimes over the lower teeth. The lower teeth are so far back that they cannot provide the necessary friction to make a good [s] or [z]. With this condition the lower jaw usually recedes.

In other cases the lower jaw protrudes and the lower front teeth project over the upper front teeth. This condition is called an underbite and is usually associated with an undershot jaw.

In still other cases a space occurs between the upper and lower teeth when they are brought together. This condition is called an open bite. Normally the upper incisor overlaps its counterpart on the lower jaw so that about one-third of the surface of the visible lower incisor is covered by the upper incisor. In an open bite [s] and [z] are most frequently defective since the narrow stream of air cannot be directed against the cutting edge of the teeth. Sometimes [ʃ], [ʒ], [θ], and [ð] are distorted. If the lips cannot be brought together [p], [b], and [m] may be defective. When the lower lip cannot touch the teeth easily, [f] and [v] may be inaccurate.

Finally, a space may occur between the central incisors or the canine teeth may be irregularly placed. In both these instances [s] may be defective. When the space occurs, too much air is allowed to escape. Where the teeth are irregularly placed, they may interfere with the tongue so that the air is allowed to escape over one or both of its sides. Frequently, however, individuals themselves, finding compensatory movements, speak well in spite of having teeth that are very irregular.

Snow (1961) did a study on articulation proficiency in relation to certain dental abnormalities; the purpose of the study was to study the articulation of six consonant sounds [f], [v], [θ], [ð], [s], and [z], for which the upper central incisor teeth are ordinarily considered important. She found that a statistically significant larger proportion of "normal" first-grade children with missing or abnormal upper central incisor teeth misarticulated [f], [v], [θ], [ð], [s], and [z], compared with children with normal teeth. However, she notes that most of the children with missing or abnormal teeth made the sounds correctly and some children with normal teeth did not make the sounds correctly.

Bankson and Byrne (1962) investigated the influence of missing teeth on the production of initial, medial, and final /s/, /ʃ/, /f/, and medial /z/. A statistically significant relationship was found between production of the initial, medial, and final /s/ and the presence or absence of teeth among children who on a pretest had used the sound correctly. No statistically significant relationship was found between the accuracy of the initial, medial, and final /ʃ/, /f/, and medial /z/ and the presence or absence of teeth among children who had produced the sound correctly on a pretest. Loss of incisors may be the cause of a defective /s/. But missing teeth will not usually permanently influence the speech patterns of children.

Tongue. The term "tongue-tied" is applied when the frenum of the tongue (the little web of tissue underneath the front part of the tongue) is abnormally short so that the tip of the tongue cannot move to points such as the ridge behind the upper teeth. This condition, where it severely disturbs articulation, is comparatively rare in children.

Other conditions may involve the tongue. The sounds that may be disturbed because of the tongue are [k], [g], [ŋ], [θ], [ð], [l], [r], [s],

[z], [ʃ], and [ʒ]. In some few cases the tongue is so large or sluggish that it cannot make the small, precise, and quick movements necessary for certain sounds. Sometimes the tongue may be paralyzed or weak. At other times, there may be poor muscular coordination. Occasionally a thyroid deficiency causes sluggishness and poor control of the tongue, the result of generally poor motor coordination.

In [l] and [r] the tongue tip points to the teeth ridge. In [s] and [z], the tongue is grooved to direct a small stream of air against the teeth. In [n], [t], and [d], the tongue touches the teeth ridge. In [ʃ] and [ʒ], the tongue directs a broader channel of air against the teeth. In the sibilant sounds the tip of the tongue may reach toward the upper gum. In teaching the sibilants, however, clinicians sometimes find it better not to have the child try to reach toward the upper gum but to have him reach toward the gum behind the lower teeth. The tongue is obviously an important articulatory agent.

Tongue-Thrust. Dentists frequently refer children to the speech clinician for a neuromuscular syndrome commonly called "tongue-thrust." Palmer (1962, p. 323) lists these synonyms for tongue-thrust: reverse swallowing, deviant swallowing, visceral swallowing, and orofacial muscle pressure imbalance. The features of the syndrome include: a deviant swallowing pattern because (1) unusual tension exists in the mouth-enclosing musculature, (2) perceptible contraction of swallowing muscles decreases or is absent, (3) the tongue is thrust forward, causing it to protrude between the teeth, and (4) the molars are separated during deglutition. As a result of one or more of the above, the structure of the oral cavity may be modified and dental irregularities produced. Associated with these modifications are sound production defects, especially of the sibilants. Fletcher, Casteel, and Bradley (1961) found that a child with a tongue-thrust swallow is more likely to have a deviant /s/ than the child with a normal swallow. They indicate that further information is needed to establish more clearly the role of the speech therapist in tongue-thrusts. Evidence of the influence of tongue-thrust on sibilants is contained in a study by Ronson (1965) who found that the incidence of visceral swallowing among a group of 60 lispers in second, third, and fourth grades was 32.

Palmer (1962, p. 323) gives a more precise symptomatology than that listed above. He categorizes its symptomatology by differences in: (1) patterns of swallowing, (2) orofacial function, (3) orofacial structure, (4) dental structure, (5) speech sound production. The swallowing involves a vigorous pressing of the tongue against or through the teeth anteriorly or laterally. He notes that research is needed to determine how basic a component of abnormal swallowing tongue-thrusting is, what directions and degrees the thrusts take, and how they are related to observed oral abnormalities. Bell and Hale (1963), in evaluating 353 five- and six-year-old children, found that 82 per cent exhibited a low forward tongue and a slightly depressed mandible during swallowing. 89 per cent of the tongue-thrusters appeared to articulate /t/, /d/, /l/, /n/, /tʃ/, /s/, /ʃ/, and /z/ in a dental and/or interdental position.

Hoffman and Hoffman (1965) give three criteria for considering tongue-thrusting as a speech problem: (1) if it interferes with or prevents the proper production of speech sounds when the child is able to make the necessary tongue movements and placements to improve or correct these sounds; (2) when tongue-thrusting persists after space is available in the oral cavity for the tongue; and (3) when tongue-thrust is observed as a concomitant of a condition that ordinarily responds to speech therapy. They admonish the clinician to remember that tongue-thrusting may be a temporary developmental manifestation occurring throughout or intermittently during the growth and development of the lower face of some individuals. It may also develop as a habit after development has taken place or as a necessary placement of the tongue if growth and development are inadequate when completed. They stress that the clinician should differentiate between tongue-thrusting as a temporary developmental phase and as a permanent practice because of insufficient oral space. They also stress that swallowing is a complex reflex action not likely to be retrained successfully and permanently.

Palate. In sounds such as [ʃ] and [ʒ], the palate plays a part. When it is abnormally high and narrow, the child's tongue may have difficulty in making the necessary contacts. When an opening occurs along the middle line of the palate, the condition is serious. This condition is discussed in a later chapter.

MOTOR ABILITY

Some children are poorly coordinated. Quite obviously some youngsters run, go up- and downstairs, and jump much more easily than others. One youngster will put a jigsaw puzzle together and fit the pieces with little or no effort. Another will struggle with it. This motor ability develops with maturation. But children of the same age vary widely in this ability. Sometimes poor coordination is evident around the mouth; the tongue, jaw, and palate are awkward. Some studies have shown that children with articulatory defects tend to score significantly lower on tests of motor ability than do children with normal speech. Not all children with articulatory defects are deficient in motor skill, but poor motor ability may be a contributing cause of the defect. Bilto

(1941) compared the muscular abilities of a group of 90 children who had articulatory defects or stuttered with a group of children with normal speech. The children with defective speech had no organic difficulties. Approximately two thirds of the speech-defective children were inferior to the children with normal speech on the test that included appropriate rhythm, coordination, and application of strength. Patton (1942) found a tendency for children with articulatory defects to show less kinesthetic sensibility than children with normal speech. He defines kinesthesia as the sense by which muscular motion, weight, and position are perceived and as the sense whose organs lie in the muscles, tendons, and joints, which are stimulated by bodily movements and tensions. A study by Karlin, Youtz, and Kennedy (1940) indicates that children with defective speech are inferior to those with normal speech in ability to perform tasks requiring motor speed.

On the other hand, Mase (1946) found no significant difference in his matched groups of intermediate elementary school children with and without articulatory defects on rate of movement of articulators and general muscular coordination. Reid (1947) concludes from her study of functional articulatory defects that the degree of neuro-muscular control and the degree of kinesthetic sensitivity are not related to articulation ability. She does point out, however, that, without doubt, there are minimum levels of maturity for these two factors. Maxwell (1953) found no difference between normal-speaking and articulatory cases in his tests of motor performance.

Jenkins and Lohr (1964) compared motor proficiency as measured by the Oseretsky Test of Motor Proficiency given to 38 first-grade children with "severe articulatory defects" and 38 normal-speaking controls matched for age, sex, and I.Q. The results of the study showed that the speech-defective group was significantly lower on the total test score and on each of the subtests administered. The tests involve maintaining bodily balance for a given period without gross movements of limbs or torso, performing coordinated hand activities within a time limit and with accuracy (cutting paper), maintaining balance while performing a given movement of the whole body, as in running or hopping, simultaneous voluntary movements, as in tapping the left and right feet alternately, or performing a given muscular activity without extraneous movements, such as clenching the teeth without wrinkling the forehead.

AUDITORY MEMORY AND DISCRIMINATION

Some children may hear very well but have difficulty in retaining auditory impressions. Others with excellent hearing may have trouble in discriminating one sound from another. Mase (1946) found no significant difference in either auditory memory or discrimination between the speech-defective group and the normal-speaking group. Reid (1947) also found that the length of auditory memory span is not related to articulatory ability. She found, however, a significant relationship between articulatory ability and the ability to discriminate between speech sounds. Hall (1938) found that children and adults with articulatory defects are not inferior to normal-speaking children and adults in auditory discrimination of either simple or complex speech patterns or in regard to auditory memory for speech sounds. Metraux (1944) in a study of the auditory span of children ranging in age from four years to 12 years determined that there are significant differences in auditory memory span among the various age groups for both the vowel and consonant sounds. The scores for recalling both the vowel and consonant sounds gradually increase with age, although the peak for the vowel test is reached at age 10 while the peak for the consonant test is reached at age 12.

Other studies emphasize that the ability of the child with an articulatory defect in auditory discrimination is inferior to that of the normal-speaking child. Bruns (1957) using the Templin modification of the Travis-Rasmus Test of Auditory Discrimination and the standardized Phonetically Balanced Kindergarten Word List found that the group of children possessing articulatory defects scored significantly lower on both the Templin test and the Phonetically Balanced Kindergarten Test than did the group of children with normal speech. Farquhar (1961), in studying the value of a battery of imitative articulation and auditory discrimination tests in predicting speech development of two groups of kindergarten children, found that children with severe speech problems had significantly inferior auditory discrimination than children with mild speech problems. Mange (1960) found that his group of normal-speaking children achieved significantly higher scores in discrimination of pitch than did his group of children with functional misarticulation of [r]. In this study, there was also a significant but low partial correlation between phonetic word-synthesis ability and the number of articulatory errors. Schiefelbusch (1958), in a study to develop a new test for sound discrimination, found that significant differences exist between the speech-defective and normal-speaking groups in relation to sound discrimination abilities in each form: rhyming, initial, and final sounds. He also found that the second-grade normal-speaking groups had significantly better sound discrimination than the first-grade normals, but a similar gain was not found for the second-grade speech-defective group in comparison with the first-grade speech-defective group.

Still other evidence supports the relationship between poor auditory discrimination and lack of articulatory ability. Wepman (1960) found that a close relationship existed between auditory discrimination and accuracy of speech sounds. Cohen and Diehl (1963) compared 20 elementary school children with articulatory problems with 30 normal-speaking children. They tested both groups with the Templin Speech Sound Discrimination Test and found that the children with articulatory problems made significantly more speech-sound discrimination errors than did the normal-speaking children. Although the speech-sound discrimination ability improves with grade level, the speech-defective group continues to perform less well than the normal-speaking group. Sherman and Geith (1967) tested 529 kindergarten children with 50 sound discrimination items of the Templin Sound Discrimination Test, and then selected from this group 18 with high speech-sound discrimination and 18 with low speech-sound discrimination. They then administered the Templin-Darley Picture Articulation Test to both groups and found that the children with the high sound discrimination were significantly superior in articulatory ability to the low speech-sound discrimination group.

Fairly recent research suggests that sound discrimination tests should be developed to measure abilities to discriminate sounds in terms of type of articulation error as manner of production, vocal component, and articulatory agents used and to discriminate sounds in a variety of phonetic contexts.

Aungst and Frick (1964) questioned whether the ability to discriminate between paired auditory stimuli presented by another speaker is related to ability to judge one's own speech utterances as correct or incorrect. They therefore studied the relationship between abilities to produce /r/ and to discriminate /r/. Each child was tested with a traditional test of auditory discrimination and with one constructed to measure ability to judge one's own speech production, to judge it when compared with the production of another speaker, and to judge it when heard on a tape recording. The researchers further tested with a 50-item deep test for production of /r/ in various contexts. Correlations with the tests of production of /r/ and the traditional test of auditory discrimination was −.03, whereas correlations with the devised test and the deep test of articulation ranged from .59 to .69. The findings suggest that /r/ errors are not related to general discrimination ability but are related to ability to discriminate /r/.

Liberman and others (1957) showed that sheer temporal duration is sometimes a cue for distinguishing speech sounds. Duration of transition distinguishes stop-consonant sounds from semivowels; duration of fricative noise is a cue for distinguishing among the classes fricative, affricate, and stop. Liberman (1961) has also shown that normal speakers are best able to discriminate minimal sound differences when the acoustic variations are phonemic, signaling a change in linguistic meaning. Liberman believes that a speaker learns to connect speech sounds with their appropriate articulatory characteristics and that eventually the articulatory movements become part of the perceiving process, mediating between the acoustic stimulus and its ultimate perception. In other words, he hypothesizes that speech-sound discrimination ability is closely related to the articulatory movement feedback that an individual receives as he speaks.

Partly because of this hypothesis, Prins (1963) decided to look among children with developmental articulatory disorders for evidence of specific relationships among the various deviations of articulation and scores on a clinical measure of sound discrimination ability. He divided articulatory deviations into three error classes: (1) phonemic sound substitutions, (2) nonphonemic sound substitutions, and (3) sound omissions. Classes (1) and (2) he further divided into: M, manner of articulation; P, place of articulation; and V, voicing. He noted whether the deviation occurred singly or in combinations and the degree to which the place of articulation was changed. The degrees were based on: (a) front—bilabial, labio-dental; (b) middle—linguadental, or alveolar; (c) back—lingua-palatal and velar; and (d) glottal.

He found significant correlations between sound discrimination test scores and articulatory errors in which only one feature of the intended phoneme was altered and in which the place of articulation was altered one degree. Thus, children who tended to confuse the place of articulation during speech-sound production also had difficulty discriminating minimal word pairs in which a single phoneme was altered in place of articulation. He suggests that sound discrimination ability is a function of articulation and the total language learning process.

According to this study (Prins, 1963, p. 385), the correlations between the total number of articulatory errors and the sound discrimination score was not significant. Furthermore, the results of correlations between selected types of articulatory deviations and sound discrimination test scores suggest a functional relationship between certain kinds of errors of articulation and sound discrimination ability as measured by the Wepman Test. Prins believes these are related to findings on normal-speaking subjects which have indicated that discrimination ability among minimal sound differences is related to the significance of these differences in the language system of the discriminator. He notes that poor sound discrimination ability is an effect of disturbance in the total language learning process rather than a primary auditory perceptual limitation which is of etiologic significance in defective articulation. Children who alter place of articulation in production of phonemes may have difficulty in using place-change information to differentiate phonemes that they hear. This is related to Liberman's hypothesis that speech-sound discrimination ability is closely related to the articulatory movement feedback that an individual receives as he speaks.

A study by Winitz and Bellerose (1963) seems to indicate that speech-sound discrimination tests may measure not only developmental skills, but the learned equivalence and distinctiveness of speech sounds. They studied the discrimination learning of 200 first- and second-grade children as a function of several pretraining conditions. Pretraining conditions were so constructed as to permit the correct or incorrect learning of /vroʊ/; that is /vroʊ/ for /broʊ/ and /broʊ/ for /vroʊ/. The findings indicate that discrimination learning was significantly impaired following the incorrect learning of /vroʊ/. It is possible that articulatory errors themselves may bring about sound discrimination difficulties. More research is needed to determine the kind of relationship that exists.

INCOMPLETE PHONEMIC DEVELOPMENT

Winitz (1969, p. 132) contends that an articulatory error persists because of an incompletely developed phoneme system which does not conform in a one-to-one fashion with the adult system. He cites two studies which hypothesize that children with articulatory defects and those without articulatory defects learn new sounds equally well when the learning does not include the particular sounds with which a child has difficulty.

Winitz and Lawrence (1961) compared kindergartners with good and poor articulation on their ability to learn three non-English sounds /x/, /œ/, and /ɛ/. They found no significant differences between the two groups. Winitz and Bellerose in an unpublished piece of research cited in Winitz (1969, p. 131) studied three groups: (1) children with normal articulation; (2) children with defective /r/ phoneme; and (3) children with defective /r/ and /s/ and other articulatory errors. They were tested on their ability to learn /vroʊ/ and /ʃmeɪ/. Learning occurred for /ʃmeɪ/ but not for /vroʊ/. The learning of /ʃmeɪ/ seems to be related to the child's ability to articulate /ʃ/ and /m/ and not to the children's errors that exist in phonemes other than /ʃ/ and /m/.

SPELLING DIFFICULTIES

Two studies show that some kind of relationship seems to exist between spelling and articulatory difficulties. A study by Ham (1958) reports that words that are misarticulated tend to be misspelled more frequently than words that are pronounced correctly, even though the spelling error is not related to the type of mispronunciation, as a [w] for [r] substitution. He notes, therefore, that the presence of articulatory problems may tend to be accompanied by problems in the areas of language skills. He makes no decision as to whether articulation problems contribute to spelling and reading problems or whether all are facets of a general language skills deficit. A study by Zedler (1956) shows the effect of phonic training on speech-sound discrimination and spelling performance. After a series of training periods with stories that emphasize sounds and listening to them, she found that the written spelling performances changed significantly and favorably and that speech-sound discrimination ability increased significantly. She notes that written spelling ability and speech-sound discrimination are significantly related variables.

FAULTY LEARNING

The child may have had no good models to imitate. One of the writers interviewed three children aged 12, 10 and six from the same family. All of them were above average in intelligence. The two older children made so many substitutions for sounds that their speech was almost unintelligible. The youngest child had normal speech. The two older children grew up in a rural environment with no playmates. Their father's speech was normal but their mother's was the original edition of the two older children. The younger child, had, however, because of the illness of the mother, lived with her grandmother in town from the age of six months to five years. The model that the two older girls imitated was in all likelihood the cause of their articulatory disorder. Another example shows the influence of the child's playmates. A small child had parents with excellent speech. She herself, however, from three until six years of age regularly played with children with a decided foreign accent. She had the same kind and amount of foreign accent as the children she played with.

Relationship of Articulatory Difficulties with Reading and Spelling Disabilities

READING DISABILITIES

Research shows that speech and reading are related, particularly where oral reading is involved. Research, however, has not shown the extent of the relationship, for the amount of research is too small to prove or to disprove assumptions. We do know that speech defects and reading difficulties occur concurrently in a certain proportion of children.

Moss (1946) showed that normal-speaking children surpassed deficient speakers in speed of reading and freedom from reading errors. Monroe (1932) in a study of 415 reading defectives (based on both oral and silent reading tests) found that 9 per cent stuttered and 18 per cent had articulatory defects. In a group of 101 nondefective readers, only 1 per cent stuttered and 7 per cent had articulatory defects. Robinson (1946) found in a study of 30 retarded readers that 20 per cent had articulatory defects. Bond (1935) in a study of the auditory and speech characteristics of poor readers compared 64 poor readers with 64 good readers in second and third grades. In silent reading, he found no relationship between speech difficulties and reading difficulties. But he noted that 35 per cent of those children who were poor oral readers but good silent readers had speech defects. No child who was a good oral reader but poor silent reader had a speech difficulty. Moore's (1942) results differed from those just cited. In a study of 123 ninth-grade children with articulatory defects, he found that as a group they ranked above the grade median on the Iowa Silent Reading Test.

Sonenberg and Glass (1965) used the Hejna Articulation Test to test 40 children enrolled in a reading clinic who had reading difficulties, according to the Durrell Analysis of Reading Difficulty. They found that only two children (5 per cent) were free from articulatory errors, whereas 38 (80 per cent) had functional articulatory errors. Forty-seven per cent had some trouble in the area of auditory discrimination; many of the sound substitutions manifested in the study showed up as reading reversals. In the comparative portion of the study, children with articulatory difficulties who received both reading and speech therapy showed discernible reading improvement over those who received reading instruction alone.

The interplay of several factors may cause both articulatory and reading difficulties. Writers in both fields mention similar causes: auditory difficulties, lack of motivation to read or to speak, poor instruction, improper materials for instruction, emotional disturbances, or delayed muscular maturation.

Irwin (1966) designed a study to identify facts or measures predicting improvement in speech, language, and auditory skills for a group of children with misarticulation. She found the following relationships between articulatory development and reading: (1) Progress in word recognition can be predicted by initial scores on Wepman's Auditory Discrimination Test. (2) Vocabulary recognition ability or improvement as measured by the raw score on the Peabody Picture Vocabulary Test can be predicted by freedom from misarticulation. (3) Proficiency or improvement in reading readiness can be predicted by freedom from misarticulation. The normal speakers made significantly higher initial scores than those with misarticulations on the reading readiness tests.

Eames (1950) thinks that both reading and speaking disabilities are likely to have a common cause. For example, he believes that a neurological lesion of the language centers or a failure or inadequacy of auditory association and discrimination may be a common cause for speech difficulty and general linguistic deficiency. Emotional reactions may increase the degree of difficulty in both reading and speaking.

Hildreth (1946) says that a large proportion of children with speech problems tend to be retarded in reading and that speech defects can be an important secondary cause of reading disability. She also makes the point that weakness in auditory discrimination is a common defect that interferes with progress in reading.

Eustis (1947) says the relationship of the speech and reading difficulties may well lie in a delayed muscular maturation. He points out that 48 per cent of children who have specific speech and reading disabilities also showed one or more of the following: left-handedness, ambidexterity, or body clumsiness. He believes that these conditions suggest a combination of symptoms, which involve, among other things, poor muscular coordination due to the slow maturations of coverings of the nerve fibers.

Weaver, Furbee, and Everhart (1960), on the basis of data obtained from administering a speech articulation test and a Gates Reading Readiness Test, conclude that reading readiness and acquisition of adequate speech are to some extent related, although the proportion of variance common to reading readiness measures and articulation measures is quite small. They say that it is possible that the Gates Reading Readiness Test measures part of an underlying variable causal to the acquisition of both reading and speech.

Studies in reading and speech point to auditory discrimination as a causal factor in reading retardation. Wepman's (1959) results of a study of the relationship of auditory discrimination to speech and reading difficulties seem to indicate that delay in the development of auditory discrimination relates positively and probably causally to poor speech articulation, poor reading ability, or both. Christine and Christine's (1964) research provides evidence that poor auditory discrimination is one causal factor of reading retardation and functional articulatory problems among primary-grade children. As noted earlier, Irwin (1966) found that initial scores in Wepman's Auditory Discrimination Test can be used to predict progress in word recognition.

Research tends to indicate that auditory training and a program to develop auditory discrimination are useful to the beginning reader. Silvorski and Wheelock (1966) found that auditory training and an auditory discrimination program helped beginning readers to discriminate more effectively the 33 basic speech sounds. The Sommers studies reported in Chapter 8 show that the effect of speech improvement (which involved analytical ear-training procedures) affected reading skills as expressed in reading factor scores in a significant way. However, higher reading factor scores for children who had speech improvement in first and second grade did not result in higher reading comprehension at the end of the second grade, as compared with those who never received the treatment.

The relationship between articulatory deficiencies and reading difficulties needs further exploration. Our personal belief is that underlying factors, which in turn hinder reading and articulatory development, are due to delays in four developmental functions: (1) sensory-motor, (2) language, (3) perception, (4) higher cognitive processes (Frostig, 1968). The sensory motor functions, developing maximally to two years, give the child an experiential background in using all his sense modalities and movements in his environment. The language functions, developing maximally from one and a half to the age of three or four, help the child to receive and express ideas through speech. The perceptual development, from three and a half to seven and a half years, helps the child to discriminate and recognize stimuli within his environment. He uses largely the modalities of hearing and seeing. His immediate perceptions determine his thought processes. In the development of the higher cognitive processes, the child develops and continues to develop abilities that deepen his awareness and understanding of the environment and of himself as a person. These processes are not limited to the recognition of stimuli that are immediately present. Frostig also names two other functions: social adjustment and emotional development (Frostig, 1968, pp. 105–107).

We believe in a developmental point of view—that a speech clinician is involved in the fostering of the development of all these functions. We believe that the speech clinician working to help the child who substitutes /w/ for /r/ and /l/ cannot separate the therapy involved in correcting the substitution from therapy in language and cognitive functions. We believe the phrase "educating the whole child" is just as applicable to the speech clinician as it is to the teacher. The speech clinician should be involved in developing all facets of language—from helping the child to transform his sentences into larger units to fostering his ability to repeat a series—whether it be numbers or days of the week. We believe, too, that the clinician must be concerned with the child's feelings—that he do what he can to build a positive self-concept in the child, as noted in Chapter 4. Lastly, we believe that the diagnosis and subsequent therapy must be followed by synthesis in the classroom. The communicative skills must exist in a larger sphere than in the therapy room; this concept calls for the kinds of cooperation by members of the school team that were indicated in Chapter 2.

References and Suggested Readings

American Speech and Hearing Association Committee on Legislation, "Need for Speech Pathologists," *ASHA*, I (December, 1959), 138–139

AVANT, V., and C. HUTTON, "Passage for Speech Screening in Upper Elementary Grades," *Journal of Speech and Hearing Disorders*, XXVII (February, 1962), 40–46. (Contains a passage to test articulation and certain aspects of voice.)

American Speech and Hearing Association Research Committee, "Public School Speech and Hearing Services," *Journal of Speech and Hearing Disorders*, Monograph Supplement 8 (July, 1961).

AMATORA, SISTER M., "Psychological Implications of Speech Problems in the Primary Grades," *American Childhood*, XLIII (January, 1958), 28–29.

ARTLEY, A. S., "A Study of Certain Factors Presumed to be Associated with Reading and Speech Difficulties," *Journal of Speech and Hearing Disorders*, XIII (December, 1948), 351–360.

AUNGST, L. F., and J. V. FRICK, "Auditory Discrimination Ability and Consistency of Articulation of /r/," *Journal of Speech and Hearing Disorders*, XXIX (February, 1964), 76–85.

BANGS, J. L., "A Clinical Analysis of the Articulatory Defects of the Feeble-Minded," *Journal of Speech Disorders*, VII (December, 1942), 343–356. (Analyzes the articulatory deficiencies of the feeble-minded. Shows correlations between speech proficiency, chronological age, mental age, and intelligence quotients. Analyzes phonetic errors, the sounds most frequently preferred as substitutions for each sound, all errors for each sound, and the sounds most frequently omitted and added.)

BANKSON, M. W., and M. C. BYRNE, "The Relationship Between Missing Teeth and Selected Consonant Sounds," *Journal of Speech and Hearing Disorders*, XXVII (November, 1962), 341–348.

BARKER, J., and G. ENGLAND, "A Numerical Measure of Articulation: Further Development," *Journal of Speech and Hearing Disorders*, XXVII (February, 1962), 23–27. (Explains the giving of a numerical measure of articulation.)

BELL, D., and A. Hale, "Observations of Tongue-Thrust Swallow in Pre-school Children," *Journal of Speech and Hearing Disorders*, XXVIII (May, 1963), 195–197. (Gives the characteristics of tongue-thrust swallow and the results of the evaluation of 353 children of preschool age.)

BERRY, M., and J. EISENSON, *Speech Disorders: Principles and Practices of Therapy*. New York, Appleton-Century-Crofts, 1956, Chap. 5. (Discusses possible causes of articulatory defects.)

BILTO, E. W., "Motor Abilities of Children with Defective Speech," *Journal of Speech Disorders*, VI (December, 1941), 187–203.

BOND, G. L., *The Auditory and Speech Characteristics of Poor Readers*. New York, Bureau of Publications, Teachers' College, Columbia University, 1935.

BRUNS, J. M., "Experimental Study of Auditory Discrimination Ability of Children with Articulatory Disorders," *Exceptional Child*, XXIII (March, 1957), 264–266.

CABRINI, M. "Auditory Memory Span and Functional Articulatory Disorders in Relation to Reading in Grade II," *Journal of Developmental Reading*, VII (Autumn, 1963), 24–28.

CARTER, E. T., and M. BUCK, " Prognostic Testing for Functional Articulation Disorders Among Children in the First Grade." *Journal of Speech and Hearing Disorders*, XXIII (May, 1958), 124–133.

CARTER, E. T., and M. BUCK, " Prognostic Testing for Functional Articulation Disorders among Children in the First Grade," *Journal of Speech and Hearing Disorders*, XXIII (May, 1958), 124–133.

CARVER, C., " The Aural Analysis of Sounds," *British Journal of Educational Psychology*, XXXVII (November, 1967), 379–380. (Shows the significance of context on ability to identify sounds.)

CHRISTINE, D., and C. CHRISTINE, " The Relationship of Auditory Discrimination to Articulatory Defects and Reading Retardation," *Elementary School Journal*, LV (November, 1964), 97–100.

COHEN, J. H., and C. F. DIEHL, " Relation of Speech-Sound Discrimination Ability to Articulation-Type Speech Defects," *Journal of Speech and Hearing Disorders*, XXVIII (May, 1963), 187–190.

CURTIS, J. F., and J. C. HARDY, "A Phonetic Study of Misarticulation of /r/." *Journal of Speech and Hearing Research*, II (September, 1959), 244–257. (Suggests that phonetic context is an important factor in the articulation process.)

CYPREANSEN, L., " The Standardization of a Speech Articulation Test with the Use of a Colored Filmstrip," *ASHA*, I (November, 1959), 103. (Presents an objective method of studying, recording, and comparing the speech articulatory differences of children.)

DICKSON, S., " Differences Between Children Who Spontaneously Outgrow and Children Who Retain Functional Articulation Errors," *Journal of Speech and Hearing Research*, V (September, 1962), 263–271. (Studies the differences in motor proficiency, auditory discrimination, and emotional characteristics of parents of two groups: (1) those who outgrew functional articulatory errors, and (2) those who did not.)

EAMES, T., " The Relationship of Reading and Speech Difficulties," *Journal of Educational Psychology*, XLI (January, 1950), 51–55.

ELBERT, M., R. SHELTON, Jr., W. B. ARNDT, Jr. "A Task for Evaluation of Articulatory Change," *Journal of Speech and Hearing Research*, X (June, 1967), 281–288. (Examines the feasibility of measuring articulation change on a lesson-to-lesson basis by administration of a brief articulation task at the beginning of every second lesson.)

EUSTIS, R. S., " The Primary Origin of the Specific Language Disabilities," *Journal of Pediatrics*, XXXI (October, 1947), 448–455. (Indicates that the relationship between speech difficulties and reading difficulties may well lie in a delayed neuromuscular maturation.)

EVERHART, R. W., " Literature Survey of Growth and Developmental Factors in Articulatory Maturation." *Journal of Speech and Hearing Disorders*, XXV (February, 1960), 59–69.

FARQUHAR, M., " Prognostic Value of Imitative and Auditory Discrimination

Tests," *Journal of Speech and Hearing Disorders*, XXVI (November, 1961), 342–347.

FERRIER, E. E., "Investigation of ITPA Performance of Children with Functional Defects of Articulation," *Exceptional Child*, XXXII (May, 1966), 625–629.

FLETCHER, S. G., R. L. CASTEEL, and D. P. BRADLEY, "Tongue-Thrust Swallow, Speech Articulation, and Age." *Journal of Speech and Hearing Disorders*, XXVI (August, 1961), 201–208.

FROSTIG, M., and P. MASLOW, "Language Training: A Form of Ability Training," *Journal of Learning Disabilities*, I (February, 1968), 105–115. (Discusses developmental functions of language.)

FRISTOE, M., and R. Goldman, "Comparison of Traditional and Condensed Articulation Tests Examining the Same Number of Sounds," *Journal of Speech and Hearing Research*, XI (September, 1968), 583–589. (Compared testers' ability to listen to and evaluate more than one sound in a word.)

GAINES, F. P., "Interrelations of Speech and Reading Disabilities," *Quarterly Journal of Speech*, XXVII (February, 1941), 104–110.

GOLDMAN, R., and M. FRISTOE, 'The Development of the Filmstrip Articulation Test," *Journal of Speech and Hearing Disorders*, XXXII (August, 1967), 256–262.

HALL, M., "Auditory Factors in Functional Articulatory Speech Defects," *Journal of Experimental Education*, VII (December, 1938), 110–132.

HAM, R. E., "Relationship Between Misspelling and Misarticulation," *Journal of Speech and Hearing Disorders*, XXIII (August, 1958), 294–297.

HEALEY, W., and W. Hall, *A Study of the Articulatory Skills of Children from 3–9 Years of Age.* Unpublished doctoral dissertation, University of Missouri, 1963. (Tells at what ages sounds are acquired.)

HILDRETH, G., "Speech Defects and Reading Disability," *Elementary School Journal*, XLVI (February, 1946), 326–332.

HOFFMAN, J. A., and R. L. HOFFMAN, "Tongue-Thrust and Deglutition: Some Anatomical, Physiological, and Neurological Considerations," *Journal of Speech and Hearing Disorders*, XXX (May, 1965), 105–120. (Covers anatomy and development of the tongue, growth of oral cavity, pharyngeal space for the tongue, deglutition and the tongue, and tongue-thrust as a speech problem.)

IRWIN, R. B. "Effectiveness of Speech Therapy for Second-Grade Children with Misarticulations: Predictive Factors." *Exceptional Child*, XXXII (March, 1966), 471–479.

————, "The Effects of Speech Therapy upon Certain Linguistic Skills of First-Grade Children," *Journal of Speech and Hearing Disorders*, XXVIII (November, 1963), 375–381. (Evaluates the effects of speech therapy upon articulatory adequacy, reading achievement, word recognition, word meaning, auditory discrimination, and sound stimulability.)

IRWIN, R. B., and B. W. MUSSELMAN, "A Compact Picture Articulation Test," *Journal of Speech and Hearing Disorders*, XXVII (February, 1962), 36–39. (Contains a picture test that checks more than one sound in a word.)

JENKINS, E., and F. E. LOHR, "Severe Articulation Disorders and Motor Ability," *Journal of Speech and Hearing Disorders,* XXVIX (August, 1964), 286–292. (Compares motor proficiency as measured by the Oseretsky Tests of Motor Proficiency of 38 first-grade children with severe articulation defects with 38 normal-speaking children.)

JOHNSON, W., et al., *Speech-Handicapped School Children,* 3rd ed. New York, Harper & Row, Publishers, 1967, Chap. 3. (Discusses causes and treatment of articulatory disorders.)

JORDAN, E. P., "Articulation Test Measures and Listener Ratings of Articulation Defectiveness." *Journal of Speech and Hearing Research,* III (December, 1960), 303–318.

KARLIN, I. W., A. C. YOUTZ, and L. KENNEDY, "Distorted Speech in Young Children," *American Journal of Diseases of Children,* LIX (June 1940), 1203–1218. (Compares ability to perform tasks requiring motor speed of children with defective speech with normal-speaking children.)

KEENAN, J. S., "What Is Medial Position?" *Journal of Speech and Hearing Disorders,* XXVI (May, 1961), 171–177.

KLEFFNER, F. R., *A Comparison of the Reactions of a Group of Fourth-Grade Children to Recorded Examples of Defective and Non-Defective Articulation.* Ph.D. thesis, University of Wisconsin, 1952.

LANDERS, M. T., "Maturation Versus Speech Correction at the Kindergarten Level," *ASHA,* I (November, 1959), 80.

LEE, L. L., "Developmental Sentence Types: A Method for Comparing Normal and Deviant Syntactical Development," *Journal of Speech and Hearing Disorders,* XXXI (November, 1966), 211–330. (Investigates the development of syntactic structure in two children, one with normal speech development and one with delayed speech development.)

LENCIONE, R. M., and N. C. Trent, "Evaluation of Articulation Testing Using Spontaneous and Imitative Procedures," *ASHA,* VII (October, 1965), 380.

LEWIS, J. A., and R. F. COUNIHAN, "Tongue-Thrust in Infancy," *Journal of Speech and Hearing Disorders,* XXX (August, 1965), 280–282. (Defines tongue-thrust. Investigates whether or not tongue-thrust swallow is normal in infancy.)

LIBERMAN, A., K. S. HARRIS, P. EINAS, L. LISKER, and J. BASTIAN, "An Effect of Learning on Speech Perception: The Discrimination of Durations of Silence with and without Phonemic Significance," *Language and Speech,* IV (October–December, 1961), 175–176.

LIBERMAN, A. M., K. S. HARRIS, J. A. KINNEY, H. LANE, "The Discrimination of Relative Onset-Time of the Components of Certain Speech and Nonspeech Patterns," *Journal of Experimental Psychology,* LVI (May, 1961), 379–388.

LIBERMAN, A. M., K. S. HARRIS, H. S. HOFFMAN, and B. G. GRIFFITH, "The Discrimination of Speech Sounds Within and Across Phonemic Boundaries," *Journal of Experimental Psychology,* LIV (November, 1957), 358–368. (Investigates the relation between phonetic labeling and discrimination in one language and within one group of phonemes.)

McDonald, E. T., *Articulation Testing and Treatment: A Sensory-Motor Approach*. Pittsburgh, Stanwix, 1964.

Mange, C. V., "Relationships Between Selected Auditory Perceptual Factors and Articulation Ability," *Journal of Speech and Hearing Research*, III (March, 1960), 67–73.

Mase, D. J., *Etiology of Articulatory Defects*. New York, Bureau of Publications, Teachers' College, Columbia University, 1946.

Maxwell, K. L., *A Comparison of Certain Motor Performances of Children with Normal Speech and Children with Defective Consonant Articulation*. Unpublished Ph.D. thesis, University of Michigan, 1953.

Menyuk, P., "Comparing Grammar of Children with Functionally Deviant and Normal Speech," *Journal of Speech and Hearing Research*, VII (June, 1963), 109–122.

———, "The Role of Distinctive Features in Children's Acquisition of Phonology," *Journal of Speech and Hearing Research*, XI (March, 1968), 138–146.

Metraux, R. W., "Auditory Memory Span for Speech Sounds: Norms for Children," *Journal of Speech Disorders*, IX (March, 1944), 31–38.

Moll, K. L., and F. L. Darley, "Attitudes of Mothers of Articulatory-Impaired and Speech-Retarded Children," *Journal of Speech and Hearing Disorders*, XXV (November, 1960), 377–384.

Monroe, M., *Children Who Cannot Read*. Chicago, University of Chicago Press, 1932. (Includes a study on relationship between reading and speaking difficulties and one on the influence of poor auditory discrimination upon reading.)

Moore, C. E. H., "Reading and Arithmetic Abilities Associated with Speech Defects," *Journal of Speech Disorders*, XII (March, 1942), 85–86.

Moss, M., "The Effect of Speech Defects on Second-Grade Reading Achievement," *Quarterly Journal of Speech*, XXIV (December, 1938), 642–654.

Nichols, A. C., "Pilot Studies of the Influence of Stimulus Variables on Articulation Test Scores," *Journal of Communication Disorders*, I (1967), 170–174. (Indicates that noise in the testing environment and the intensity of the responses of the person tested affect the scores.)

Oyer, H. J., "Speech Error Recognition Ability," *Journal of Speech and Hearing Disorders*, XXIV (November, 1959), 391–394. (Assesses speech error recognition ability of two groups of college seniors: 20 majoring in speech and hearing therapy and 20 majoring in elementary education. Finds there is no significant difference in speech error recognition ability between seniors in elementary education and seniors in speech and hearing therapy.)

Palmer, J. M., "Tongue-Thrusting: A Clinical Hypothesis," *Journal of Speech and Hearing Disorders*, XXVII (November, 1962), 323–333. (Defines tongue-thrust. Gives its symptomatology in detail.)

Patton, F. E., "A Comparison of the Kinaesthetic Sensibility of Speech of Defective and Normal Speaking Children," *Journal of Speech Disorders*, VII (December, 1942), 305–310.

PENDERGAST, K., "Articulation Study of 15,255 Seattle First-Grade Children with and Without Kindergarten," *Exceptional Child*, XXXII (April, 1966), 541–547. (Shows that those children who attended kindergarten did not appear to have fewer sound errors when they entered first grade than those who did not attend kindergarten.)

POOLE, I., "Genetic Development of Consonant Sounds in English," *Elementary English Review*, XI (June, 1934), 159–161. (Includes the ages at which boys and girls normally attain the mastery of certain speech sounds.)

PRINS, D. T., "Abilities of Children with Misarticulations," *Journal of Speech and Hearing Research*, V (June, 1962), 161–168[a]. (Compared subgroups of children with different types of functional articulatory difficulties with normal-speaking children on variables such as intelligence as measured by receptive vocabulary and motor skills.)

———, "Analysis of Correlations Among Various Articulatory Deviations," *Journal of Speech and Hearing Research*, V (June, 1962), 152–160[b]. Correlated aspects of subjects with a high proportion of interdental lisping errors, those with a high proportion of omissions, and those with a variety of other errors with aspects of normal-speaking children.)

———, "Relation Among Specific Articulatory Deviations and Responses to a Clinical Measure of Sound Discrimination Ability," *Journal of Speech and Hearing Disorders*, XXVIII (November, 1963), 382–387. (Evaluates sound discrimination in relation to sound production.)

REID, G., "The Efficacy of Speech Re-Education of Functional Articulatory Defectives in the Elementary School," *Journal of Speech Disorders*, XII (December, 1947), 303–312. (Tells how children with functional articulatory defects are inefficient in intellectual self-expression until they learn to speak correctly.)

———, "The Etiology and Nature of Functional Articulatory Defects in Elementary School Children," *Journal of Speech Disorders*, XII (June, 1947), 143–150.

ROBINSON, H., *Why Pupils Fail in Reading*. Chicago, University of Chicago Press, 1946.

ROE, V., and R. MILISEN, "The Effect of Maturation upon Defective Articulation in Elementary Grades," *Journal of Speech Disorders*, VII (March, 1942), 37–50.

RONSON, I., "Incidence of Visceral Swallow Among Lispers," *Journal of Speech and Hearing Disorders*, XXX (November, 1965), 318–324. (Determines the incidence of visceral swallow and explores the validity of certain diagnostic procedures developed by investigators for determining visceral swallow.)

SAYLER, H. K., "The Effect of Maturation upon Defective Articulation in Grades 7–12," *Journal of Speech and Hearing Disorders*, XIV (September, 1949), 202–207. (Indicates sounds most commonly missed. Shows a slight decrease in the mean number of articulatory errors from Grades 7–10.)

SCHIEFELBUSCH, R. L., and M. J. LINDSEY, "A New Test of Sound Discrimination," *Journal of Speech and Hearing Disorders*, XXIII (May, 1958), 153–159.

SCHLANGER, B. B., and G. I. GALANOWSKY, " Auditory Discrimination Tasks Performed by Mentally Retarded and Normal Children," *Journal of Speech and Hearing Research*, IX (September, 1966), 434–440. (Compared a group of 85 institutionalized mentally retarded children with 65 normal children on a battery of auditory discrimination tests. The subjects were matched for mental age.)

SCHNEIDERMAN, N., "A Study of the Relationship Between Articulatory Ability and Language Ability," *Journal of Speech and Hearing Disorders*, XX (December, 1955), 359–364.

SHERMAN, D., and A. GEITH, " Speech-Sound Discrimination and Articulation Skill," *Journal of Speech and Hearing Research*, X (June, 1967), 277–280. (Compared a group of kindergartners with high speech-sound discrimination with a group with low sound discrimination on various measures: intelligence, articulation.)

SHRINER, T. H., M. S. HALLOWAY, and R. G. DANILOFF, " The Relationship Between Articulation Deficits and Syntax in Speech-Defective Children," *Journal of Speech and Hearing Research*, XII (June, 1969), 319–325.

SIEGEL, G. M., " Experienced and Inexperienced Articulation Examiners," *Journal of Speech and Hearing Disorders*, XXVII (February, 1962), 28–34. (Studies the ability of the inexperienced to test after they have been given minimal training.)

SIEGEL, G. M., H. WINITZ, and H. CONKEY, " The Influence of Testing Instruments on Articulatory Responses of Children," *Journal of Hearing and Speech Disorders*, XXVIII (February, 1963), 67–76. (Investigated the effects of test construction and of method of presenting word stimuli during articulatory testing.)

SILVAROLI, N. J., and W. H. WHEELOCK, " Investigation of Auditory Discrimination Training for Beginning Readers," *Reading Teacher*, XX (December, 1966), 247–251.

SMITH, C. R., "Articulation Problems and Ability to Store Articulation and Process Stimuli," *Journal of Speech and Hearing Research*, X (June, 1967), 348–353. (Compares the performance of children with nonorganic articulatory problems with children with normal speech as to the short-term storage of auditory and visual stimuli.)

SMITH, M. W., and S. AINSWORTH, " The Effects of Three Types of Stimulation on Articulatory Responses of Speech-Defective Children," *Journal of Speech and Hearing Research*, X (June, 1967), 333–338. (Studied whether children with defective articulation produced the same number of articulatory errors when their speech was stimulated by three different methods: picture stimulus, auditory stimulus, and auditory-visual stimulus.)

SNOW, K., "Articulation Proficiency in Relation to Certain Dental Abnormalities," *Journal of Speech and Hearing Disorders*, XXVI (August, 1961), 209–212. (Studies the articulation of six consonant sounds for which the upper central incisor teeth are ordinarily considered important.)

SNOW, K. A., "A Detailed Analysis of Articulation Responses of 'Normal' First-Grade Children," *Journal of Speech and Hearing Research*, VI (September, 1963), 277–290. (Reports on the frequency of substitutions for various sounds.)

SOLOMON, A. L., "Emotional and Behavior Problems of First-Grade Children with Functional Defects of Articulation." *ASHA*, II (October, 1960), 378.

SOMMERS, R. K., W. J. MEYER, and A. K. FENTON, "Pitch Discrimination and Articulation," *Journal of Speech and Hearing Research*, IV (March, 1961), 56–60. (Investigates pitch discrimination in school children with functional articulation errors in grades 3 to 12.)

———, "Factors Related to the Effectiveness of Articulation Therapy for Kindergarten, First and Second Grade Children." *Journal of Speech and Hearing Research*, X (September, 1967), 428–437.

SONENBERG, C., and G. G. GLASS, "Reading and Speech: An Incidence and Treatment Study," *The Reading Teacher*, XIX (December, 1965), 197–201. (Compared children with reading difficulties who received speech therapy with those who did not receive speech therapy.)

SPRIESTERBACH, D. C., "Research in Articulation Disorders and Personality," *Journal of Speech and Hearing Disorders*, XXI (September, 1956), 329–335. (Reviews literature which shows the relationship or lack of it between articulation disorders and personality.)

STEER, M. C., and H. G. DREXLER, "Predicting Later Articulation Ability from Kindergarten Tests," *Journal of Speech and Hearing Disorders*, XXV (November, 1960), 391–397.

TEMPLIN, M. C., *Certain Language Skills in Children: Their Development and Interrelationships*, Minneapolis, University of Minnesota Press, 1957.

———, "Norms on a Screening Test of Articulation for Ages 3–8," *Journal of Speech and Hearing Disorders*, XVIII (December, 1953), 323–331. (Compares articulatory ability of boys and girls. Indicates when boys and girls reach approximately mature articulation.)

———, "Spontaneous Versus Imitated Vocalization in Testing Articulation in Preschool Children," *Journal of Speech Disorders*, XII (December, 1947), 293–300.

———, "A Study of the Sound Discrimination Ability of Elementary School Pupils," *Journal of Speech Disorders*, VIII (June, 1943), 127–132. (Contains a short test of sound discrimination. Indicates the relationship of position of discriminative element to error.)

THOMAS, B. M., "Informational Processing Ability of Children with Articulation Problems as Compared with Normal Children," *ASHA*, I (November, 1959), 106. (Compares the informational processing ability of children with articulation problems with children with normal speech.)

THORNDIKE, E. L., and I. LORGE, *The Teacher's Word Book of 30,000 Words*. New York, Bureau of Publications, Teachers' College, Columbia University, 1944.

VANDEMARK, A. A., and M. B. MANN, "Oral Language Skills of Children with Defective Articulation," *Journal of Speech and Hearing Research*, VIII (December, 1965), 409–414. (Investigates the oral language achievement of children with defective articulation to determine if such children differ from children with normal articulation, as indicated by quantitative language measures.)

VAN RIPER, C., *Speech Correction: Principles and Methods*, 4th ed. Englewood Cliffs, N.J., Prentice-Hall, Inc., 1963. Chap. 7.

———, and R. Erickson, "A Predictive Screening Test of Articulation," *Journal of Speech and Hearing Disorders*, XXXIV (August, 1969), 214–217. (Describes a test designed to identify children who have articulatory defects but who will overcome these difficulties without speech therapy.)

———, and J. V. IRWIN, *Voice and Articulation*. Englewood Cliffs, N.J., Prentice-Hall, Inc., 1958.

VENTURA, B. P., G. INGEBO, and P. WOLMUT, "A Comparative Evaluation of Speech Correction Techniques in the Primary Grades and the Role of Maturation on Misarticulation," *ASHA*, II (October, 1960), 378.

VOEGELIN, C. F., and S. ADAMS, "A Phonetic Study of Young Children's Speech," *Journal of Experimental Education*, XIII (December, 1934), 107–116. (Studies the substitution of sounds made by children. Shows the inconsistency existing in children's articulatory errors.)

WARD, M. M., SISTER H. D. MALONE, and G. R. and H. W. JANN, "Articulation Variations Associated with Visceral Swallowing and Malocclusion," *Journal of Speech and Hearing Disorders*, XXVI (November, 1961), 334–341.

WEAVER, C. H., C. FURBEE, and R. W. EVERHART, "Articulatory Competency and Reading Readiness," *Journal of Speech and Hearing Research*, III (June, 1960), 174–180.

WEPMAN, J. M., "Auditory Discrimination, Speech, and Reading," *Elementary School Journal*, LV (March, 1960), 325–333. (Shows the relationship between auditory discrimination and speech accuracy of articulation and between poor reading ability and auditory discrimination.)

———, "Relationships of Auditory Discrimination to Speech and Reading Difficulties," *ASHA*, I (November, 1959), 96.

Wilson, F. B., "Efficacy of Speech Therapy with Educable Mentally Retarded Children," *Journal of Speech and Hearing Research*, IX (September, 1966), 423–433. (Evaluates the articulatory abilities of 777 educable mentally retarded children. Indicates the types of errors that exist in this group.)

WINITZ, H., *Articulatory Acquisition and Behavior*. New York, Appleton-Century-Crofts, 1969. (Includes material on prelanguage articulatory development, phonetic and phonemic development, variables related to articulatory development and performance, articulatory testing and predicting, articulatory programming.)

———, "Temporal Reliability in Articulatory Testing," *Journal of Speech and Hearing Disorders*, XXVIII (August, 1963), 247–251.

———, and B. BELLEROSE, "Effects of Pretraining on Sound Discrimination Learning," *Journal of Speech and Hearing Research*, VI (June, 1963), 171–180. (Studies discrimination learning of 200 first- and second-grade children as a function of several pretraining conditions.)

———, "Phoneme-Cluster Learning as a Function of Instructional Method and Age," *Journal of Verbal Learning and Behavior,* IV (April, 1965), 98–102. (Determines whether the development of an articulatory response would be facilitated in a familiar speech unit that did not evoke a previously learned word, and what the effects of chronological age are on sound learning.)

———, " Sound Discrimination as a Function of Pretraining Conditions," *Journal of Speech and Hearing Research,* V (December, 1962), 340–348.

WOLFE, W. D., " The Nature and Frequency of Misarticulation Relationship to Method of Eliciting Speech," *ASHA,* II (October, 1960), 374. (Measures and compares articulation responses of children during oral reading and conversation.)

WOOD, K. S., "Parental Maladjustment and Functional Articulatory Defects in Children," *Journal of Speech Disorders,* XI (December, 1946), 255–275.

YEDINACK, J. G., "A Study of the Linguistic Functions of Children with Articulation and Reading Disabilities," *Journal of Genetic Psychology,* LXXIV (March, 1949), 23–50.

ZEDLER, E. Y., " Effect of Phonic Training on Speech Sound Discrimination and Spelling Performance," *Journal of Speech and Hearing Disorders,* XXI (June, 1956), 245–250.

Articulation Tests

Arizona Articulation Proficiency Scale, by J. Barker. (Provides a measure by percentage of correctly articulated speech sounds.) Western Psychological Services, 12035 Wilshire Boulevard, Los Angeles, California 90025.

Articulation, Testing and Treatment: A Sensory Motor Approach. A Deep Test of Articulation by E. T. McDonald. (Based on constructs derived from motor and acoustic phonetics, control theory, developmental psychology, and linguistics.) Stanwix House, Pittsburgh, Pennsylvania.

Developmental Articulation Test, by R. F. Hejna (Revised Edition). (Assesses articulatory development of children.) Speech Materials, Box 1713, Ann Arbor, Michigan.

The Lardon Articulation Scale, by W. Edmonstron. (Developmental analysis of articulation.) Western Psychological Services, Los Angeles, California.

Photo Articulation Test, by K. Pendergast, S. E. Dickey, J. W. Selmar, and A. L. Soder. (Tests all consonants, vowels, and diphthongs. Final series used to elicit story to assess language.) The King Company, Chicago, Ill, 60625.

The Riley Articulation and Language Test, by G. D. Riley. 2½ mins. (Provides an Articulation loss score.) Western Psychological Services, Los Angeles, California.

Screening Deep Test of Articulation, by E. T. McDonald. 5 mins. (Tests nine commonly misarticulated sounds in 10 contexts.) Stanwix House, Pittsburgh, Pennsylvania.

The Templin–Darley Test of Articulation, by M. C. Templin and F. L. Darley. Bureau of Education Research and Service, Division of Extension and University Services, University of Iowa, Iowa City, Iowa.

Language Tests

Houston Test for Language Development, by Margaret Crabtree. (Tests language abilities in children through six years.) Houston Test Company, Houston, Texas.

The Illinois Test of Psycholinguistic Abilities, by S. Kirk and J. McCarthy (Revised Edition). (Assesses aspects of linguistic behavior. Designed as a diagnostic instrument.) University of Illinois, Urbana, Illinois.

Peabody Picture Vocabulary Test. Forms A & B, by L. M. Dunn. Tests recognition vocabulary. Can be converted to M. A. American Guidance Service, Nashville, Tenn.

Utah Test of Language Development, by M. J. Mecham, J. L. Jex, and J. D. Jones (1967 Edition). (Tests both receptive and expressive language from one year to 15 years.) Communication Research Association, Salt Lake City, Utah.

Full Range Picture Vocabulary Test, by R. B. Ammons and H. S. Ammons. (Intelligence test based on verbal comprehension.) Psychological Test Specialists, Box 1441, Missoula, Montana.

Verbal Language Development Scale, by M. J. Mecham. American Guidance Service, Minneapolis, Minn.

Auditory Discrimination Tests

Auditory Discrimination Test, by Joseph M. Wepman. (Tests to determine child's ability to recognize fine differences that exist between sounds in American English. Measures ability to hear accurately.) 950 East 59th Street, Chicago 37, Ill.

A Picture Type Speech-Sound Discrimination Test, by W. Pronovost and C. Dumbleton. (This test is based on pictures with word pairs phonetically balanced so that only one sound varies in each word of a pair.) *Journal of Speech and Hearing Disorders,* XVIII (1953), 266.

Templin Auditory Discrimination Tests, by Mildred C. Templin, in *Certain Language Skills in Children.* Minneapolis, University of Minnesota Press, 1957, p. 159.

Problems

1. Give an articulatory test to four children. How many of the children appear to have articulatory difficulties?
2. Give the test on sound discrimination from one of the sources suggested on page 235 to five children of the same age. Indicate differences in their levels of ability.
3. Visit a high school or elementary school class. Indicate how many articulatory defects you heard and the kind of defects they were.

4. Visit a class conducted by a speech clinician. List the substitutions, omissions, or distortions of sounds of one of the observed children.
5. If a case history of a child with an articulatory defect is available to you in a school or clinic, check from it the information relative to the child's intelligence, hearing ability, emotional health, and structural abnormalities of the speaking mechanism.
6. Plan and have a group discussion on the relationship of reading, spelling, and articulatory difficulties.
7. Read and report on one of the following: Aungst and Frick, 1964; Bell and Hale, 1963; Cabrini, 1963; Cohen and Diehl, 1963; Frostig and Maslow, 1968; Sherman and Geith, 1967; Siegel and others, 1963; Silvaroli and Wheelock, 1966; Snow, 1963; Vandemark and Mann, 1965.

Chapter 11

Defects of Articulation (11)

Treatment of Articulatory Difficulties

We have already discussed the possible causes for articulatory difficulties. Some of these causes point to the need for the assistance of other specialists in solving the problems of the youngster with an articulatory difficulty. The teacher, his supervisor, principal, and the speech clinician must be aware of this need, for the child's defective articulation may be but the symptom of another difficulty.

Finding the Cause

Both the teacher and the clinician take into account the stage of development of the child. The child of six who substitutes a [w] for an [l] is probably in no need of immediate speech help, for in all likelihood maturity alone will take care of the difficulty. But when a child of the same age confuses [p] and [b], he is in need of help, because by six years of age he should be distinguishing accurately between these two sounds. As the child is learning to speak, he frequently omits sounds, distorts them, or substitutes one sound for another. These conditions in the young child are often part of a particular step in his development. The teacher and the clinician must decide whether a child needs speech therapy. In the preceding chapter we discussed the part that maturation plays in articulation and cited the studies that take it into account in making a prognosis on an articulatory defect.

Because in some instances the child's speaking mechanism may be inadequate, the clinician should observe it. He finds out whether the child has an underbite, overbite, or malocclusion that is an obstacle to his making certain sounds easily. As a result of his examination, he may recommend the child's seeing his dentist or orthodontist. The importance of organic factors should not be overemphasized. As noted in the previous chapter, many children with oral anomalies such as marked overbites nevertheless do articulate proficiently. In many instances, oral structural deviations constitute a contributing rather than a sole cause for speech difficulties. The clinician also examines the child's health record to see whether another medical problem exists or has existed. The incidence of such problems as polio, cleft palate, cerebral palsy, or a thyroid deficiency may appear on his record. Furthermore, when obvious difficulty with muscular coordination or symptoms such as constant colds or listlessness suggest a poor physical condition, the clinician refers the child to his doctor through the health officials of the school.

When an emotional difficulty causes or partly causes the defective speech of a child, he may or may not respond to treatment for the articulatory disorder alone. If he does respond, the symptom, but not the cause, may be removed. In such instances, the school psychologist helps the child; his help may come before the child's speech correction or be given concurrently with it. The psychologist administers intelligence and personality tests to the child that assist the other persons who are teaching him to understand him and his problems. He advises those teaching the child how to handle him. Frequently the psychologist works with the child himself and with his parents to help them better understand themselves and those around them. With the aid of the psychologist, their adjustment to one another and to society improves.

No obvious reason for the many articulatory errors of an eight-year-old girl of average intelligence was evident. But as the school psychologist talked with the family, he found the mother to be oversolicitous and a sister, four years older, overprotective. The mother, confined to a wheel chair, wanted both girls to do well and set very high standards for them. She was a kind, likeable person, anxious to do all she could for her children. The psychologist conferred with the mother and helped the teacher and the clinician to understand the child and the parents. He suggested to all three ways of assisting the child to develop self-confidence. The child began to take and accept responsibility. The older sister learned to let the younger child work out her own problems and to allow her to play and live with other youngsters more normally. Concurrently with the psychological help, the speech clinician worked with the child's speech and the teacher reinforced the work. The psychologist's help made the work of both the clinician and the teacher more effective. Not all children and perhaps not even most children with articulatory defects are so badly adjusted that they need help from a psychologist. Many of them use incorrect sounds simply because of faulty learning. When needed, however, psychological help is important and uniquely effective.

As noted earlier, children with functional articulation difficulties are likely to be deficient in language functions. Research seems to indicate, however, that children with certain specific articulatory difficulties may not have language deficits. Prins' research (1968) raises the probability that children with an interdental /s/ and children whose substitutions involve only one phonetic feature distinct from the correct sound will not be deficient in language abilities; these children are not below normal-speaking children in intelligence, as measured by a verbal test, and in socioeconomic status. Again using Prins' research as a guide, children with omissions and substitutions involving differences from the correct sound of more than one phonetic feature would seem likely to be deficient in language; their I.Q. scores and socioeconomic statuses are lower than those of normal-speaking children. For those children, language should be evaluated. The Illinois Test of Psycholinguistic Abilities may well be administered to children with functional articulatory difficulties who seem to be deficient in language. With this information, the clinician can plan therapy that will help to build the needed language abilities. For instance, the child who does not do well in expressing ideas verbally but who *does* do well in expressing ideas through gesture may at first be provided with opportunities to express ideas largely through pantomime. After communication through pantomime is successful, the expression will then become more and more verbal.

Interpreting the Articulatory Test

The examiner gains considerable information about the child's articulatory difficulty through articulation testing. He finds out which sounds are omitted or distorted and what sounds are substituted for what other sounds. He discovers whether the deviant sound occurs before stressed or unstressed vowels, between vowels, in initial or final position of a syllable, or in a cluster as /r/ in *street* or /s/ in *lips*; he finds out whether the sound is ever correctly uttered and if so, where. That such a preliminary analysis is important is evident from a study by Wentland and Minific (1965) who in testing 25 first grade children with functional /r/ difficulties for their utterance of /r/ in 211 different phonetic contexts found that the most successful production occurred in clusters and the least successful in intersyllabic vocalic formations. Such information, the result of a deep test of articulation, is of value in articulation therapy. The correctionist also compares the phonetic features of the deviant sound with the phonetic features of the correct sound. This information is helpful in determining the kind of involvement of the articulatory difficulty. He discovers whether categories of defects occur. For example, whether the unvoiced sounds are used for voiced sounds, whether stops are used for fricatives, whether the place of articulation of several sounds is moved forward. He learns whether the child can say the sound accurately in nonsense syllables. For example, he says to the child who does not make *k* correctly, "Repeat after me."

kay may	[ke me]
meekeem	[mi kim]
fawk	[fɔk]

When the child makes the sound correctly in certain positions, or when he makes it accurately in nonsense syllables, retraining is usually easier.

The speech clinician considers various other factors. For example, he finds out whether the sounds the child is missing are those that he should have acquired early or late. This information helps him to determine in part the influence of maturity. He checks to see whether or not the sounds the child says incorrectly are those readily visible. He learns whether they are high- or low-frequency sounds, for a hearing loss may cause the lack of perception of these sounds for a particular individual. He ascertains whether other members of the same family make the same substitutions, distortions, or omissions.

Finally, the examiner finds out which incorrect or omitted sounds influence the child's pattern of speech the most. Bud, a 10-year-old boy who made a [θ] sound for [s], said, "The kith thay I talk like a thithy. My th'th, you know." He realized that his speech sounded out of place. This boy, who liked to box, ride a bike fast, and play baseball, was "all boy." Although he said [t] and [d] for [θ] and [ð], [t] and [d] for [tʃ] and [dʒ], [w] for [l] and [r], he himself was most concerned about his [s]. To his listeners the [w] for [l] and [r] was also a part of the "sissy speech." Bud went on to tell the speech clinician that almost every word has an *s* in it; he pointed out that he lived on Sycamore Street. In this instance, the clinician attacked the [s] first. Bud was so strongly motivated that his improvement was rapid.

Some sounds occur more frequently than others. Mader (1954) indicates the relative frequency of consonant sounds in the speech of children in the primary grades. Five sounds, [n], [t], [d], [r] and [s], make up 40 per cent of the total occurrence of all sounds.

The factors just mentioned help the clinician to determine whether he will work with categories of sounds and to determine the order in which he and the child will attack the categories or the individual sounds. In general the clinician works first with the sounds or categories of sounds the child can correct most easily, for success brings approval and a feeling of well-being to the child. As the child hears his corrected speech recorded, he is happy. Sometimes, however, the sounds most easily corrected are not the sounds that distort the child's speech the most—or they are not the sounds about which the child is most concerned. In such cases the clinician and the teacher must use their best judgment.

Motivation for Correction of Sounds

Not all children are as strongly motivated as Bud, the 10-year-old lisper. Some children do not even know that they are making sounds incorrectly. Others seemingly do not care. As in all learning, children must want to speak acceptably. The classroom teacher, particularly in the lower grades, can build an attitude that acceptable speech, like good manners, is a personal asset. After a speech clinician had worked several years with both children and teachers in a small school system, the principal of the school said, "I am *most* pleased with the improvement of speech at the basketball games. The boys and girls sound grown up." The comment not only reflected the attitude of the principal and his teachers but also showed that their attitudes had influenced the children.

Because children do not hear themselves accurately, a recording device proves helpful. At first, they may not believe their own ears, but as they listen to the recordings of the speech of others, they become convinced that the recording of their own speech is accurate. When for the first time a seventh-grade girl heard herself making [f] and [v] for [θ] and [ð], she did not believe that it was herself speaking. As she became convinced that the recording was accurate, she was astonished and hurt. She wailed, "Nobody ever told me." As she was strongly motivated and intelligent, she improved rapidly. When she left the school, her teacher offered her the record on which her speech was recorded. Her response, "I don't ever want to remember I talked like that," was revealing.

Correcting the Sound

CASES THE CLASSROOM TEACHER HANDLES

When the distorted or incorrect sound is the result of structural or organic difficulty, the classroom teacher needs the help of the speech clinician. For example, if the malocclusion of the teeth is such that a wide space is apparent between the two sets of teeth, the classroom teacher will rely on the clinician to teach the *s*. The clinician will teach the child a compensatory way of making the sound. He will find out how the child attempts to produce the sound and discover what structures the child does have that he could use for the essential mechanics of the sound. By explaining to him how to make the sound, using a mirror, and showing him how to manipulate his mechanism, the speech clinician helps the child to make the sound. For such correction, specialized knowledge and training are necessary.

Where, however, the child does not need to be taught compensatory movements and where he can make the sound correctly by imitating the teacher's nonsense syllable, the teacher can retrain him. But the teacher must be careful to remember that his own way of making a sound may be unorthodox and that variations occur in the making of a sound. *S*, for example, may be made with the tongue pointing to the teeth ridge or to a point behind the lower teeth. In fact, the teacher must have training and practice before working with children with speech difficulties. Furthermore, it is advisable that the classroom teacher's speech correction work be done under the supervision of a speech clinician.

Steps in Correcting the Individual Defective Sound

The steps in correcting the individual defective sound frequently are:

1. Teaching the child to recognize both his error and the correct sound.

2. Teaching the correct sound in syllables.

3. Teaching the correct sound in a limited number of commonly used words.

4. Teaching the child to carry over the correction into his everyday speech.

TEACHING THE CHILD TO RECOGNIZE HIS ERROR AND TO PERCEIVE THE CORRECT SOUND

In teaching the child to recognize his error and the correct sound, the speech clinician must work from an assessment of the child's discriminatory ability. Not all children with defective articulation need discrimination training, but many seemingly do. Discrimination tests are listed at the end of the preceding chapter.

In general research shows that discrimination errors tend to occur in phonetic contexts that contain the child's deviant sound. Thus, types of articulatory errors may be related to specific discrimination abilities or the learning that took place in learning the deviant sound may be reflected in the discrimination tests. Winitz and Bellerose (1962a), as cited in the previous chapter, would seem to support the second premise. At any rate, the research indicates that sound discrimination training involving the particular deviant sound is imperative.

The speech clinician, therefore, stresses discrimination between the acceptably uttered sound and the deviant one. He first helps the child to identify the sound. For example, with three children, one with a deviant /s/, one with a deviant /l/, and one with a deviant /r/, he might ask each to raise his hand as *his* sound is uttered. With small children he would label the sound as the hissing sound, the lollipop sound, and the airplane sound. He might then read this sentence: "I'm going to serve for dinner: celery soup, left-over roast beef made into stew, Lyonnaise potatoes, rolls, a salad of lettuce, lima beans, a relish—and, finally, for dessert, a choice of raspberries or strawberries with ice cream." Or he may ask the child to read the sentence and encircle his sound. Or he may provide pictures asking the child to encircle the pictures that contain his sound. Or in a simple short sentence like "For lunch I had a roast beef sandwich, lemonade, and rice pudding," he may ask the children to count the /r/'s, /s/'s, and /l/'s and then indicate which words contain the sound.

Secondly, he helps the child to discriminate between the acceptably uttered and the deviant sound. He can read the same sentence making errors on some of the sounds; when he makes an error, the child can tap the table or raise his hand. The speech clinician can also say a word with the sound uttered acceptably and the same word with its deviant sound, asking whether the first or second is right. He can then reverse the procedure.

The clinician or teacher does well to remember Ritterman's (1969) finding that ability to produce an unfamiliar sound may develop as a function of the ability to contrast that sound with other sounds; hence discrimination ability is more a function of the number of available cues (distinctive features) than of the type of cues available. In discrimination teaching the teacher can point to these clues: manner of production, articulatory position, and the vocal component. As the child works on distinguishing /θʌm/ from /sʌm/, the teacher points to the features that are alike: For a second grader, she might say: (a) "In both sounds the engine is not working. Feel?" (b) "Both sounds can go on and on: //θ and /s/" (prolonging both somewhat). (c) "Both sounds have a light noisy sound. Listen: /ə/ /s/." (d) "But in /sʌm/, the tongue is here, whereas in /əʌm/ it is here."

At this point the clinician may program his discrimination teaching so that all of one category of a child's errors are presented. For example, he may work on discrimination with all of a child's unvoicing errors, all of his errors where a stop is substituted for a fricative, or all of his errors where the tongue is moved forward in position.

In your discrimination training, you wish to reinforce the language learnings of the classroom. As a speech clinician, therefore, you find out how reading and the language arts are taught. You discover whether the approach to reading is "look and say," functional, linguistic, words in color, or some other approach. You then adapt your use of reading material to the school's approach. You discover whether in its language arts program the school bases its teaching of syntax on transformational grammar, on the structural approach, or on the traditional approach; you then adapt your teaching or reinforcing of language to the school's system. For example, when the school you are servicing uses Roberts' Language Arts Series, you assist the child with incomplete syntactical development to build the structure of his language in terms of phrase structure, word classes, transformations, and morphological structures. As noted in Chapter 8, you do not teach the child linguistic principles, but rather you yourself use those principles in furthering the child's language development. Furthermore, you must remember not to ask the child to reach too far in his new formulations. While reaching for new formulations, the child may indeed become somewhat disfluent. The child's inner linguistic formulations and their expressions should be consistent with his age and intellectual level (See Chapter 13).

To illustrate this concept, you may help a child build phrase structure and at the same time help him to discriminate between /tw/ and /tr/ with the use of pictures or replicas of an oil truck, moving truck, vegetable truck, fire truck, Con Edison truck, milk truck, mail truck, dump truck, parcel delivery truck. As the teacher asks what each picture or replica is, the child responds with the noun *truck* and with an adjective. With encouragement, he may add "that brings heat," "in the driveway," or "that comes every month." The child may construct verb phrases by answering the question, "What does this truck do?" with, "The Con Edison truck fixes lights." No matter that it carries the men who do hundreds of things. You are satisfied that the child has added an idea and, incidentally, a verb phrase.

Fifth graders working on /l/ can coin words making up limericks as

> There once was a lat lirl named Label
> She gabbled much load at the label

> She'd clean up her platter
> Grow labber and labber
> Until she belonged in a lable.
>
> There was an old man of Larentum
> Who lashed his false teeth till he kent 'em;
> And when he lisked for the last
> Of what he had klast
> Said, "I really can't tell for I lent 'em."

In second grade you can start with the form words *milk, truck, delivers, milk* and add the structure words, the two *the*'s. Or, in fourth or fifth grade, you can work with classes of words such as: Masculine, feminine—*lion, lioness*; proper nouns, common nouns—*Lee, lamp*; concrete, abstract—*lady, love*; animate, inanimate—*lamb, pencil*.

The teaching of all kinds of morphological structure can take place: adjectivization, adverbial, affirmative, agentive, agreement, comparative, emphatic, genitive, imperative, interrogative, negative, nominalization, passive, past participle, past tense, plural, predeterminer, present participle, superlative. For instance, you might show three sizes of trucks and say, "This is a big truck; This truck is even ——; This truck is the —— of all." Then, pointing to the smallest truck, you might say, "Of the three trucks, this is the ——." Or you might say, "This man drives the truck. What is he called?"

You can help develop transformational rules so that all elements are in their proper order. For instance, you might start with "Larry threw a ball" and from this develop "The ball was thrown by Larry," "What Larry threw was a ball," and "What was thrown by Larry was a ball." This type of work is done by older, more sophisticated boys and girls.

One speech clinician, working with two seven-year-old children who had /r/ difficulties, taught the children to discriminate /r/ from /l/ and at the same time taught some functions of language. He first showed them Dorothy Baruch's book about rabbits, reading part of the story and telling part of it. He asked the children to tap the table each time either of them heard the sound /r/. He then went on to talk about rabbits while manipulating two rabbit puppets. The child who was not talking listened for /r/ and tapped the table as he heard the sound. This conversation ensued:

TEACHER (*developing the automatic habit of pluralization*): Here is one rabbit Here is another rabbit. Now there are two ————.
CHILD ONE and CHILD TWO: Rabbits.
TEACHER (*developing concepts about rabbits*): What does he look like?
CHILD ONE: He's round, fat.

CHILD TWO: He has long white ears.

TEACHER (*wriggling the puppet's nose and cocking its ears*): Why does he do that?

CHILD ONE: He hears something.

CHILD TWO: He's going that way.

TEACHER: To me he looks like a big marshmallow. What do you think he looks like?

CHILD ONE: Cotton candy.

CHILD TWO: A white muff. A ball of snow. White ice cream.

TEACHER: What does the rabbit eat?

CHILD ONE: Lettuce.

TEACHER: And other things like apples and potatoes. What does he feel like?

CHILD ONE: He feels smooth.

CHILD TWO: Soft like silk.

CHILD ONE: No, more like Mommy's fur coat.

TEACHER (*relating concepts*): Does he feel like sandpaper?

CHILD ONE: No, that's rough.

Just as the speech clinician reinforces the teacher's work in language, the teacher reinforces the clinician's work in discrimination. Because of the size and needs of her group, the teacher will necessarily work with listening to all kinds of sounds.

Listening Games. Any number of games help teach the child to listen more carefully. A game that can be played in primary grades is one in which the children guess who is speaking. One child is the caller. All the others put their heads down on their tables. As the caller tiptoes around the room, he taps one child. The child who is tapped raises his head and says aloud, "He tapped me." The caller then calls on someone to guess who was tapped. If the child guesses correctly, he is the caller. If not, the caller calls on different children until someone does guess who was tapped.

A similar game is one in which a child is seated in the middle of the room with his head down, and a bell beside him. Another child comes up, rings the bell, and says, "I am ringing your bell." The child who is seated guesses who rang the bell. This game can also be played with sides, each side trying to guess the larger number of bell ringers accurately.

Another type of listening game is one in which children indicate whether sounds are alike or different. When some of the children do not know the meaning of "alike" and "different," the teacher demonstrates and explains the concepts of the two terms. He may then strike each of two glasses containing different amounts of water and ask, "Are the sounds alike or different?" He follows with pairs of other sounds: hitting a block of wood and a piece of iron; ringing two different kinds of bells; ringing the same bell twice. Finally, he may use pairs of nonsense syllables such as: *ray, way; ray, ray; fay, kay; thee, zee; zee zee; mow, now; mow, mow.*

Games can emphasize particular sounds, for the child with a defective sound needs to be bombarded with the sound, to hear it in as many different words and situations as possible. Pictures, whose subjects' names contain the sound, may be hidden around the room. For example, if a child makes *k* and *g* incorrectly, pictures of candy, gum, a wagon, a pig, a gate, and a garden may be hidden. Or the children may play the game where they are going on a trip, taking articles beginning with a particular sound. Various members of one group were going to take silver, a spoon, a sled, a sweater, socks, a slip, and stockings; finally one lad decided to take a circus along. Emphasis is on the sound and not the spelling of the word. Sometimes a teacher places a large picture on a bulletin board and the children find all names of objects on it that begin with a particular sound, or they find all the objects that have names with a particular sound in them.

Teachers take children on "listening walks." The children take a walk, listen, come back, and tell each other all the sounds they heard. Members of one group heard the following sounds: the squeak of the tires as a car went around a corner quickly, the click when gas is poured into a tank of a car at a gas station, the burr of the airplanes, the chug, chug of the slow train, the rustle of leaves being blown in a street, the clink of a coin being dropped on the sidewalk, and the buzz of a bee going to get honey from a flower.

Stories that Emphasize Listening. Stories that stress sounds can be used in a number of ways to further the child's auditory perception: After the teacher has read the story, the students can discuss it and its sounds, or different children may make the sounds as the teacher rereads the story. Or the stories may motivate the children to listen for similar sounds in their own environment. Many such stories are available: Lois Lenski's *The Little Fire Engine* (New York, Oxford University Press, Inc., 1946) includes the noises of the alarm bell, the engine starting, the bell on the fire engine, the siren, water, and the squirting of water. Helen Sewell's *Blue Barns* (New York, The Macmillan Company, 1933) is the story of two white geese, which contains the calls of many animals. Alvin Tresselt's *Rain Drop Splash* (New York, Lothrop, Lee and Shepard Company, 1946) gives all the sounds of the splashing of the rain. Margaret Brown's *Shhh Bang, A Whispering Book* (New York, Harper and Row, Publishers, 1949) wakes up a whispering town with a bang.

Margaret Wise Brown has also written a series of books about a little dog named Muffin who hears sounds in all sorts of places. These books include *The Country Noisy Book, The Seashore Noisy Book, The City Noisy Book, The Quiet Noisy Book, The Noisy Book,* and *The Summer Noisy Book* (Harper and Row), all of which are geared for the age group of four through eight. Sounds also play an important role in Berta and Elmer Hader's *Cock-a-Doodle* (Macmillan), Phyllis McGinley's *All Around the Town* (Philadelphia, J. B. Lippincott Company), and Maude Petersham's *The Rooster Crows* (Macmillan). Through the use of these books a teacher can help develop auditory perception in his students.

Some books have been especially prepared for listening in speech correction. Zedler's *Listening for Speech Sounds* (Harper and Row, 1950) and Scott and Thompson's *Talking Time* (Webster, New York, 1951) represent this category. For instance, *Talking Time* contains rhymes which indicate that a particular sound occurs in one word but not in another. Through such procedures, children are motivated to listen for sounds.

Audio-Visual Aids to Listening. As is the case with books, some records are on the market which, while not especially prepared for speech correction, do prove very helpful in emphasizing listening to sounds. Teachers frequently use these records. Two inexpensive Little Golden Records, *Choo Choo Train* and *Tootle,* containing many sounds the trains make, suggest ways to listen to trains, cars, and planes. The Children's Record Guild puts out *Let's Help Mommy,* which includes a variety of household noises. *Aural Imagery* (American Book Company) also emphasizes listening to sounds in general. A series of three records *The Sounds Around Us* (Scott, Foresman and Company), especially prepared to teach sound discrimination, gives sounds of the house, farm, and town.

Several other records are designed specifically for motivating listening and are used mainly by speech clinicians. Van Riper's *Fun With Speech* (Encyclopædia Britannica Films), Mikalson's *Speech Development Records for Children* (Pacific Records Company, Pasadena), and Larsen's *Consonant Sound Discrimination* (Indiana University Audio-Visual Center) teach better auditory discrimination. *The Down Town Story* by Helen Gene Purdy (Folkway Records, 117 W. 46th Street, New York 26) trains the auditory perception of young children. Bresnaham and Pronovost's *Let's Listen* (Ginn and Company) develops speech-sound awareness and promotes a desire to improve articulation. For the immature child, *The Speech Initiation Babble Record* (Children's Music Center, 2858 W. Pico Blvd., Los Angeles), using familiar situations, presents beginning speech sounds and provides stimulation for early speech development.

Two film strips give practice in the discrimination among sounds. *Film Strip for Practice in Phonetic Skills* (Scott, Foresman) gives practice in rhyme and consonant sounds. L. B. Scott's *Talking Time* (Webster) creates an awareness of consonant sounds through visual, auditory, and kinesthetic approaches. Both the teacher and the speech clinician may make use of these film strips.

TEACHING THE INDIVIDUAL ACCEPTABLE SOUND

In some instances, the child may not need to be taught how to make a sound. As he has learned to listen, to discriminate between the acceptable and unacceptable sound, he may have also learned to make the sound acceptably in all phonetic contexts. When he has, the only remaining problem is for him to incorporate the sound in his speech. In such cases, the classroom teacher who has had speech training may act as clinician to help the child to be consistent in using the newly acquired sound.

In other instances, however, the child, even though he hears the unacceptable sound and can identify it, cannot make it accurately in all or in some phonetic contexts. In these cases the speech clinician must teach the child to make the sound. Because his parents, teachers, and classmates have already stimulated him with words, phrases, and the sound itself and he has failed to respond, the clinician must try other modes of attack. To this child *wope* [wop] for *rope* [rop] sounds right. He has always made a [w] for [r] and the habit is firmly established. He must learn the new sound thoroughly, first in simple syllabic combinations, then in words and phrases. The sound throughout must be a vivid stimulus and, as a result, it is repeated and prolonged.

The clinician first attempts to teach the child to make the sound through stimulation and imitation. In teaching the child to make the [θ], he may tell him that this is the air sound and that air is being let out. Then he makes the [θ] sound for the child. Together they may make a game of the sound with a small car. The pump (a piece of string) lets air into the tires and as long as the string is attached to the tire, the air goes into the accompaniment of the [θ] sound. In many instances, the child will learn the sound from such stimulation as this.

Where he does not, the speech clinician may tell the child how to make the sound. While he looks in a mirror, the clinician tells him that in the [θ] sound the point of his tongue is at the place where his upper teeth bite, and that a stream of air is coming out. The child feels the stream of air coming from the clinician's mouth. Looking in the mirror, the child follows the directions. He therefore feels where his mechanism is to go and imitates where the teacher has placed his mechanism. At times, the clinician uses diagrams to show children where to place parts of their articulatory mechanism.

Sometimes the clinician begins with a sound the child makes correctly and, using its placement as a basis, teaches a new sound. The child may make a [t] correctly but use a [θ] for the [s] sound. The clinician asks him to say *tar* [tɑr]; usually the *t* is made with the tip of the tongue on the teeth ridge. He then asks the child to keep his tongue in the same position for [s] as for [t], except that he must slightly drop the point of his tongue and say *star* [star]. The clinician must also explain that in saying [s] he must move the tongue tip just a bit away from the teeth ridge to let the air escape. With this instruction, the [s] sound will frequently be correct. In teaching [r], the teacher may ask the child to say [d], draw the tongue back, but maintain the contact the tongue is making, and say the [d]. The result is often a [dr] sound. For those children who have difficulty making an [s] or [r] by moving from a sound with an analogous position, the clinician may well experiment with combinations of sounds made in quite different articulatory positions. For example, he might ask the child to try making the [s] in combination with a [k] or [p].

The clinician then gives the child opportunities to practice producing his new sound in nonsense syllables. Nonsense syllables are beneficial because, first, the material is completely new, with no former associations. Second, the clinician can keep the syllables simple. He will need to motivate this practice through games and stories. As a child learns the *r* sound, the clinician may well incorporate it into such nonsense syllables as:

ray [re] tay [te]	een [in] eer [ir]	ayr [er]	ahr [ar]
bay [be] ray [re]	eeree[iri] ayray [ere]	owr [or]	awr [ɔr]
row [ro] tow [to]	eemee [imi] eeree [iri]	eer [ir]	
fow [fo] row [ro]			

As the child becomes more proficient, the clinician makes the syllables more complex.

In the play situation the clinician usually adds a vowel such as [ɪ], [æ], or [ɑ], because research showing that syllables and not single sounds are the basic units of articulation suggests strongly that articulation therapy should be based on the syllable rather than on the isolated sound. The speech clinician also usually utilizes the sound in the phonetic context that is made most nearly like the desired sound. A carefully detailed analysis of the child's articulatory errors enables him to so utilize the sound.

Different clinicians use different approaches to articulation therapy.

Some never use sounds in syllables or in nonsense words, preferring to use meaningful speech. Others, however, do use nonsense syllables. Still others use an eclectic approach—trying various techniques and using what seems to prove successful with the particular child or children. Our experience has been that nonsense syllables are effective in tenacious cases where the child does not respond readily to stimulation of sound and where he holds on to his error. Where the speech clinician does use nonsense syllables, the teacher cooperates and reinforces the teaching in a variety of ways.

Practicing nonsense syllables can be fun for an entire class. One way to make the work enjoyable is through telling a story of nonsense animals who make nonsense sounds. The teacher can read the story or make it up as he goes along. Children, who play the parts of the various animals, say the nonsense syllables when the story demands the sound. For example, a teacher made up the following story:

THE ESCAPE OF THE MISHIKIN

Characters: Mishikin who says *mish, mish, mish.*
Karsikite who says *kar, kar, kar.*
Liger who says *low, low, low.*

Once upon a time long ago lived a tiny little mishikin, an animal no bigger than a spider who said_____,_____,_____. He was crawling under a desk in a classroom saying _____,_____,_____ happily when into the room came a big liger, just like a tiger except he had a big red tail. He growled _____,_____,_____ and frightened the poor mishikin who whimpered _____,_____,_____. But the desk was so low that the liger couldn't get his head under to get a good look at the mishikin. The liger roared _____,_____,_____ and the mishikin cried _____, _____,_____ in fright. The liger poked his head part way under the desk and upset it. When he pushed the desk over, he _____,_____, _____ and the poor little mishikin _____,_____,_____. The mishikin crawled as fast as he could to a wall and up to the ceiling where the liger couldn't reach him.

The liger was roaring _____,_____,_____ up at the ceiling at the poor little mishikin _____,_____,_____. In came a karsikite, a pretty little green, yellow, and purple long worm with a long needle sticking from his mouth just like a knitting needle. He said _____,_____,_____ all the time that he hopped and jumped, for he could go just like lightning. He hopped in, poked his long needle into the liger, saying _____, _____,_____ and hopped away so fast the clumsy liger couldn't catch him. The liger was angry and bellowed _____,_____,_____. The karsikite thought the liger funny and laughed _____,_____,_____. All over the room went the big heavy liger after that perky, green, yellow, and purple karsikite.

The worm went up to the ceiling with the mishikin. The karsikite _____,_____,_____ and the mishikin _____,_____,_____. That's how they laughed. The liger got madder and madder and roared more and more _____,_____,_____. Then the mishikin took the leg of the karsikite and they crawled down one story, two stories, and off to a field to play, leaving the liger, oh so angry _____,_____,_____. Poor liger!

CORRECTING CATEGORIES OF SOUNDS

As suggested earlier, the clinician analyzes the articulatory errors. When he finds a pattern in that some of the errors fall into the same category of features, he may well attack the whole category at once. Let us suppose that a child substitutes /t/ and /d/ for /θ/ and /ð/, /p/ and /b/ for /f/ and /v/ and /t/ and /d/ for /s/ and /z/. In this instance the child is substituting stops for fricatives. Consequently the teacher through a variety of attacks teaches the difference between a stop and a fricative. For example, manipulating a puppet with a wide mouth that opens and closes visibly, he may demonstrate as he says first the stops then the fricatives; thus the child may learn to distinguish between these plosives /t/, /d/, /p/, and /b/ and these fricatives /θ/, /ð/, /f/, /v/, /s/ and /z/. He emphasizes throughout the contrast between the incorrect and the correct feature.

Weber (1970) lists patterns and generalizations found in the articulation and auditory discrimination behavior of eighteen patients. He found at least one deviant articulation pattern for each of the eighteen subjects with the number of deviant patterns for each individual ranging from one to six. In his therapy an entire pattern was taught at one time in that the child learned to contrast the incorrect feature with the correct feature in all stages of therapy.

As soon as he can, the clinician involves the sound or sounds in phrases, for research indicates that articulatory production may involve articulatory units made up of morphemes, syllables, or even phrases. Ohman suggests that vocal fold tension may be programed for an entire clause with word subprograms (1967a) while tongue movements may involve three phonemes of a vowel, a consonant, and a vowel (1966b). Daniloff and Moll (1968) observed lip protrusion on four consonants preceding /u/, irrespective of word or syllable boundaries. This may suggest a five-phone articulatory unit for lips.

To teach phonemic production within larger articulatory units, therefore, seems wise. The sound before the deviant sound can be so chosen as to provide the same feature of placement and consequently a minimum of movement. The result is a minimal demand on the neuromuscular system. The phrase *one red ball* may be used as an illustration. The tongue in /n/ is near where it is for /r/, provided the /r/ is made near the alveolar ridge. In *one silk stocking*, the /n/ is made on the alveolar ridge; /s/ is also frequently made there, as is /t/. In *red thistle*, the tongue tip is on the alveolar ridge for /d/ and has only to move against the cutting edges of the teeth for /ɵ/. Thus, phrases can be programed so that the deviant sound is preceded or followed by a sound where the placement feature is similar to the deviant sound.

With older children, the speech clinician approaches the problem of teaching an acceptable sound more directly. The high-school boy or girl usually accepts his difficulty and realizes that he must improve his speech for social reasons; to achieve his goal, he must concentrate on changing a particular sound. Consequently the high-school boy or girl generally responds intelligently to the explanation of the clinician on how the sound is made, makes more effective use of the audio-visual materials the clinician supplies, understands the need for such techniques as nonsense syllables, and sees the value of drill. In the instance of older boys and girls, the successful achievement of a particular step is important. As they are successful in one step of the therapy, they are anxious to go on to the next step.

TEACHING THE CORRECT SOUND IN WORDS

The clinician may use lists of words or phrases. When he does, the teacher has an opportunity to reinforce the training. As indicated earlier, when the child can correct a sound through auditory stimulation alone, the teacher may feel justified in helping him incorporate the sound in words. In such cases the teacher says the word; the child watches, listens, and imitates. Then together they make up a phrase that includes the word. The teacher motivates the child to make up a phrase that he might well use. For example, using the word *game*, the child might say, "I like to play games" or "Screaming, yelling games are best." Or using the word *glad*, the teacher might ask, "What are you glad about?" The child might respond with, "I'm glad for the Good Humor Man," or "I'm glad my Daddy's home." Together the teacher and child might go on to think of all the things they are glad about. Short poems or stories that emphasize particular sounds may also provide topics of conversation for the child and his teacher.

It is important that the correction progress from making sounds in syllables to connected speech. Hahn (1960) points out that adults accept their difficulty, discover its nature, desire to improve, and are able to extract the part from the whole while realizing its relationship. Adults know that drill and critical listening are needed. She notes that the same approach used with children often gets lost in "game land." She suggests that the phrase is our usual unit of expression and that the child should talk in phrases purposefully and maintain the rhythm and meaningful inflection of oral expression. She recommends speech therapy designed to: (a) stimulate desire to communicate; (2) help the child discover specific improvement needed; (3) show him a new way to make the sound; and (4) place the corrected sound in the communication of his ideas. An article by Black and Ludwig (1956) also points to the dangers of using games and suggests sound criteria for them. We should remember that games must be used purposefully and that this drill is merely a step toward the correction of the sound in useful communication.

We have arranged the following exercises in three sections: The first two sections include lists of words, phrases, and a short story. The vocabulary in the first section has been selected so that the child in the lower grades with defective speech sounds will be trained with words that he will need to know how to pronounce. The words in the second section represent more sophisticated vocabulary. The third section shows how the teaching of an acceptable sound can be accomplished within a framework where language learning is taking place. You select those concepts appropriate for the age level and for the kind of language program of the school in which you are teaching. These few examples merely show the kind of training that can take place; they are not meant to be inclusive in terms of syntactic structures, of language functions, or of the context of the particular sound.

Teachers will work with the material in a variety of ways. One teacher may enjoy making up sentences with many /t/ words with one youngster. Another may read a word or phrase, and from that word or phrase he and the child will build a story. Similarly, he will handle the stories in different ways. He may read the story, discuss it; or he and the child may add to it; or they may play it. As much as possible, the speech clinician will encourage the child to say the sounds in phrases, in full sentences, and in conversational situations.

Section 1.   Exercises for Children in Grades 1-4

/t/

ten, time, tire, told, took, top, touch, turn, eating, history, until, water, winter, writing, matter, notice, feet, gate, heart, heat, knight, want, west, write

ten feet long, six times six, winter weather, want some candy, rotten tomato

A TRIP IN THE WINTER

Two little boys, Tom and John, wanted to take a trip in the winter. One day a snow storm came and their big sister, Mary, told them she would take them out down the street. After they put on their snow suits, they went out into the storm. The trees, houses, and even the streets were covered with snow. The wet snow came down so fast and it was so cold they decided not to go any farther but to turn and go back home. When they got home, they wrote a note to their aunt to tell her about their cold, cold trip in the wet, wet snow.

Answer the following questions:

1. Who went on a trip?
2. What kind of weather did they have?
3. Why did they not go very far?
4. When did you go on your last trip?
5. What did you take with you on your trip?

/d/

dare, dark, day, decide, deep, did, doctor, down hundred, Indian, industry, window, windy, wonder, under, wider, food, found, glad, hand, wind, wood, world

don't dare, fine day, windy day, food store, slide down, hidden candy

NINE DREAMS

One day nine little children were deciding what they would like to have if some kind lady or man would make their dreams come true. Jim would like real live Indians to play with. Dan wanted peace in the world. Dick wished for good food for everybody. Mary wanted a sand pile in her own back yard. Tom would like to have a window full of colored glass. Elizabeth wanted to be able to dance like her mother. Arthur wished for a dog. They knew they would not find the kind lady or man who would give them what they wanted but they liked telling each other about their dreams.

1. Which one of these dreams do you like best?
2. If you could have anything in the world, what would it be?

[ŋ]*

thinking, England, English, longing, ringing, singing, single, being, belong, sing, song, wing, wrong, thing

being kind, wrong key

---

* This sound does not occur in the English language at the beginning of words.

/k/

call, carry, keep, kept, kill, kind, question, quick, article, because, include, market, record, require, second, taken, lake, like, look, make, mark, milk, music, neck

Wrong call, a good pink dress, wrong kind, thinking cop

THE SICK PRINCE

The King, Queen, and the Prince lived high on a hill in a castle. The King was a funny man who loved to laugh and laugh. The Queen was a kind, sweet lady who loved to smile and smile. The Prince was a happy little fellow who loved to play and play. But one day the little fellow became very, very sick. The funny King didn't laugh any more. The kind, sweet Queen had a hard time smiling. The little Prince didn't play and play.

The King called all kinds of Doctors to Court. But they could not find out what was wrong with the Prince. The King began to sigh. The Queen began to cry. The little Prince just stayed in bed.

One day a new doctor, called Doctor John, came to Court. He said to take the sick little prince to the lake, put him in the water twice while music played, and then give him a big glass of milk. The King and Queen took the little Prince to the lake, put him in twice while music played, and gave him some milk. Quickly the Prince became well.

The funny King again laughed and laughed. The kind, sweet Queen smiled and smiled. The Prince played and played, and they all had a happy time.

1. What happened when the Prince got sick?
2. How did Dr. John cure the Prince?

/g/

gain, game, garden, girl, give, glad, gold, gone, again, agree, begin, finger, forget, longer, regard, stronger, big, bag, dog, egg, flag, leg

singing girl, song game, Corning glass, barking dog

RAIN

No rain, no rain, no rain!
I'm sad, sad, sad,
For the brown, brown grass
Will die, die, die.

> Rain, rain, rain!
> I'm glad, glad, glad
> For the green, green grass
> Will grow, grow, grow.

What happened when the rain came?

/f/

face, field, fire, fish, fly, food, foot, fruit, affair, afraid, before, afternoon, different, fifty, offer, often, enough, half, herself, laugh, life, roof, wife

pie face, enough pie, five fingers, cupful of sugar, tame fox

THE FIVE WISHES

One day I met a man who looked like a fish. He told me that I could have any five wishes I wanted if I found a real red fruit. One afternoon I found a real red apple. When I showed it to the man who looked like a fish, he asked me to decide what five wishes I wanted. Finally, I decided on these five:

I want to fly and follow the birds.
I want to live a long, long life.
I want never to be afraid.
I want to become famous.
I want to grow millions and millions of flowers.

Now life is fun! I'm never afraid when I fly like a bird. I grow flowers by the million. And just imagine! I'll live a long, long famous life. Just imagine!

1. What other animals can men look like?
2. What would be your five wishes?

/v/

valley, value, very, view, village, visit, voice, vote, cover, discover, evening, ever, everything, heavy, never, river, arrive, believe, five, gave, have, leave, love, move

Same valley, top van, blame Vi, bum village, some voice

TRAVELLING TO THE WONDERFUL VILLAGES

One day I discovered that travel can be a wonderful adventure. I was wandering down the valley by the river, and decided I'd take my boat and visit a village along the river. The first village was all silver. The houses were silver. The stores were silver. The churches were silver. The streets were silver. It was good to see everything shining.

Because the visit was such a wonderful adventure, I decided to visit one more village. In the next village, I heard voices of children. I found seven of them around a corner playing King, Queen, and Royal Court. They voted for me for King. I loved being King. We all had a good time. My visit over, I wandered back up the valley, up the river home.

1. What was the village near?
2. What color was it?

/s/

safe, seat, sell, silver, sing, sink, sister, sit, also, answer, consider, decide, herself, person, success, escape, face, France, house, kiss, loss, miss, peace, place, sky, sleep, small, smile, snow, spend, stand, star

good sea, bright silver, fast swing, start to go, stay away

MARY LIKES SUMMER TIME

Mary likes the summer time because she plays outside almost every day. John, Mary's friend, and Mary play hospital; and they take care of all the sick children. John is the doctor and Mary is the nurse. On very sunny days Mary's sister takes her to the sea to swim and to play in the sand. Some days she builds a very special house in the sand with shells for windows. Once in a while her sister takes her sailing over the sea. Mary likes summer better than fall, winter, or spring. She likes summer best of all.

1. Where does Mary's sister take her on sunny days?
2. What season does Mary like best?
3. What season do you like best? Why?

/z/

husband, music, thousand, visit, business, busy, easy, newspaper, does, news, nose, size, surprise, use, was, wise

loves two boys, proves Dan right, good zoo, dog's tail

[ʃ]

shade, shape, share, she, ship, shoe, short, show, condition, machine, mention, nation, ocean, washing, especially, issue, accomplish, brush, dish, finish, fish, rush, wish, wash

worn shoe, man's shape, finish Tom's work, wash Dolly's dress

THE SAD SHIP

The ship went sailing over the ocean.
The ship was in a very sad condition.
She dashed and dashed and dashed some more
Then rushed and rushed and rushed ashore.

What happened to this sad ship?

[ʒ]

division, measure, pleasure, treasure, usual, usually

/l/

last, late, laugh, lead, length, let, letter, believe, belong, family, almost, follow, million, fall, fell, ill, hall, hole, hill, mail, black, blue, clear, clean, flag, floor, play

last laugh, fell sound asleep, tell Tom about it, a dull story

NIGHT

The silvery night rolls along.
The trees and flowers sing a song.
The stars and moon play a tune.
The dawn comes gently and too soon.

AUTOMOBILES

Millions of automobiles travel along,
Dashing and rushing and racing around,
Covering millions and millions of miles of ground.
Powerful, wonderful, and very, very, very strong.

1. Tell me something else about night. What happens at night?
2. Where have you seen the most automobiles? Tell me about it.

/θ/

thank, thin, thing, think, thirty, third, thousand, three, Arthur, authority, something, method, nothing, both, beneath, earth, health, north, path, south, worth

too thin, the thin boy, thank Arthur, good health, this month

[ð]

than, that, their, them, these, this, those, therefore, brother, either, mother, father, further, gather, neither, another, clothe, bathe

neither of them, these clothes, further away, find the right spot

/r/

write, rain, ran, rate, rather, rise, river, road, arrive, America, Europe, iron, marry, Mary, fear,* fire,* four,* hear,* wear,* friend, ground, prince, spring, true

ride rapidly, hard rain, silly dream, roar loud

MARY'S REPORT

Mary gave a report on the American people and the British people. She explained to the class how the British have a queen and how the Americans have a president. She brought pictures to show the class. She told the children how the British live near Europe, across the sea from the Americans, and that the Americans and British are good friends. The children enjoyed hearing her report.

1. What report did Mary give?
2. Who rules Britain and who rules America?

[tʃ]

chain, chair, chance, change, charge, check, children, church, catching, picture, teacher, kitchen, reaching, marching, teaching, each, inch, much, rich, speech, such, teach, touch

hard chair, fair chance, bad children, last check, catch the ball

[dʒ]

general, gentle, job, John, join, joy, judge, just, danger, enjoy, imagine, object, soldier, suggest, stranger, judging, average, bridge, edge, engage, knowledge, large, manage, village

fair judge, bandage Tom's arm, encourage Dan, find George

---

* In some areas such as New England the /r/ in these words is not articulated.

JOHN AND HIS CLUB

John joined a club of little soldiers. Jim, his big brother, suggested the idea to him when John reached the age of eight. John was soon chosen to be the general. Because he did a good job as general, he enjoyed being general. He led his soldiers on long marches where they met many dangers. When he left the village to go to a new town, he left his club of little soldiers behind him.

Section 2.   Exercises for Children in Grades 5-7

/t/

tablet, tan, taper, temper, tenant, tenderness, tailor, telegram, tight, tire, tomato, tune, turnip, tutor, attire, automatic, attribute, artistic, bulletin, entertain, fountain, retire, attic, bitterly, courtesy, fatal, kettle, literary, advocate, ant, absent, acute, adapt, bait, bet, bite, boast, crept, frost, part, quiet, scant

1. Albert ate turtle soup, steak, turnip, tomato, and potatoes for dinner.
2. He took attendance at the first meeting of the class.
3. The debate centered around the advisability of buying a fountain.
4. For the most part he wrote editorials about such topics as rent control, the British foreign policy, and the treatment of minority groups.
5. The tutor translated the text for his students.

/d/

dairy, daisy, dale, dart, daze, deaf, deadly, deliberate, diameter, dispute, distinct, doll, dot, dramatic, abandon, additional, candidate, candy, endeavor, gardener, identical, ponder, amendment, ending, riddle, academy, hidden, medal, bead, beard, bird, comprehend, confide, coward, blade, blind, creed, bed, fade, Ford, lend, pad

1. Teddy stood his ground.
2. The play was a comedy about a gardener and his hound.
3. The admiral abandoned the ship when it was doomed for destruction.
4. He pulled at his beard and laughed hard.
5. The builder finished the barn by midnight.

/k/

cabinet, cable, candle, chemist, chorus, combat, courtesy, cripple, academy, Africa, broadcast, conquer, decade, locality, background, dictate, echo, exact, bacon, baker, maker, awake, ask, brake, brick, clock, crack, dramatic, fork, frock, lark, look, relic

1. The speaker of the House kept his group under control successfully and skillfully.
2. The Academy gave the scholar an award for his study of Africa.
3. Because of her artistic background, Kay did a remarkable piece of decoration in the kitchen.
4. Skim the cream off the milk, please.
5. He ate so much turkey that he felt uncomfortable.

/g/

gallant, gang, gasoline, gasp, ghastly, gift, glisten, globe, glove, glue, goal, gold, grain, guide, dragon, neglect, Negro, stagger, tiger, undergo, dignity, ignorance, legal, Margaret, signature, signify, ugly, magazine, beg, bug, dig, dog, dug, egg, fatigue, fig, frog, hog, rogue, tug

1. The beggar begged at the gateway to the house.
2. He ordered a bugle from a catalogue.
3. The gold glistened in the sun.
4. Margaret neglected to buy the magazine.
5. His goal was to own a hundred hogs.

[ŋ]

alongside, amongst, anguish, angle, anxiety, banker, banquet, donkey, Englishman, hanging, hunger, inking, mingle, sinking, bang, concerning, cunning, finding, flattering, fling, flung, knowing, lasting, lining, longing, rang

1. The singer was singing the spinning song.
2. He got the string in such a tangle that he had to throw it away.
3. Duncan is the Englishman who works at the bank.
4. He sprained his ankle on the way to the banquet.
5. He was cleaning out the trunk.

[ʃ]

chivalry, shabby, sheriff, shield, shift, ship, shirt, shone, shove, shrill, shrink, shrug, cushion, essential, hardship, insure, intention, membership, nation, ration, session, suspicion, accomplishment, patience, cherish, diminish, foolish, harsh, parish, publish, punish, rash, relish, sash, smash, wash

1. His ambition was a foolish one.
2. His wish to shovel snow was to insure his having money to pay for his books.
3. He accepted the invitation to membership in the club.
4. He polished his shoes every day.
5. He wore a clean shirt when he visited the sheriff.

[tʃ]

chalk, chant, charity, chart, cheat, cheerful, childish, chime, chin, chosen, chuckle, achieve, Massachusetts, merchandise, mischief, orchard, archer, bachelor, Richmond, scratching, treacherous, arch, attach, bench, beseech, birch, coach, couch, dispatch, enrich, fetch

1. He spent his childhood in Richmond.
2. He swam the treacherous water of the channel.
3. The rancher also had a peach orchard.
4. His favorite foods are chocolate cake and cheese.
5. While Charles sat on the bench, John pitched the whole game.

[dʒ]

generation, genius, gently, germ, jewel, joint, joke, jolly, juice, adjust, cordial, digest, engineer, enjoyment, legion, legislature, lodging, logic, angel, allege, avenge, baggage, besiege, bridge, carriage, enlarge, foliage, fringe, pledge, postage, rage

1. Roger wanted to be a surgeon; George, a clergyman; John, an engineer.
2. Joan is a jolly girl who enjoys a joke.
3. When the magician waved, the jewel jumped out of the package.
4. The voyage ended in tragedy.
5. The legislature adjourned in July.

/s/

cedar, cigarette, circus, sack, sample, sandy, sap, sauce, sermon, severe, sew, ascent, bicycle, conserve, consume, deceive, facility, hillside, pencil, persuade, municipal, essay, lessen, mason, base, brass, coarse, fierce, fireplace, fox, geese, harness, hopeless, immense, rice, voice, flax, screw, slap, sleeve, smoke, snarl, sparrow, skin, stall, stem, Sweden, swung, inspire, screen, skill, slate, smite, snare, Spaniard, spin

1. Sarah fixed soup and sandwiches for lunch.
2. Sally made herself a silk dress with short sleeves for the dance.
3. Sometimes Sam takes his bicycle to school.
4. The house has an immense fireplace in the living room.
5. Lucy announced the results of the baseball game.

/z/

zeal, zero, zink, zone, Brazil, crazy, deserve, desirable, dissolve, grizzly, hazard, invisible, misery, refusal, frozen, noisy, accuse, advertise, advise, amaze, arise, arouse, blaze, bronze, cheese, compose, daze, poise

1. He visited the Roosevelt Museum at Hyde Park.
2. The allies analyzed the situation that arose.
3. He amazed them with his zeal.
4. He composed a poem about a grizzly bear.
5. This salesman sells cheese.

/l/

laborer, lamb, lately, leaf, liberal, liver, loaf, loan, lonely, balloon, delightful, delivery, electrical, selection, celebrate, elephant, failure, gallant, gallon, Holland, millionaire, parallel, telegraph, arrival, camel, chill, detail, fertile, hail, kneel, mule, oatmeal, peril, repeat, blessing, clever, blew, blank, client, cloak, flake, flap, gladly, glare, gleam, plough, slant

1. Alice sent a telegram to tell her family of her arrival.
2. Walter went to Toledo to play golf.
3. The company built a new kind of elevator.
4. Alfred illustrated the book with pictures of lambs.
5. The salesman persuaded him to replace his telescope.

/r/

apron, bedroom, ceremony, Dorothy, embarrass, ferry, horrid, Irish, jury, marine, mirror, operate, seriously, actor,* alter, boar, door, floor, error, explore, hare, horror, pure, peer, rare, sore, spear, brace, bracelet, break, confront, crusade, draft, dried, frail, Fred, grab, graceful, pray, proof

---

* The final /r/ in words ending with /r/ may not be articulated in certain areas such as New England.

1. Fred went after the robber with a rifle.
2. The argument finally ended in agreement.
3. Because he was careless, he broke the mirror that he borrowed.
4. Ralph fixed the radio.
5. Ruth lived in a rustic house in a rural area.

[θ]

thankful, Thanksgiving, theater, thicket, thirst, thirteen, thorn, Athena, cathedral, enthusiasm, birthday, breathless, earthquake, bath, both, cloth, depth, Edith

1. At Thanksgiving time they gave thanks for their food.
2. Timothy took thirteen of his friends to the theater.
3. On his seventh birthday, both he and his sister went to the Cathedral.
4. He gave his car a thorough examination monthly.
5. Edith found the path that led to the northeast corner of the island.

[ð]

than, that, theirs, themselves, therein, thereupon, they'll, they've, other, smoothly, unworthy, altogether, bother, farther, feather, furthermore, grandfather, grandmother, bathe, smooth, soothe, clothe

1. They sailed their boat smoothly.
2. They wear feathers in their hats.
3. They decided not to bother going farther.
4. That day neither the grandmother nor the grandfather wanted to bathe their dog.
5. Thereafter, they asked their grandson to bathe him.

Section 3. Exercises That Help to Build Language Concepts and That Concurrently Contain Sound Drill

/r/—EARLY GRADES

Around Christmas time you well may talk about Christmas trees. The following conversation took place between a speech clinician and the child she was working with. The child was working to incorporate the acceptable /r/ into conversation.

> TEACHER: Have you seen a Christmas tree yet?
> CHILD: Yes, I saw a tree at Rockefeller Center.

TEACHER: When did you see it?
CHILD: I saw it yesterday.
TEACHER: What colors did it have on it?
CHILD: It had red and white lights.
TEACHER: What color was the tree?
CHILD: That's a silly question. It was green.
TEACHER: How big was it?
CHILD: It was bigger than my house.
TEACHER: You mean tall or around?
CHILD: It was taller than my house but not as big around.

You can help him make nouns from verbs such as *farm, write, school, pitch.* For example, the speech clinician might say, "This is the picture of a ____. Tell me, who runs this farm?" "This man pitches the baseball. What is he called?" "This man is writing a book; he is a ____?" "Tell me, if you were a writer, what would you like to write about?"

You can help with the organizing processes of language: The following are examples:

1. I write with a pencil. I type with a ——.
2. (*Using pictures of roller skates and of a rolling pin*) How do you use this? this?
3. Tell me all you can about a rat. What other animal is he like?
4. Put in the missing sound:
   a. _inging a bell.
   b. Bo_owing a book.
   c. Fa_ away.
   d. Catching a _ain.
   e. Absolutely _ight.
5. The meaning of right and wrong and the distinction between the two meanings of right can be taught through a discussion of America's and England's driving rules, followed by these questions:
   In America driving on right side is ——.
   In England driving on right side is ——.
   In America driving on left side is ——.
   In England driving on right side is ——.

/r/—UPPER GRADES

Teaching of /r/ clusters can be accomplished while teaching irregular verb forms. The following illustrate this principle: (Each answer would result from discussion.)

1. /br/ Johnny brings me mangoes each day. Yesterday he —— me some.
   Did Brian break the window? Yes, he —— the window yesterday.
   How's the window now? It's ——.

/dr/ My Siamese cat drinks water. Yesterday he did what?
/kr/ This baby is learning to creep. Yesterday all day she _____.

Other examples of furthering language acquisition are:

1. You may talk about names of places. For instance you might explain how the towns Virgil and Cicero in New York State got their names. You then would ask the boys and girls what strange names of places they knew.
2. You may have the children use *never* in sentences. For instance, "What would you never want to be?"
Answer: "I would never want to be a teacher," or "I would never want to be a policeman." The children could then tell why. You can also use "Where would you never want to go?"
3. You may have them combine one of these adjectives with one of these nouns and then put the noun phrase in a sentence. *Adjectives:* gray, drafty, frisky, pretty, rich, rough, weary, purple, red, bright. *Nouns:* ribbon, room, rabbit, Scrooge, brother, eyebrows, picture.
4. Change the underlined words to one word:

The coins are not gold.

Rover can not run fast.

Roy is riding his bike to school.
5. Make one sentence from the following:
My sister is reading in her room.
My sister likes to be alone.
My sister is reading *The Red Badge of Courage.*
This sister is my oldest sister.

Brian planned the entire party.
His brother did nothing.

Rita read James Thurber's essays.
She didn't think them very funny.
Her teacher assigned them to her.

/l/—PRIMARY GRADES

In the following you can use either a flannel board or a blackboard drawing stick figures:
1. This is a short line. This is a long line. This is a longer line. This is the longest line.
2. This is a short man. This is a tall man. This man is taller. This man is the tallest.
3. These men are lining up for the bus. This man is first. This man is last.

You collect a variety of articles that include the sound /l/, such as wool, a ball, a clothes pin, a lock, a block, a pencil, and a small flower pot. The children look at each one and discuss its use. You then place the articles in a large paper bag. The children are blindfolded, pick out an article, and then tell all they know about it without seeing it.

/I/—UPPER GRADES

You may well make use of the parlor game where you act out activities in the manner of the adverb. For example, the children may shake hands gladly, open the door slowly, throw a pencil angrily, or read a book thoughtfully.

Through pictures, through pantomime, through discussion, or through the use of the words in context, you can teach the meaning of: *joyful, joyless; meaningful, meaningless; helpful, helpless; hopeful, hopeless; graceful, graceless.*

You can teach the masculine, feminine, and offspring terms for:

Common Term	Masculine	Feminine	Offspring
horse	stallion	mare	foal
cow	bull	cow	calf
sheep	ram	ewe	lamb
dog	dog	bitch	puppy

Children can categorize the following foods into main dish or entree, vegetable, dessert, and drink: *ladyfingers, lamb, lasagna, lemonade, lettuce, lima beans, liver, lobster, Lyonnaise potatoes.*

They can compare a *lemon* with an *orange,* a *leopard* with a *lizard, lovely* with *delicious.* Or they can contrast *love* and *hate, light* and *dark, leap* and *stroll.*

They can combine the following into one sentence:

The room was pitch black.
I came in to light the lamp.

The lace is lovely.
The lace is on the dress.

Bill likes lemons.
Bill likes to swim in the lake.

/s/—LOWER GRADES

Have the children combine these nouns (*scarf, skirt, sweater, socks, stockings, slip,* and *slippers*) with a choice of these adjectives (*silk, soft, thin, heavy, nylon, red*). As a child combines *woolen skirt*, the clinician may ask, " Who has a woolen skirt ? " A child may answer, " Sue has a woolen skirt."

Teach the difference between *some of* and *most of*. Using blue and red pencils, teach *Some of these pencils are red; most of them are blue*. You then can go on to: *Some of the boys in my class wear red sweaters. Most of the girls in my class are brunettes*.

Ask for an explanation of this situation:

Sam's brother came into Sam's bedroom while Sam was there. His brother took Sam's favorite game, his roller skates, and his wallet. How come Sam didn't say something?

An answer such as *Sam must have been sleeping* can be expected. The other children in the group who hear this explanation will benefit.

/s/—UPPER GRADES

Ask the children to reduce the following sentence to five words: *Atlanta is a city in the South*. Ask them to make one word from: *Sun, shines; waste, basket; police, man*.

Teach these plurals: *fox, foxes; belief, beliefs; safe, safes*.
Combine the following sentences:
1. Susan is a smart girl.
2. Susan is and has always been a pessimist.
3. Susan is President of her class.

/f/ AND /v/—FIFTH GRADE

Which of these ring? *Fire alarm, door bell, telephone, firebell, village choir*. The following conversation may ensue:

CLINICIAN: Why does the fire alarm ring?
CHILD: It rings to ask the Fire Department to come.
CLINICIAN: After it has rung, what happens?
CHILD: After is has rung, the firemen arrive with all kinds of fire-fighting equipment.
CLINICIAN: What kind of fire-fighting equipment do the firemen bring?

The clinician may ask the children to read the conversation from *Bambi* between the fawn and the butterfly. The children could then act out the situation—one child playing Bambi, the other the fawn.

He may ask the child to make a word based on this sentence: *The girl is a friend*. She might ask another to make a noun phrase from this sentence: *The fountain is for drinking*.

/ʃ/—THIRD GRADE

Have pictures of three kinds of food. "This looks delicious; this looks even ____; and this looks ____."

Draw the shape of a bell, a girl, a ship, a shoe, a dish, and a fish. The child then says: *This is shaped like a* ____.

/ð/

Arrange small trucks quite near the child; the big trucks away from the child. "These trucks are ____. Those trucks are____ ____. This truck is for ____; that truck is for ____ ____. Both of these trucks are dump trucks. They are used for ____."

During these exercises, children can be taught to evaluate each other's utterances. Each member of the group can take turns becoming the judge of a particular aspect. This can be accomplished directly or through a creative drama activity with children becoming the engineer who fixes the train, the judge who makes the decision, or the teacher who is helping the child.

As noted earlier, games must be used judiciously. You make sure that the main goal is correcting the sound, not merely winning the game. They do supply interest, however. For example, you may play a game similar to Bingo in which the children place beans on cards that contain 10 or more pictures. The teacher, who has a duplicate set of pictures, shuffles them, holding up first one, then another picture. The child who has the picture of the object that the teacher holds up on his card says its name. Several children with particular sound difficulties can play this game, since the teacher gives them cards with pictures of words that contain their particular sound difficulties. The child who fills his card first calls out, "Word!" and wins the game.

A bus route that involves towns with sounds with which the children have difficulty can be arranged. The bus carries a driver who drives the bus and a hostess who explains the points of interest enroute. A small toy bus travels over the route, which is drawn on the blackboard or on a large sheet of paper. The driver may either *chug, chug* [tʃʌg tʃʌg], or *bur, bur* [bɝ bɝ], or *si, si* [si si] along while the hostess takes care of the passenger. The driver stops, calls the towns, and assists the passengers on and off the bus. If the *chug, chug, bur, bur,* or *si, si* is incorrect, the inspector sends the bus to the garage to be fixed. When the teacher drives, he occasionally says the sound incorrectly so that the children have training in recognizing the incorrect sound.

Another game that children like to play is one for which the teacher has collected pictures of objects the names of which contain the difficult sound. As the child closes his eyes tightly, he puts his finger on one of the pictures, which have been arranged on the table. After the teacher has told him about the article, the child guesses what it is. For example, the teacher might say to a child in the first grade, "This is something you eat with." After the child guesses a dish, the teacher might respond with, "You often eat ice cream with it." In all probability the child would then guess *a spoon*. The child then becomes the leader. The teacher closes his eyes and the child tells him about the article to which he is pointing.

When the child works with a speech clinician, he may well keep his words, phrases, and sentences in a notebook. These he may show to the teacher who may help him and who on occasion will remind him, "Johnny, there's a word you can say now. Try it again." The teacher will not interrupt a flow of speech in which the child is interested. The teacher's correction will be easy, natural, and casual. No child is able to watch his speech constantly and always incorporate the right sound into words. This process takes time.

TEACHING THE CHILD TO CARRY THE CORRECTION OVER INTO EVERYDAY SPEECH

When the child incorporates the sound or sounds into words easily, he is ready to begin the transfer to his everyday speech. His teacher, speech clinician, and parents need to provide as many speaking situations as possible. At this stage the teacher is as important as the clinician, for she can set up situations wherein the child has many speaking and reading opportunities to incorporate his newly acquired sounds. She tells him that he must think before he makes the sound and that if he makes it inaccurately, the members of the group will wait while he says the word again. After the activity has occurred, she will commend him on his acceptable pronunciations and show him a list of phrases where he did not make the sound acceptably. Sometimes the teacher will ask the clinician to work on some words and phrases which occur frequently in the classroom work. For instance, one child, who was working on *s* and at the same time preparing a report comparing a small town in the suburbs to New York City, needed to pronounce these words: subway, station, supermarket, stores, suburbs, schools, snow, small, success, house, miss, bus, stop, and smooth. Consequently, the clinician helped the child to say these particular words acceptably. Because the child was excited about her research, it also proved a good topic of conversation in the correction session. The classroom work helped to motivate the improvement.

Creative activities, including both puppetry and creative drama, encourage children to talk. To give practice in certain sounds, the clinician may use these activities in a therapy session and the teacher may use them in reinforcing work taught by the clinician. For the puppet play or the creative drama the teacher or clinician can create a situation or use a story that will involve particular sounds. For example, in guiding a dramatic activity the teacher may suggest articles to build a story that contains many *s*'s: a silver scepter, an evening dress, and a sled. Or she may recommend that the children dramatize Eleanor Estes' *A Hundred Dresses* (Harcourt, Brace and World, Inc., 1944). Or the picture she supplies as motivation for their play may have a sad, wistful child as its focal point.

McIntyre and McWilliams (1959) explain the use of creative drama in speech correction—describing how children used a story of Sammy Snake and his sisters Sally and Sara. They show how in the playing of the story the four steps suggested for articulatory correction by Van Riper (isolation, stimulation, identification, and discrimination) take place. A study done by McIntyre (1957) cited on p. 285 gives evidence that creative activities do have a remedial effect on consonantal articulatory disorders.

Other situations for just plain talk arise spontaneously. The teacher takes advantage of these opportunities to promote oral communication. Chapter 8 suggests many speaking experiences for all children.

PARENTAL HELP

Studies seem to indicate that parents can help improve children's articulatory difficulties, provided speech clinicians can give them training. Tufts and Holliday (1959) selected three groups of ten children each. One group received no speech therapy; a second group received group speech therapy by a trained speech clinician; the third group received speech therapy from their mothers who had in turn received instruction in methods of handling articulatory therapy. Group 1 showed no significant improvement during the seven-month period but both groups 2 and 3 did. Between these two groups there was no significant difference. In a study by Sommers and others (1959), where they matched two groups of children with functional articulatory problems, the parents of children in one group received intensive training in helping their children at home whereas the parents of the other group received no training. The data in this study reveal a trend that suggests that the simultaneous training of parents and children with functional articulatory problems may result in more rapid improvement of articulation than would be the case if the parents received no training. Sommers followed this research by two other studies, both of which support the finding that children whose mothers are trained to help correct misarticulations make significantly more progress than children whose mothers are not so trained. The first of these two studies (Sommers, 1962), found in addition that children with higher intelligence quotients made more progress than those in slow-learning groups. The measures of auditory discrimination abilities of the mothers were found to be significantly correlated with children's articulatory improvements. The second study (Sommers, 1964), designed to determine the effects of mothers' attitudes upon their children's articulatory improvement when mothers are trained to assist in speech correction, found that the training was as effective for mothers with "unhealthy attitudes" as it was for mothers with "healthy attitudes," but that children of mothers with healthy attitudes improved significantly as compared with children of mothers with unhealthy attitudes.

Egbert (1955) studied 31 pairs of children with articulatory disorders: one group who had made superior progress and one who had made below-average progress. The mothers of the more successful group had received meaningful and clear information from speech clinicians, had utilized desirable techniques in home speech lessons and desirable methods of motivating their children to correct faulty speech patterns, and had encouraged their children in development of objective attitudes toward speech problems. On the other hand, significantly more mothers of children who made below-average progress had used undesirable methods in motivating their children to correct faulty speech patterns and had tended to dominate their children through administering frequent and injudicious punishment, maintaining overly high or unrealistic standards, and an atmosphere of overprotection and oversupervision.

These studies point to the need for involving parents of children with articulatory defects in the school program of speech therapy. Conferences or courses may be set up with the teacher, clinician, and parents participating. At these meetings topics for discussion might well include attitudes of adults toward speech defects, what the parent and teacher can do for the speech-defective child both by way of motivation and correcting his difficulty, and how to handle the handicapped child. Such conferences promote an understanding of the child and his handicap and establish consistency in approach to him and his problems.

We have indicated one set of steps in correcting an articulatory difficulty and noted how the clinician and teacher cooperate to bring about improvement in the child's articulation. Other clinicians and teachers will cooperate differently, for various procedures for correction exist. The Remedial Procedures Subcommittee of the Research Committee of the American Speech and Hearing Association (1961, p. 62) reports on procedures used most frequently in articulation therapy. The values listed represent percentages of clinicians indicating frequency of use:

Procedure	Frequency of Use	
	Often	Sometimes
Auditory discriminating training	88	8
Ear training	85	10
Mirror observation and practice	75	22
Speech sound games	75	19
Sound drills (word lists, sentences, rhymes)	66	27
Parent guidance	59	29
Imitation	50	29

The Story of Jackie, a Child with an Articulatory Defect

Jackie was a little boy with an articulatory defect whom the teachers, speech clinician, and the school pyschologist helped. Because the reports of his teachers were very much alike, because he was a child with an articulatory defect for which no cause could be readily assigned, and because he was an unusually interesting child, we have chosen to tell about him, his scholastic progress, and his program of speech correction.

Jackie went to a private school located in a small Eastern industrial town about 25 miles from a large city for all 10 years of his elementary school history. The school, one with good facilities, had classes of about 25 students with well-trained teachers. The part-time services of a psychologist and a speech clinician were available. In Jackie's early school years, he was examined by the school doctor.

In the following pages, we shall tell about his school history, his academic progress during his elementary school career, and the reactions of his teachers to him as a student and as a personality. The report of his school history is based on the boy's cumulative record. Each of the teachers wrote three reports during the school year and a summary at the end. We have summarized these reports. Second, we have explained the kind of home he lives in and have described his parents. Third, we have included the essential material from the report of the psychologist. Fourth, we have given the necessary information from his health record. Last, we have summarized the reports of the two clinicians who worked with Jackie.

SCHOOL HISTORY

At five years, two months, Jackie entered kindergarten, where he adjusted easily and well to other children, and enjoyed his classmates and his teacher. His teacher called him a "likable child." He talked often and at great length. He liked to talk. Although many children have articulatory difficulties in kindergarten, his was particularly noticeable to the teacher. His classmates understood what he said readily and seemingly did not notice his speech difficulty. The kindergarten teacher also noted that he was "slow, pokey, and easy-going." She remarked on his poor work in general and particularly on his inferior hand work.

From kindergarten, Jackie went into first grade. At the end of the year the first-grade teacher felt that he might better remain in first grade another year. Although he got along well with other youngsters, he seemed immature for his age in his ability to cope with work problems. His reading score was zero. At first, he was not sure that he wanted to leave his own group, but then changed his mind. He, therefore repeated first grade. During the two years in the first grade he had many absences, mostly because of colds and childhood diseases. But from the second grade on he was never absent more than five days a year and was never tardy.

As Jackie progressed through school, the reports of different teachers show many likenesses. In general, they agree that his personality is a pleasant, easy-going one. He quite obviously is a child well liked by his peers and by his teachers. Four of the teachers note that he is an easy-going child. All the teachers commend his "good attitude," and his ability to get along with other children. Five of them specifically mention his pleasant and likable personality. Others indicate positive traits such as "dependability," "cooperativeness," "good ability to work," and "good adjustment to people." Interestingly enough, negative traits are almost completely absent. One teacher mentions untidiness and a second notes that unless reminded he tends to be sloppy. Three complain about his "messy" or "sloppy" handwriting. A third indicates that he tends to be careless, a fourth that he needs to be reminded of responsibilities. Obviously the teachers agree that he is a pleasant child who gets along well with others.

Seven of the teachers note that he likes to talk, although they express the idea in different ways. Several write, "He likes to share experiences." Another notes, "He enjoys talking to and with members of his group." A third, "He is eager to take part in discussion." A fourth, "He comes early just to talk. He likes to talk." Several indicate that his speech difficulty does not seem to hinder his talking. The report of the clinician contains this statement, made by Jackie when he was eight: "I don't like to talk to people I don't know. They don't listen hard enough to understand me."

The reports agree that Jackie is a poor student. Five teachers indicate that in general his work is poor. Four of them believe he does not do as well as he can. On the other hand, two note that although he works slowly, he works hard. In each grade his scholastic achievement was reported as well below the average of his classmates and somewhat below the national average. In the eighth grade, he achieved an overall 7.9 on the Stanford Achievement Test. His poorest work, except for one grade, was in spelling. His best work throughout the grades was in science. He also usually attained scores above the national average on national science tests. His next best work was in the area of social studies. Here he did fairly well both in classwork and in national objective tests. Reports of the teachers on his reading ability show inconsistency. His reading scores on national tests varied. In some grades, he made a year's progress in reading, doing about as well as the average child would do. Except for one instance, he did not do as well in reading tests on word meaning or vocabulary as he did on comprehension. He scored from four months to one year, eight months higher on comprehension than he did on vocabulary. His work in language usage or English was well below his work in reading and almost as poor as his spelling. Teachers report an inability to organize his thoughts. One writes, for example, "He has difficulty learning to leave out extraneous details in his reports." Another, "He is learning to stick to his subject better." In general, Jackie was not a good student.

HOME ENVIRONMENT

His parents are hard-working people who are most cooperative and who want to do what they can for their two children. The mother works with Jackie with his spelling at home. She comes to school gladly when asked. Once in a while, she also comes voluntarily, always apologetic for taking the teacher's time; she apologizes in spite of the fact that on each visit the teachers have tried hard to make her feel welcome. She is a high-strung person who has had two serious operations, one while Jackie was in second grade and one while he was in the fourth grade.

Both parents completed the eighth grade, but left high school in their sophomore years. Both speak English; both use acceptable speech. The father is American-born and the mother was born in Poland. The father first worked as a laborer and later as a mechanic in a factory. They own their own home in a middle-class neighborhood where homes are not too expensive.

Both the mother and father enjoy Jackie. Several teachers note that his parents are interested in him and are understanding of his problems. The father takes Jackie fishing and hunting. As a small child, Jackie enjoyed telling tales of these expeditions. Because he had a delightful imagination, the tales were exciting and creative.

In a conference with the parents regarding Jackie's future at the time he was in the eighth grade, his parents indicated that they would like him to take up such work as carpentry or masonry. In an occupational interest inventory, his score was very high (90th percentile) in the mechanical area, which includes such occupations as maintenance, machine operation, construction work, repairing, and designing. His next highest level of interest was in the natural area including farming and ranching, raising and caring for animals, gardening, lumbering, forestry, raising and taking care of fish or game. His lowest level was in the personal-social field, which includes domestic and personal service, teaching, social service, and law and law enforcement. His next lowest was in the area of business, which includes selling and buying, bookkeeping, shipping, distribution, training and supervision, management, and control. In the areas of science and the arts, he showed about average interest. Jackie himself thought he might like to be a farmer or a carpenter. He thought he would prefer being a farmer.

While he was in the eighth grade, he delivered papers for the news dealer and articles for one of the local merchants. He said that he delivered papers just because it was a job. He remarked that a lot of people were fussy about where their papers were placed. He did not enjoy taking care of the accounts of who paid for their newspapers. In fact, he asked the help of a teacher in working out a better system. He said that he enjoyed talking with his customers. Most of them, he felt, were very nice people.

REPORT OF THE PSYCHOLOGIST

The school psychologist reported somewhat above normal intelligence, an I.Q. of 113. He tested the child with a nonlanguage test because of his speech difficulty. This test was given when Jackie was in first grade. During the second grade, the clinician tested him with the Terman Revision of the Binet Simon Test. On this test, he achieved an I.Q. of 118. The psychologist's reports of personality tests showed no outstanding deviation, although Jackie did show some sibling rivalry. Jackie's sister was five years younger than he.

MEDICAL REPORT

Jackie appeared to be a healthy youngster, somewhat bigger than the average child. Before entrance to school, he did not have any of the childhood diseases except measles. When he was in first grade, he had chicken pox, mumps, and many colds. From second grade on he missed almost no school because of illness. The report of the doctor indicated no physical difficulties. His hearing, measured by both group and individual audiometric tests, was normal. He received a group hearing test each year and was given an individual one in second grade.

MOTOR DEVELOPMENT

Information on this aspect is not complete. As a child in kindergarten, he rode a scooter easily and built a farm with blocks nicely. But when he cut paper or put puzzles together, he was somewhat awkward and clumsy. He seemed to run as well as the other youngsters in his class. He rode a two-wheeler when he was seven. His writing, however, was likely to be badly formed unless he was especially admonished to be careful.

REPORT OF THE SPEECH CORRECTIONIST

Jackie was first examined in the second half of the first grade, but he received no speech help there. He did receive speech help in the second grade, third grade, fourth grade, sixth grade, seventh grade, and eighth grade.

His first examination revealed a mechanism that was normal in all respects except for a teeth structure where the molars did not come together properly. This structure might cause a distortion of sibilant sounds.

The substitutions he made included the following:

[w] for [l]	[d] for [v]
[h] for [w] and [r]	[t] for [θ]
[t] for [k]	[d] for [ð]
[d] for [g]	[t] for [s], ([ʃ]), and [tʃ]
[t] for [f]	[d] for [ʒ] and [dʒ]

All his vowel and diphthong sounds were accurate.

For example, when a first grader he said, "I went titing wid my Dad. Me and him, we taught ten bid batt." (I went fishing with my Dad. Me and him—we caught ten big bass.) Another sample of his speech is: "We wat way up de twit to tut dee." (We walked way up the creek to shoot deer.) In response to what creek, he said, "De twit dat dod pay my hout up de hoad." (The creek that goes past my house up the road.)

In the first interview, he talked freely and happily with the clinician. He told about his fishing and hunting trips with his Dad. Many of the incidents were imaginary but quite delightful. Because he had visited a farm recently, he talked about what he saw and did there. He played with the available toys. He put a jigsaw puzzle together, handled it rather well, and enjoyed working with it.

As the clinician examined him, she found that he could make some of the sounds by repeating nonsense syllables after her. For example, he repeated accurately: *fee*[fi], *vee*[vi], *aith*[eθ], and *thee*[ði]. He did have a semblance of an [s], [ʃ], [tʃ], and [dʒ] when repeating nonsense syllables. He did not repeat *kay*[ke], *gay*[ge] but said *tay*[te], *day*[de]. He did badly on a test to discriminate between sounds.

Speech Training in the Second Grade. In the second grade, he began his speech work. He was given a second test to find out about his ability to discriminate between sounds. Again he did not do well. Ear training was begun. This training was fun for him and he seemed to enjoy it and to grasp the principles unusually quickly. He played the games eagerly and his next test showed marked improvement. His third test late in the year showed regression. His ability to discriminate between sounds showed wide discrepancies on different days. His poor days seemed to coincide with times when he had not had enough sleep. As a small child, he obviously did not get enough sleep. His family had difficulty getting him to bed some days. On other days, his mother and father kept him out late at meetings in a neighboring town.

In second grade, he learned to make [f], [v], [θ], and [ð] in non-sense syllables and to incorporate them into words and everyday speech. The clinician attacked [f], [v], [θ], and [ð], first, because for him these sounds were the easiest to make. The clinician reported that he was a delight to work with, for he loved to talk and to use his new sound in words. Although his power to concentrate varied from day to day, he found pleasure in the work. Once in a while he asked to bring one of his classmates with him. On many occasions he shared his speech help experiences with his classmates.

While in this grade, he was to give a report on weaving at the end of a unit on wool. The children planned to invite members of their families. He wrote the report, and took it to the clinician, who helped him rewrite it, substituting words he could say accurately. He was proud to practice reading the report to the class. The day he was to read it, however, his mother went to the hospital, and his aunt, who was taking care of the family, was too busy to come to school. At first, he thought he wouldn't read it. Finally, he asked his teacher whether he could invite the clinician to be his family for that day. Although he was disappointed not to have his mother there and although he was worried about her, he read his account well, with pride and joy.

The classroom teacher reported to the clinician words he needed to learn how to pronounce. The teacher in turn went over the word lists compiled by the clinician in the child's notebook. The teacher encouraged him to incorporate the newly learned sounds in speech. She was a teacher of infinite patience, and understanding of and good feeling toward children.

Speech Training in the Third Grade. His speech work in the third grade was begun in November. The clinician and he continued work on ear training. During this year he learned to make the sounds [k], [g], [s], [ʃ], [tʃ], and [dʒ]. In the sibilants, lateral emission was obvious. The clinician, however, preferred to wait until later to help the child control the sibilant sounds, since they were at least recognizable. Work on [l] and [r] was begun. At the end of the year he could make these sounds in nonsense syllables. Although he now could make all the sounds, he did not always incorporate them into his speech. During this grade he again was particularly fortunate in having a teacher who encouraged him to do his very best and who was particularly understanding of him and his problems. She was able to give him many opportunities to feel successful.

Speech Training in the Fourth Grade. In the fourth grade ear training was still continued. A report of the clinician indicates, "A test on sound discrimination was given four weeks apart and showed wide discrepancy in ability to discriminate between sounds." During this year, the clinician concentrated on [r] and [l]. The clinician notes: "His *s*[s], *sh*[ʃ] are still poor. His *r* and *l* he can make accurately. In clusters, such as [pl], [bl], [pr], [br], [sl], and [tr], the [r] and [l] tend to be poor. He still does not consistently incorporate his new sounds in words." Until the fourth grade all the teachers complained that they could not understand what he said and that frequently the other children translated for him. The fourth-grade teacher understood him from the first day he was in her class. She was particularly helpful in giving him opportunities to succeed in speaking situations.

Speech Training in the Fifth and Sixth Grades. In the fifth grade, no speech help was available for Jackie. In the sixth grade, he was again given ear training. Here he was working with a different speech clinician. She noted that preliminary ear training to improve his ability to discriminate, analyze, and synthesize sound sequences had occupied a major part of Jackie's time in speech help and that his response was such as to indicate that his difficulties were the result of poor training. In this grade he was taught a type of compensatory mechanics for his particular mouth deformity, in teaching the [s] and [ʃ]. He was also given training on [bl], [pl], [br], [pr], and [sl].

Speech Training in the Seventh and Eighth Grades. In the seventh grade, his difficulty with clusters was largely eradicated. His phonetic discrimination became more accurate. Progress in teaching an acceptable [s] and [ʃ] continued to be slow. In this grade, however, his speech was such that an adult said, "Why, there's nothing wrong with that child's speech. He sounds all right to me." There was no report for the eighth grade.

COMMENTS ON JACKIE'S PROGRESS

Several factors are noteworthy. Jackie's largest gain in reading was made between the fourth and fifth grades. It was at the end of the fourth grade that his speech showed the greatest amount of improvement. The success of his speech work depended on his ability to concentrate and this ability varied from day to day. He did not move forward steadily in his ability to speak. His test scores in academic subjects showed the same kind of progress and at times retrogression.

Jackie's story is particularly interesting, because his environment at home and at school, his own adjustment, and his intelligence seem conducive to at least average ability in speech. Attempts to form a hypothesis as to the possible organic cause were unavailing. His motor coordination may have been poor for tasks that needed fine, exact coordination. At one point, it was felt that his difficulty might be one of perception. A neurologist's examination indicated that he felt that this was not the cause of the difficulty.

A conclusion that can be drawn rather readily is that his speech work should have started in kindergarten rather than in second grade. His teachers felt that if the speech work had been started earlier, his spelling and reading would not have been as difficult for him.

Another interesting aspect is that Jackie remained an alive, outgoing child who got along well with his peers and adults. It appeared that his speech difficulty did not affect his relationships with others. That he did accept his defect and that his classmates also did so are a credit to his teachers and to his family. One time an adult in his neighborhood said, "Jackie's stupid—the way he talks." A small friend of his, overhearing, said, "Ah, he's good at a lot of things." One day Jackie brought to school a small tool that he had built to show his classmates and teacher. When he showed it to the clinician, she remarked, "I couldn't make that." Jackie replied, "Well, everybody can't do everything. Lotta things I can't do—like spelling."

Jackie's progress in learning to make all the sounds was not rapid. But he finally learned to speak so that his difficulties were not apparent to his listeners. That he did learn to speak well is in a large part due to the help given him by his elementary school teachers and the speech clinicians. They accepted him as he was, and encouraged him to speak well and to participate in a variety of experiences.

Bibliography of Children's Books That Provide Practice Material for the Indicated Sounds

[t]	3, 4, 12, 16, 21, 23, 33
[d]	3, 4, 5, 12, 16, 21, 23, 33
[k]	5, 11, 12, 25, 26, 30, 32, 40
[g]	6, 12, 25, 32, 40
[p]	20, 33
[b]	8, 20, 33
[s]	1, 4, 7, 9, 15, 17, 20, 29, 36, 38, 39, 41
[z]	4, 16, 22
[ŋ]	22, 24
[ʃ]	3, 5, 12
[tʃ]	3, 7, 17, 20, 33, 41
[dʒ]	5, 14, 21, 30, 33, 35, 38
[f]	14, 20, 24, 30, 32, 33
[v]	24, 32, 33
[θ]	11, 16
[ð]	11, 16
[l]	8, 10, 13, 16, 20, 22, 28, 30, 41
[r]	16, 17, 18, 20, 24, 28, 30, 33, 38
All sounds	19, 26, 27, 34, 37, 39

1. ADELSON, LEONE, *Who Blew That Whistle?* New York, William R. Scott, 1946. (The story of Officer Chuffey and the use of his whistle in directing traffic.)
2. BANNON, LAURA, *Baby Roo.* Boston, Houghton Mifflin Company, 1947. (Story of the kangaroo's friendship with other animals.)
3. BEIM, JERROLD, *Shoeshine Boy.* New York, William Morrow and Company, Inc., 1954. (A story of how Teddy earned money shining shoes.)
4. BEIM, LORRAINE, and JERROLD BEIM, *Two Is a Team.* New York, Harcourt, Brace & World, Inc., 1945. (The story of how two little boys play together.)
5. BENÉT, WILLIAM ROSE, *Timothy's Angels.* New York, Thomas Y. Crowell, Inc., 1947. (A story of how the angels found their ball.)
6. BETTINA, *Cocolo Comes to America.* New York, Harper & Row, Publishers, 1948. (The separation of Cocolo the donkey from his friend Lucio.)
7. BISHOP, CLAIRE HUCHET, *The Five Chinese Brothers.* New York, Coward-McCann, Inc., 1938. (A story of a particular ability of each of the Chinese brothers.)
8. BROWN, MARGARET WISE, *The Little Cowboy.* New York, William R. Scott, 1948. (A tale of cowboys—where they lived—what they did and sang.)
9. BROWN, PAUL, *Silver Heels.* New York, Charles Scribner's Sons, 1951. (The story of a pony and his owners.)

10. DE BRUNHOFF, JEAN, *The Story of Babar*. New York, Random House, Inc., 1933. (The story of the life of Babar, the elephant, and his fine new clothes. Tells of his life in the forest and of his going to town and finally coming back to the forest.)

11. BURTON, VIRGINIA LEE, *Katy and the Big Snow*. Boston, Houghton Mifflin Company, 1943. (The story of how Katy, the snow plow, saved the city in a snow storm.)

12. ————, *Mike Mulligan and His Steam Shovel*. Boston, Houghton Mifflin Company, 1939. (The story of a steam shovel, outmoded, digging a cellar in a new house.)

13. CAMPBELL, BARBARA, *Barbara Lamb*. New York, Roy Publishers, no date. (The tale of the lamb Barbara and her life in the city and on the farm.)

14. CARROLL, RUTH, and LATROBE CARROLL, *Tough Enough*. New York, Oxford University Press, Inc., 1954. (Set in Smoky Mountains. Tale of the mischief of Tough Enough, Beanie's dog.)

15. FENNER, PHYLLIS R., *Circus Parade*. New York, Alfred A. Knopf, Inc., 1954. (A collection of stories about animals and circus.)

16. GÁG, WANDA, *Nothing at All*. New York, Coward-McCann, Inc., 1941. (The story of three little orphan dogs.)

17. ————, *Snippy and Snappy*. New York, Coward-McCann, Inc., 1931. (A tale of two little field mice.)

18. GOUDEY, ALICE, *The Good Rain*. New York, American Book Company, 1950. (An explanation of all the good rain does for us and for nature.)

19. HUGHES, LANGSTON, *First Book of Rhythms*. New York, Franklin Watts, 1954.

20. JOHNSON, ELEANOR M., *Our Houses*. Columbus, Ohio, Charles E. Merrill Books, Inc., 1942. (An explanation of different kinds of houses and how they are made.)

21. KARASZ, ILONKA, *The Twelve Days of Christmas*. New York, Harper & Row, Publishers, 1949. (A song telling what my true love sent to me. A partridge in a pear tree is always included.)

22. LENSKI, LOIS, *I Like Winter*. New York, Oxford University Press, Inc., 1950 (Description of the fun of winter—Christmas, snow, and the cold, cold weather.)

23. ————, *The Little Train*. New York, Oxford University Press, Inc., 1940. (A tale of Engineer Small and his engine.)

24. ————, *Now It's Fall*. New York, Oxford University Press, Inc., 1948. (A story of what children do in the fall.)

25. LIPKIND, WILLIAM, *The Two Reds*. New York, Harcourt, Brace & World, Inc., 1950. (The narration of how a cat and a dog learned to get along together.)

26. LOVE, KATHERINE A., *Pocketful of Ryhmes*. New York: Crowell-Collier Publishing Company, 1946.

27. McGINLEY, PHYLLIS, *All Around the Town*. Philadelphia, J. B. Lippincott Company, 1948 (A tale of city sights beginning with A and ending with Z. Good for almost all sounds. For example, words containing the *k* sound include crocus, crows, crackerjack.)

28. ——, *The Plain Princess*. Philadelphia, J. B. Lippincott Company,1945. (The Princess becomes beautiful through a change in personality.)
29. MARIANA (Marian C. Foster), *Miss Flora McFlimsey's Christmas*. New York, Lothrop, Lee & Shepard Company, Inc., 1949. (A tale of a doll long hidden in the attic now placed under a Christmas tree.)
30. PARKER, BERTHA MORRIS, *Fall Is Here*. New York, Harper & Row, Publishers, 1953. (Contains a picture dictionary at end. An explanation of fall—its flowers, berries, wild life, weather, harvest of fruit and vegetables.)
31. ——, *Winter Is Here*. New York, Harper & Row, Publishers, 1948. (An explanation of winter—its snow, weather, trees, birds, animals, sky, stars, and sleigh riding. Includes a picture dictionary.)
32. READ, HELEN S., *Mr. Brown's Grocery Store*. New York, Charles Scribner's Sons, 1929. (An explanation of the operation of a grocery store—where groceries come from and how they are sold. Tells about children playing store.)
33. REED, MARY, ed., *Counting Rhymes*. New York, Simon and Schuster, Inc., 1946. (Rhymes having to do with numbers.)
34. SALAFF, ALICE, *Words Are Funny*. Garden City, N.Y., Doubleday & Company, Inc., 1952. (A book of riddles including word games and puzzle rhymes.)
35. SAWYER, RUTH, *Journey Cake, Ho!* New York, The Viking Press, Inc., 1953. (How Journey Cake became a Johnny Cake.)
36. ——, *Roller Skates*. New York, The Viking Press, Inc., 1936. (Exploration of New York City on roller skates.)
37. SEATTER, MINNIS, *Romp in Rhythm*. Cincinnati, Ohio: Willis Music Company, 1944. (For kindergartners.)
38. SLOBODKIN, LOIS, *Clear the Track*. New York, The Macmillan Company, 1945. (A story of playing at traveling.)
39. STEINER, CHARLOTTE, *Charlotte Steiner's A B C*. Garden City, N.Y., Garden City Books, 1946. (An A B C book.)
40. TRESSELT, ALVIN, *Autumn Harvest*. New York, Lothrop, Lee & Shepard Company, Inc., 1951. (Description of autumn with its harvest time, Hallowe'en, and Thanksgiving.)
41. ——, *Sun Up*. New York, Lothrop, Lee & Shepard Company, Inc., 1949. (The description of the day with sun, wind, rain and night.)

References and Suggested Readings

American Speech and Hearing Association Research Committee, "Public School Speech and Hearing Services," *Journal of Speech and Hearing Disorders*, Monograph Supplement 8 (July, 1961.)
BERRY, M., and J. EISENSON, *Speech Disorders: Principles and Practices of Therapy*. New York, Appleton-Century-Crofts, 1956, Chaps. 6, 7. (Includes carefully planned drill material.)
BLACK, M. E., and R. A. S. LUDWIG, "Analysis of the Games Technic,"

Journal of Speech and Hearing Disorders, XXI (June, 1956), 183–187. (Gives criteria for using games in treatment of articulatory difficulties.)

BRICKER, W. A., " Errors in the Echoic Behavior of Preschool Children," *Journal of Speech and Hearing Research*, X (March, 1967), 67–76. (Notes that: (1) errors are inversely related to the frequency of the sounds in the repertoire of infants and to the frequency of the sounds in the English language; (2) stability of specific errors increases with age while total frequency of errors decreases; and (3) more errors are associated with the placement of articulation than with either the manner of articulation or the voiced-voiceless dimension.)

BURKLAND, M. " Use of Television to Study Articulatory Problems," *Journal of Speech and Hearing Disorders*, XXXII (February, 1967), 80–81. Discusses the effectiveness of ultilizing videotape equipment for simultaneous viewing of a student's phoneme production by the speech clinician and his student.)

CROCKER, J. M., "A Phonological Model of Children's Articulation Competence," *Journal of Speech and Hearing Disorders*, XXXIV (August, 1969), 203–213. (Explores the possibility of constructing a theoretical linguistic model of children's developing consonantal phonological competence.)

CYPREANSEN, L., J. H. WILEY, and L. T. LAASE, *Speech Dvelopment, Improvement and Correction*. New York, The Ronald Press Company, 1959.

DANILOFF, R., and K. MOLL, " Coarticulation of Lip Rounding," *Journal of Speech and Hearing Research*, XI (December, 1968), 707–721. (Investigates the extent of co-articulation of lip rounding in selected string of morphemes in constructed sentences with sequences of one to four consonants preceding /u/.)

EGBERT, J. H., *The Effect of Certain Home Influences on the Progress of Children in a Speech Therapy Program*. Unpublished Ph.D. thesis Stanford University, 1955.

GOTT, S. R., and R. MILISEN, " Functional Articulatory Disorders," *Education*, LXXX (April, 1960), 468–470. (Tells how classroom teacher can help the child with an articulatory disorder.)

HAHN, E., " Communication in the Therapy Session: A Point of View," *Journal of Speech and Hearing Disorders*, XXV (February, 1960), 18–23.

JACOBS, R., *On Transformational Grammar: An Introduction for Teachers*. Monograph 11, New York State English Council, Oneonta, New York, 1968.

JOHNSON, W., et al., *Speech-Handicapped School Children*, 3rd ed. New York, Harper & Row, Publishers, 1967. (Describes retraining and states the classroom teacher's responsibility for it.)

LLOYD, G. W., and S. AINSWORTH, " The Classroom Teacher's Activities and Attitudes Relating to Speech Correction," *Journal of Speech and Hearing Disorders*, XIX (June, 1954), 244–249.

McINTYRE, B. M., " The Effect of Creative Activities on the Articulation of Children with Speech Disorders," *ASHA*, I (November, 1959), 80.

———, *The Effect of a Program of Creative Activities upon the Consonant Articulation Skills of Adolescent and Pre-Adolescent Children with Speech Disorders*. Ph.D. Dissertation, University of Pittsburgh, 1957.

————, and B. J. McWilliams, " Creative Dramatics in Speech Correction," *Journal of Speech and Hearing Disorders*, XXIV (August, 1959), 275–279.

Mader, J. B., " The Relative Frequency of Occurrence of English Consonant Sounds in Words in the Speech of Children in Grades One, Two and Three," *Speech Monographs*, XXI (November, 1954).

Ohman, S. E. G., "Numerical Model of Co-Articulation," *Journal of Acoustical Society of America*, XXXXI (1967), 310–320.

Ohman, S. E. G., " Coarticulation in VCV utterances: Spectographic Measurements," *Journal of Acoustical Society of America*, XXXIX (1966), 151–168.

Prins, D. T., "Abilities of Children with Misarticulations," *Journal of Speech and Hearing Research*, V (June, 1962), 161–168. (a)

————, "Analysis of Correlations Among Various Articulatory Deviations," *Journal of Speech and Hearing Research*, V (June, 1962), 152–160. (b)

Ringel, R. L., and S. J. Ewanowski, "Oral Perception: 1. Two-Point Discrimination," *Journal of Speech and Hearing Research*, VIII (June, 1968), 389–398. (Discusses the concept that knowledge of the perceptual abilities of certain oral structures may yield insights into the role of tactile feedback in the total speech-monitoring system.)

Ritterman, S. I., *Practice Variables and Speech Sound Discrimination in Learning.* Ph.D. thesis, Case Western University, 1969.

Scott, D. A., and R. Milisen, "The Effect of Visual, Auditory, and Combined Visual-Auditory Stimulation upon the Speech Responses of Defective Speaking Children," *Journal of Speech and Hearing Disorders*, Monograph Supplement, IV (1954), 37–43. (Reports differences between an imitative nonsense syllable test and an imitative word test, with the nonsense test yielding fewer errors in both instances.)

Sommers, R. K., " Factors in the Effectiveness of Mothers Trained to Aid in Speech Correction," *Journal of Speech and Hearing Disorders*, XXVII (May, 1962), 178–186.

————, et al., " Effect of Maternal Attitudes Upon Improvement in Articulation When Mothers Are Trained to Assist in Speech Correction," *Journal of Speech and Hearing Disorders*, XXIX (May, 1964), 126–132.

————, " The Effectiveness of Group and Individual Therapy," *Journal of Speech and Hearing Research*, IX (June, 1966), 219–225. (Finds that individual and group therapy are equally effective, independent of either the grade level or the degree of articulatory defect.)

Sommers, R. K., S. P. Shilling, C. D. Paul, F. G. Copetas, D. C. Bowser, and C. J. McClintock. "Training Parents of Children with Functional Misarticulation," *Journal of Speech and Hearing Research*, II (September, 1959), 258–265.

Templin, M. G., *Certain Language Skills in Children.* Minneapolis, University of Minnesota Press, 1957.

————, "A Study of the Sound Discrimination Ability of Elementary School Pupils,' *Journal of Speech Disorders*, VIII (June, 1943), 127–132.

Thomas, O., *Transformational Grammar and the Teacher of English.* New York, Holt, Rinehart & Winston, Inc., 1965.

Thorndike, E. L., and I. Lorge, *The Teacher's Word Book of 30,000 Words.* New York, Bureau of Publications, Teachers' College, Columbia University, 1944.

Travis, L. E., *Handbook of Speech Pathology.* New York, Appleton-Century-Crofts, 1957.

Tufts, L. C., and A. R. Holliday, "Effectiveness of Trained Parents as Speech Therapists," *Journal of Speech and Hearing Disorders,* XXIV (November, 1959), 395–396.

Van Riper, C., *Speech Correction: Principles and Methods,* 4th ed., Englewood Cliffs, N.J., Prentice-Hall, Inc., 1963, Chap. 7.

Van Riper, C., and J. V. Irwin, *Voice and Articulation.* Englewood Cliffs, N.J.: Prentice-Hall, Inc., 1958.

Weber, J. L., "Patterning of Deviant Articulation Behavior," *Journal of Speech and Hearing Disorders,* XXIV (May, 1970), 135–41. (Indicates how entire pattern of articulation can be taught at once.)

Webster, E. J., "Procedures for Group Parent Counseling in Speech Pathology and Audiology," *Journal of Speech and Hearing Disorders,* XXXIII (May, 1968), 127–131. (Discusses use of group discussion and role playing in parent counseling.)

Weiss, H. H., and B. Born, "Speech Training or Language Acquisition? A Distinction When Speech Training Is Taught by Operant Conditioning Procedures," *American Journal of Orthopsychiatry,* XXXVII (January, 1967), 49–55. (Reports on behavior modification in teaching speech to a seven-and-a-half-year-old boy with success in several learning paradigms within limits of circumscribed training sessions, but failure to generalize learned speech patterns outside of experimental settings. Suggests this may be an important distinction between speech and language.)

Wentland, T. J., and F. D. Minifie, "The Effect of Phonetic Environment on the Consistency of Misarticulations of /r/," *ASHA,* VII (October, 1965), 387.

Winitz, H., *Articulatory Acquisition and Behavior.* New York, Appleton-Century-Crofts, 1969, Chap. 5. (Discusses articulatory programing.)

————, and B. Bellerose, "Sound Discrimination as a Function of Pretraining Conditions," *Journal of Speech and Hearing Research,* V (December, 1962), 340–348.

Materials for Articulation Therapy

Alphabet of Sound Pictures and Word List. (Contains 24 identification pictures for the consonant sounds and pictures for isolating sounds in words. A set of 35 copies of the pictures, composites, and word lists: $2.00.) Sound Materials.*

An Automated Program in Speech Therapy, by J. Ervin, M. Grundman, E. Pea-

---

* An alphabetical list of publishers of this material, with addresses, is given on page 290.

body, and G. Sterns. (Consists of tapes for 44 programed lessons designed for the correction of faulty articulation of kindergarten and primary school ages. Provides auditory discrimination of minimal differences between paired sounds. $121 for set of 44 tapes (3¾ ips).) Institute of Modern Languages.

The Best Speech Series, by Jack Matthews, J. W. Birch, E. J. Burgi, and E. R. Wade. (Made up of seven student " My Sound Books," one each for /s/, /r/, / θ/, /l/, /k/, /g/ and /ʃ/ sounds. Presents each sound in hundreds of contexts. $1.25 per copy.) Stanwix House.

Captain Good Speech and Mr. Mumbles, by J. M. Sayre and J. E. Mack. (Contains six full-color film strips, three 33⅓ rpm records, 58 sequence cards, individual student activity book with flip-out mirror, and teacher's manual. Designed to improve listening skills of the preschool and primary child.) Eye Gate House.

City Rhythms, by A. Geufalcone. (Explores sounds and rhythms of the city for young children. Film strip, recording, and book.) Hudson Photographic Industries.

Dig for Gold, by M. R. Kodama. (Helps children recognize and pronounce single consonants in various positions in word. Contains 75 cards. $2.95 per deck.) Interstate Printers and Publishers.

Equipment Checklist for Preschool, Kindergarten, and the Early Grades. (Contains list of materials useful in Headstart Centers. Free.) Creative Playthings, Inc.

ID Cards. (Contains 12 characters that help children identify with their particular sound difficulty. $7.50 per set.) Speech and Language Materials.

Hand Puppets, created by H. Beeckler. (Can be used as visual aids to show tongue placement for sound production. $2.00 each.) Hazel Beeckler.

Hear, See and Tell Stories by M. F. Perritt. (Presents auditory, visual, and kinesthetic aspects of speech sound recognition, discrimination, and production. Written for young children. $2.00.) American Southern Publishing Company.

Language Lotto by L. G. Gotkin. (Consists of six games which elicit words, phrases, and sentences from children. Helps to teach sound discrimination. $43.50.) Appleton-Century-Crofts.

Let's Talk About. (Consists of a record and film strip which discusses child's life in the city—big-city housing, animals, travel, and food in the city.) Hudson Photographic Industries.

Listen and Speak to Read, by B. J. Ortiz, H. S. Beck. (Contains materials to be used as a training program developing sound discrimination and articulation needed for reading. 44 pages of lessons on liquid duplicator master sheets. $3.50 per copy.) Hayes School Publishing Company.

Louie the Lazy Listener and *Holiday Activity Stories,* by G. L. Smith and V. P. Call. (The first contains three listening activity stories incorporating /r/, /l/, /s, and /s/ clusters. The second is a collection of seasonal, language-oriented stories. For K-3. *Louie*—$5.95; *Holiday*—8.95.) Selected Creative Communication.

Louie the Listener in Garble Glen and *S'More Holiday Activity Stories. Louie* emphasizes /s/, /z/, /ʃ/, /tʃ/, and /dʒ/. *S'More* emphasizes /s/, /l/ and /r/. $4.95 each.) Selected Creative Communication.

Pape Series of Speech Improvement Books, by D. L. Pape. (Provides sound identification, sound stimulation, and carryover practice for children in elementary grades. Series of six books, $3.48 per volume.) Oddo Publishing Company.

Peabody Language Development Kit, Level #1 and #2. (Stimulates overall language and cognitive development. Lessons were developed cooperatively by speech clinicians, educators, psychologists, and were tested in the field. Kit #1 contains 180 lessons, 430 color stimulus cards, 10 large "story" and "I wonder" cards in color, colored plastic chips, two hand puppets, a tape of fairy tales and songs and music for "Language Time." Housed in a metal container. Kit #2 contains similar material. $48.00 per kit.) American Guidance Service, Inc.

Peel and Put Speech and Language Activity Program. (Set 1 (sibilant phonemes set), Set II (Dialectal phonemes set), and Set III (/r/ and /l/ phonemes set). 240 pictures in each set. $9.85 per set.) Communication Skill Builders.

Play and Say It, by B. L. Mellencamp. (Covers sounds that present the most difficulty for the child with a functional articulatory defect. $3.75.) Expression Company.

Programmed Articulation Sequences, by D. E. Mowrer, R. L. Baker, and R. E. Schutz. (Contains instructional script and necessary stimulus materials for modifying the frontal lisp. $24.50 for complete kit.) Educational Psychological Research Associates.

Read-the-Picture-Story Books, by E. Dunlap. (A series of sound-centered stories.) Word Making Production.

See and Say, by Joseph Michel. (Contains material for students who are beginning their study of a second language, English. $1.00.) W. S. Benson and Company.

Snoopy Snake and Other Stories. (Contains 31 sound-centered stories for use in ear training. $3.50.) Word Making Productions.

Sound Clown. (A set of 18 spirit masters that progresses from sound discrimination to the production of the sound in isolation, in words, in sentences, and in poems. $7.50.) Interstate Printers and Publishers.

Speech Correction Series, by R. Hendricks. (A manual and a series of 31 dual track tape recordings for practice. Deals with sounds most frequently misarticulated. $110.00.) General Electronic Laboratories (Learning Material Division).

Speech Sound Series, by K. Mosier. (Contains perceptual training materials oriented to sound and functional language. Consonant series: 15 books, $21.75; Vowel Series: 6 books, $8.75.) Keystone View Co.

Spin-a-Test, by Cecil Alberts. (Consists of a 15-inch counterbalanced indicator wherein pictures can be arranged around the circumference of the circle. $5.00.) Spin-a-Test Company.

Spoken Word Count, by L. V. Jones and J. M. Wepman. (Contains lists of the most frequently used words in spoken language, presented in order of frequency of use, in alphabetical order, and alphabetically by part of speech. $3.00.) Language Research Associates.

Stimulation Cards and Conversational Stimulation Cards. (Elicits one word and phrase and sentence responses. Set of 30 for /r/, /θ/, /l/, and /ʃ/ sounds. Each set contains 15 stimulation and 15 conversational stimulation cards. $6.00 per set.) Speech and Language Materials.

Talking Magic, by E. Marquardt. (Promotes listening. $3.25.) Interstate Printers and Publishers.

Think, Listen and Say, by J. M. Sayre and J. E. Mack. (Consists of 8 filmstrips, four 33⅓ rpm records, and four sets of story sequence cards designed to improve listening skills.) Eye Gate House.

Time for Phonics, by L. B. Scott. (Teaches phonics through listening, speaking, reading, and writing. Under $1.00. Other publications by the same author include *Phonics* and *Flashcards,* $4.00 to $5.00 per set.) McGraw-Hill, Inc. (Webster Publishing Division).

Tony Plays with Sounds, by Jane R. Aponner. (Includes stories, rhymes and exercises for sounds from simplest to the more difficult. $2.95.) John Day.

When People Talk . . . on the Telephone, Book A and Book B. (Involves realistic situations with adults or teenagers. $0.60 each.) Bureau of Publications, Teachers' College, Columbia University, New York.

Addresses of Companies Supplying Material for Speech Therapy

W. H. Acton Company, 392A Hillside Avenue, Williston Park, New York.

American Guidance System, 720 Washington Avenue, S.E., Minneapolis, Minneapolis 55414.

American Southern Publishing Company, Northport, Alabama.

Appleton-Century-Crofts, 440 Park Avenue South, New York, New York 10016.

Genevieve Arnold, University of Houston, Houston, Texas.

Hazler Beeckler, 122 Kennedy, San Antonio, Texas.

Bureau of Educational Research Services, State University of Iowa, Iowa City, Iowa.

Children's Press, Chicago, Illinois.

Chronicle Guidance Publishing Company, Moravia, New York.

Communication Skills Builders, 234 East Pasadena Avenue, Phoenix, Arizona 85012.

Continental Press, Elizabethtown, Pasadena.

Creative Playthings, Princeton, New Jersey 18540, or 5757 West Century Block, Los Angeles, California.

The John Day Company, 62 West 45th Street, New York, New York.

Developmental Learning Materials, 3505 North Ashland Avenue, Chicago, Illinois 60657.

Educational Psychological Research Associates, P.O. Box 741, Tempe, Arizona 85281.

Expression Company, P.O. Box 11, Magnolia, Massachusetts.

Eye Gate House, 146–01 Archer Avenue, Jamaica, New York 11435.

Follett Library Book Company, 1018 Washington Boulevard., Chicago, Illinois 60607.

General Electric Laboratories, Inc. (Learning Materials Division), 1085 Commonwealth Avenue, Boston, Massachusetts.

Ginn and Company, 125 Second Avenue, Waltham, Massachusetts.

Go-Mo Productions, Box 143, Waterloo, Iowa.

Golden Press, 850 Third Avenue, New York, New York.

J. L. Hammett, 2393 Vauxhall Road, Union, New Jersey.

Harper & Row, Publishers, 49 East 33rd Street, New York, New York.

Hayes School Publishing Company, Wilkensburg, Pasadena.

Hudson Photographic Industries, Irvington on Hudson, New York 10533.

IDA, P.O. Box 55, Citrus Heights, California 95610.

Institute of Modern Languages, 1666 Connecticutt Avenue, N.W., Washington, D.C. 20009

Interstate Printers and Publishers, Danville, Illinois, 61832

Instructional Materials Association, 175 Fifth Avenue, New York, New York 10010.

Keystone View Company, Meadville, Pasadena, 16335

Language Research Associates, 300 North State Street, Chicago, Illinois, 60610

McGraw-Hill, Inc. (Webster Division), Manchester Road, Manchester, Missouri 63062.

Oddo Publishing Company, Box 833, Mankato, Minnesota 56002.

Phonovisual Producers, P.O. Box 5625, Washington, D.C.

Pollywood Publishing Company, 5548 West Gladys Avenue, Chicago, Illinois 60644

Primary Playhouse, Sherwood, Oregon.

Selected Creative Communication, Box 6723, Long Beach, California 90815.

Scott, Foresman and Company, 99 Baver Drive, Oakland, N.J., 07436.

Simon and Schuster, Inc., 1 West 39th Street, New York City.

Sound Materials, P.O. Box 453, Knoxville, Tennessee.

Speech and Language Materials, P.O. Box 721, Dept. A., Tulsa, Oklahoma 74101.

Spin-a-Test Company, 627 Rose Avenue, Pleasanton, California 94556.

Stanwix House, 3020 Chartiers Avenue, Pittsburgh, Pennsylvania.

Teachers' College, Columbia University, New York, New York.

Warnock Medlen Productions, P.O. Box 305, Salt Lake City, Utah 84110.

L. L. Weans Company, Beltagh Avenue, Wantagh, New York.

Word Making Productions, P.O. Box 305, Salt Lake City, Utah 84110.

Problems

1. Visit a school or clinic where you may observe a specialist working with a child with an articulatory difficulty. Indicate how you can reinforce in

the classroom some of the learning that took place in the speech class or clinic.

2. Indicate ways other than those mentioned in the chapter of helping a child to listen to a specific sound.

3. How, as a classroom teacher, can you make use of some of the drill material listed in this chapter?

4. Find children's books that emphasize a particular sound. How can these books be used in the classroom?

5. Make up a story involving nonsense syllables.

6. Indicate ways you, as a classroom teacher, could help a child like Jackie (page 274) to speak better.

7. Read and report on one of the following: Daniloff and Moll, 1968; Prins, 1962 (b); Sommers, 1964; Webster, 1968; Wentland, 1965, Weber, 1970.

Chapter 12

Voice
Disturbances

Before considering disturbances of voice we suggest that the student review the material on the vocal mechanism in Chapter 5. As supplementary reading, we recommend the chapters by Curtis (1967) and Van Riper (1958). Although much in these chapters covers the same areas as does our discussion, they will provide a firm introduction and some essential concepts for our study.

The incidence of voice disturbances in school-age children, especially in the primary grades, is much lower than for articulatory defects or for stuttering. For every child with a vocal disturbance we are likely to find from 10 to 15 who have defective articulation or who show signs of stuttering. Thus, the study of voice disturbances is not as important for its total incidence as it is for its possible significance as a reflection of the child's personality, or perhaps of the personality of the individual with whom the child is identifying and imitating. Another reason for us to study voice disturbances is that they may be associated with a physical condition that may require medical attention.

Before considering vocal disturbances, we ought first to appreciate the characteristics and potentialities of a normal voice.

Characteristics of a Normal Voice

A normal voice should be able to communicate reliably the feelings and thoughts the speaker wishes to convey to his listener. When well controlled, the voice should reveal rather than betray the types and shades of feeling that color the speaker's thinking. Through appropriate changes in pitch, force, duration, and quality a speaker's voice should be able to command attention, maintain interest, and convey changes and emphasis in meaning.

The ability of a speaker to communicate intellectual and affective content will be enhanced if the speaker's voice attracts no attention to itself because of the manner in which it is produced or because of any undesirable characteristics. Vocalization should take place without apparent effort or strain. The acoustic results should be appropriate to the speaking situation. The voice should, in addition, be appropriate to the age and sex of the speaker. Little children may sound like little children, but older ones should not be mistaken for them. Neither should first graders sound like their parents or their teachers.

From the point of view of the listener, a normal and effective voice is one that is pleasant, clear, and readily audible. It should be heard without listener effort, provided, of course, that the listening conditions are not unfavorable for the purpose.

TYPES OF VOICE DISTURBANCES

The defects of voice most frequently heard are: (1) inadequate loudness; (2) faulty volume (loudness) control; (3) loudness inappropriate to the speaking situation or speech content; (4) defects of quality, especially nasality and denasality, breathiness, and huskiness; (5) faulty pitch range or too narrow a range of pitch; and (6) inappropriate rate. Each of these will be considered in some detail in our discussion of therapy for voice disturbances.

CAUSES OF VOCAL DISTURBANCES

At the outset, it should be pointed out that the *diagnosis of a voice disturbance should be made by a specialist.** Where a physical condition may be

---

* By a specialist we mean a professional person whose training and experience qualify him for making diagnoses and for treating persons who present vocal difficulties when speaking. Such a person should have considerably more than the usual exposure to voice problems as part of his general training.

the underlying cause, treatment should not be undertaken without medical clearance and approval. Fortunately, even where the cause is physical, treatment may help to prevent aggravation of the disturbance and often may improve the condition as well as the voice.

Vocal disturbances may be present for a variety of reasons. Among the most numerous are: (1) poor physical health; (2) anomalies in the structure or condition of the voice mechanism; (3) pathologies in the neurological control of the mechanism; (4) glandular conditions or other physical conditions that may affect the growth or the tonicity and the responses of the muscles involved in voice production; (5) defects of hearing that impair the individual's ability to respond to and monitor his own voice as it is being produced; (6) disturbances of personality that reflect themselves in voice; (7) the presence of poor models which the child is imitating, so that he acquires a vocal defect through normal processes of learning; and (8) poor habits of vocalization.

The speech clinician and classroom teacher are most likely to be directly concerned with the last two of the listed reasons. To a lesser degree, defects of hearing may also directly concern them. Vocal disturbances that have a physical basis, as already suggested, are the therapeutic concern of the specialist in voice problems. The teacher, however, is frequently the first to have an opportunity to recognize that something may be wrong which is causing the child to have a vocal difficulty, and so has a responsibility for bringing the condition to the attention of the parent and speech clinician.

Poor Physical Health. Most of us are able to recognize that "something is wrong" with a friend or relative by the way he sounds. Sometimes "what is wrong" may be temporary and a matter of momentary mood; occasionally, it may be physical and a matter of health. The interested and sensitive listener, who may be parent, friend, or teacher, is often the first to suspect that a speaker may not be well. Voice, because it is a product of the physiological as well as the emotional and intellectual state of the speaker, is the mirror that reflects the speaker's state of health. The expert speaker may, with awareness, control his voice and so succeed in disguising this condition. The school-age child, less practiced in concealment and control, frequently reveals both his affective state and the state of his general physical health through his vocalization.

Physical Anomalies. Perhaps the most frequent cause of vocal disturbances is the common cold. When we suffer from a cold, any or all of the following modifications of the voice mechanism may be present. The nasal cavities may be filled with mucous and so prevent adequate reinforcement of voice. The mucous membranes of the nose, throat, and larynx may be inflamed, and so modify the normal resonating activity of the voice mechanism. The vocal bands may themselves be inflamed and swollen, and so prevent normal vocal activity. The general "rundown" condition of the individual may impair normal functioning and control of the voice mechanism. If the cold is accompanied by a persistent cough, the general condition may be aggravated by the vocal abuse that is caused by coughing.

Persistent coughing may produce laryngitis. The condition of laryngitis may, however, be caused by vocal abuse not associated with either a cough or a cold. Continued overloud talking, or yelling under conditions of competing noise, may also produce a laryngitis.

Sometimes vocal difficulties are associated with abnormalities of the structure of the larynx. The laryngeal cartilages may, for congenital reasons or through injury, be so constructed that the vocal bands may not be able to approximate normally, or the reinforcement of vocal tones may be impaired because of the change in the size and shape of the larynx. More frequently, the vocal bands may have developed nodules on the inner edges as a result of vocal abuse. Sometimes the vocal bands become thickened because of chronic incorrect vocalization. The effect is usually a voice characterized by low pitch, breathiness, and effort in production. Fortunately, these conditions usually improve through a combination of voice rest and a program of training to modify the incorrect vocal behavior of the speaker. Occasionally, the edges of the vocal bands may have slight irregularities, which impair normal activity. Any of the conditions described can be determined only through an examination of the larynx by a competent physician. The treatment of these conditions will call for the active cooperation of the classroom teacher. Voice therapy, if it is indicated, is a problem for the speech clinician working in cooperation with the physician.

Hearing Loss. Because we learn to vocalize as well as to articulate "by ear," hearing loss, especially in the low-pitch ranges, is likely to be manifest in vocal inadequacies. If the hearing loss is appreciable, and of the type that does not permit the child to check on the voice he produces, he may speak in a voice too loud, or not loud enough, for the specific speaking situation. Sometimes the loss may be temporary, and associated with the effects or aftereffects of a cold. Occasionally, as a result of middle-ear involvement, there may be prolonged hearing loss. With proper medical attention, this situation should clear and the vocal disturbance disappear.

Glandular Disturbances. Thyroid gland deficiency is associated with a falling of the basal metabolic rate. Frequently, though not invariably, decrease in metabolic rate is causally associated with sluggish physical and mental activity, and with a general reduction of body tone. This condition is likely to reflect itself in a colorless, poorly modulated voice.

In contrast with thyroid deficiency, the presence of an excess of thyroid hormone generally results in making the individual hyperactive and "nervous." The condition is likely to be reflected in a rapid rate of speech and in a tense, high-pitched voice.

The teacher and speech clinician who observe what appear to be significant changes in the general activity and mental alertness of a child, in association with vocal changes, should refer the child to the school nurse or physician for a medical examination to determine the possibility of a glandular involvement. Caution, however, should be exercised that no hasty conclusion be made. Comparable changes in the voice of a child may result from conditions not related to glandular disturbances. Vocal changes may sometimes merely indicate a temporary indisposition on the part of the child.

Pubertal Changes. With the coming of physical adolescence and associated physiological and growth changes, many children have marked vocal difficulties. These are more likely to be present among boys than among girls. In males, the size and structure of the larynx undergo considerable change, so that boys have to adjust to longer vocal bands as well as a larger larynx. Girls, with a longer and slower pubescent period, and with a smaller amount of laryngeal growth, have less modification and more time for adjustment. The little girl soprano may, during adolescence, become a woman mezzo-soprano or perhaps an alto. The boy soprano may become a tenor or a baritone.

Often the difficulty during puberty is aggravated by problems of social adjustment. The shy youngster may be so embarrassed by his voice "breaks" that he withdraws from his groups or finds excuses for not talking. Some of the difficulties may be related to self-consciousness resulting from a poor skin condition, or an awareness of physical awkwardness. Occasionally, overly passive adolescents may try to vocalize within a pitch range determined for them by their parents or older siblings, or other influential members of their environment. In some instances, dependent and infantile boys and girls may try to maintain their preadolescent voices as an aspect of their general wish to continue to be young children. In other instances, both boys and girls may try to show how mature they are by attempting to establish low, deep-pitched voices inconsistent with their amount of laryngeal growth and general physical change.

It should be apparent that the influence of the speech clinician and the classroom teacher in helping the adolescent through his period of voice change can hardly be overestimated. The teacher can ward off taunts and help the adolescent build up his defenses. If the adolescent has prolonged difficulty in arriving at his "new voice," referral to a speech clinician may be of help. If there is reason to believe that psychological problems may be part of the difficulty, referral of the adolescent for proper guidance is in order.

Personality Disturbances. Few of us question the general observation that the voice is a mirror of the personality. Temporary emotional upsets are likely to be reflected in the speaker's voice. Similarly, chronic emotional disturbances and maladjustments of attitude are likely to be manifest in disorders of voice.

Early in his experience, the classroom teacher may have had to urge some child to "speak up" because of a weak and apologetic voice. Some other child may frequently need to be reminded to "tone down" because his classmates are close to him and shouting is not necessary. Both these children may be revealing attitudes toward their classmates in particular and their environment in general that are suggestive of a significant degree of maladjustment. So does the child whose voice is a constant whine; so also does the child whose breathless voice and breathtaking rate suggest that he is afraid that someone may interrupt him if he pauses, and that once interrupted he may not be able to resume his talking.

Although the vocal defects briefly described are not important in themselves, they are of importance if they are symptoms of chronic personality maladjustments. Occasionally, the child's voice may be reflecting not his own maladjustments but one of an older member of his environment whom the child is unconsciously imitating. Whatever the case may be for the individual child, appropriate treatment calls for determining and dealing with the underlying cause as well as with the vocal symptoms of the cause. With the young child, the voice symptoms are likely to disappear without direct treatment provided that the basic personality problem is relieved. The older child, who may have established his vocal traits so that they are fixed and habitual, may need direct treatment for voice even if the personality problem is treated.

Imitation of Poor Models. The child learns both his language and the manner in which his language is produced by ear. The mother who teaches her child the name of something also teaches him the manner in which the naming is done. If mother shouts, so will the child; if mother speaks as though she were not worthy of the evocation, the child is apt to develop the same tone. As the child grows up, other models become subjects for imitation. Friends, liked or respected adults, who frequent the home, and teachers, when the child is of school age, become likely models. Usually the imitation is unconscious; occasionally a child's urge or need to identify with another person is so strong that the imitation may be conscious. Imitation that begins early may continue into and beyond adolescence.

Often a parent will be aware that there is something wrong with a child's voice but have no awareness that the fault is parent-centered. We have frequently pointed out to complaining parents that they must have children who love them because the children spoke so much like them. And we have frequently suggested to parents that they accept treatment for their own voices as the best device for improving the voices of their children.

Teachers, obviously, have a great responsibility for the voices of their classroom children. If the teacher is liked, the children may imitate him unconsciously or consciously; if he is not liked, he may be mimicked in manner as well as in voice. Before the teacher turns to other sources for his pupils' vocal traits, he should listen to himself or have an objective appraisal of his voice made by a professionally competent person. He may then conclude that the "epidemic of hoarseness" is a tribute to his influence in the classroom and followed his own recovery from laryngitis. He may in some instances have to conclude that his own habit of breathiness, denasality, low pitch, or rapid rate needs attention if he is to hope that the children in his class are to vocalize without these specific defects.

Poor Habits of Vocalization. The professional speech clinician often treats persons whose vocal habits are poor and are not apparently associated with any present disturbance of personality or any specific or general physical condition. It is possible, of course, that the faulty vocal habits have outlived the cause of their origin, that in a given instance the speaker is presenting the residual of an adolescent "crush," or a once-serious personality maladjustment, or a vocal manner that began with an illness and has persisted long after all physical evidence of illness disappeared. Not infrequently vocal habits may be interpreted as lingering memories of what used to be. If, however, "what used to be" is no longer in need of treatment, the vocal symptoms, or the vocal habits with which the symptoms are associated, may be directly treated. Chief among faulty vocal habits are unsuitable pitch level, inappropriate nasal reinforcement, and poor breath control for speech.

Vocal pitch and vocal range are not to be selected by the individual as he might choose his clothes. Pitch, as we pointed out earlier, is determined by the size, shape, and normal functioning of the vocal bands and the resonating cavities. Each of us is potentially intended for a given "optimum pitch" and range of pitch according to individual vocal equipment. Most of us arrive at this without special instruction by doing "what comes naturally." Some of us make the most of our potential by special motivation or by competent instruction. A few of us succumb to pressures to vocalize in a manner not consistent with nature's intentions for us, and difficulties may arise. One of these pressures is the contemporary one of admiring women's voices that are low-pitched and somewhat breathy in quality. The not infrequent result of employing a voice pitched too low for the physical mechanism is hoarseness. Although there is considerable variability in regard to the consequences of the constant use of a voice pitched too low for the mechanism, there is a growing body of evidence indicating that undesirable physical consequences can frequently be expected. Among these consequences are thickening of the vocal bands and chronic irritation of the larynx.

Boys, as well as men, are not at all exempt from the cultural pressure for the low-pitched voice. Unfortunately, just so many women are born to have soprano voices, and only a few to be altos; so it is that many boys and men are by nature intended to be tenors and high baritones, just as some are to be low baritones and basses. The result of confusing physical virility with vocal depth is frequently low pitch and poor quality. On occasion, chronic hoarseness can result from attempts to pitch the voice at a level too low for the optimum functioning of the vocal apparatus. Strain and fatigue may also occur.

Our emphasis thus far has been on the abnormally low-pitched voice. This does not mean that some persons do not speak at a pitch level too high for their vocal mechanism. Among speakers with inappropriate pitch they are, however, likely to constitute a small minority. Cultural pressures in the United States place a premium on the low-pitched voice and are inclined to penalize the high-pitched voices. Unless there is a strong psychological drive to maintain an abnormally high-pitched voice, the individual is likely to yield in the direction of cultural pressure. Interestingly enough, persons who persist in vocalizing at high pitch levels, unless they are also shouters, are usually not as susceptible to some of the physical changes that frequently accompany abnormally low-pitched vocalization. We may appreciate some of the reasons for this by intentionally, but briefly, talking considerably below and then considerably above our normal pitch range. In talking at the low end of our range, we will find that it takes appreciably more effort to produce a loud voice than within our normal range, or at a relatively high pitch. Fatigue is likely to set in quickly, and a feeling of vocal strain will follow if vocalization is continued. We are not, incidentally, referring to the use of a high-pitched falsetto or of a pitch range associated with laryngeal hypertension.

Habitual use of pitches much below or above our natural pitch range is often accomplished at the expense of the abuse of the vocal mechanism. We have worked with preschool children who developed nodules on their vocal bands as a result of vocal abuse. Typically, these children were high-pitched screamers (Wilson, 1961). There are always, of course, some individuals who are able to vocalize either above or below normal pitch range without suffering physical consequences. Perhaps these persons are kin to those who do not develop calluses despite poorly fitted shoes, or who do not become sunburned despite what would be overexposure to the sun for most of us. Our only suggestion is that these hardy persons be considered exceptions rather than models for the more susceptible of us to follow. Most of us do better vocalizing within a pitch range suited to our vocal apparatus. How to determine this range will be considered later in our discussion of optimum pitch in the section on vocal therapy.

Caution needs to be exercised when judgments are made about pitch levels and ranges. Schneiderman (1959) found that judgments about pitch, including those by listeners with "trained ears," are not always valid. Other aspects of voice—quality or loudness—may produce an erroneous impression as to the "perceived" pitch. This observation emphasizes the need to determine optimum pitch level and range rather than to make arbitrary judgments as to the appropriateness of the speaker's pitch.

Inappropriate Nasal Reinforcement. The movements of the soft palate largely determine whether the produced voice is characterized by the presence or absence of nasality. Normally, when vocalization occurs with a relaxed soft palate that permits the stream of breath to enter the nasal cavities, the voice is reinforced there and becomes characteristically nasal. Of course, some nasal reinforcement occurs whether or not the soft palate is relaxed or elevated, so that a degree of nasality is likely to be present even when nasality is not the characteristic quality of the produced voice.

The American-English sounds *n*, *m*, and *ng* are normally produced with a relaxed soft palate and "open nasal cavities." All other sounds of English are normally produced with the soft palate elevated so that the stream of breath is directed and emitted orally. If an individual has a weakened soft palate, he will tend to speak with more than a normal amount of nasal emission, and so have a voice quality characterized by *positive nasality*. The same quality may result from sluggish palatal control and from related activity of the mouth, throat, and nasopharynx in their functions as resonators. Positive nasality may also arise as a result of imitation. The French-speaking child quite properly nasalizes some of his vowels as well as the nasal consonants of his language. The American- or English-speaking child may do the same if he is imitating the speech of a member of his environment who nasalizes more than most American or English speakers do.

Denasality, or an absence of appropriate nasal resonance, occurs when there is too little reinforcement by the nasal resonators. This may result from a blocking within the nasal cavities themselves, or a partial blocking within the area of the nasopharynx. The result is a pinched, flat quality that suggests the voice of a person with a head cold or an allergic condition involving the nasal cavities. The quality is more than an absence of nasality when it is anticipated in the production of the nasal consonants. It is an overall effect recognizable on sounds that are normally emitted orally. We can produce what approaches a denasal voice by pinching our nostrils in the articulation of such a sentence as "Who is that tall boy with a black coat?" The result, even though the sentence does not contain nasal consonants, should be different in quality if the sentence is articulated without pinched nostrils.

Techniques for recognizing and improving nasal reinforcement will be considered in our discussion of voice therapy.

Breathing Faults. It is unusual for a physically normal child to breathe incorrectly while speaking unless he has somehow been trained to do so. Such training may be the result of a child's efforts to be obedient to the direction, "Take a real deep breath before you begin to speak," or "Raise your chest high and pull your tummy in before you begin to speak." Occasionally, but really rarely, a child may speak with a too shallow breath, or attempt to speak while inhaling rather than or in addition to exhaling. In such instances investigation is likely to show that we are dealing with an insecure or anxiety-ridden child who is apprehensive that if he stops for a normal breath someone will interrupt him, or he may forget what he has to say and be embarrassed or penalized for his forgetting. The same factors are likely to operate with the child who tries to speak on inhalation as well as exhalation, or the child who forces himself to continue to speak on breath he must strain to emit when the normal "tidal breath" has been expired. We must not, of course, overlook the possibility that in a rare instance we are dealing with a normal child with normal psychological dynamisms, who is simply imitating a member of his environment whose breathing habits for speech are faulty.

We are inclined to agree with Curtis (1967, pp. 193–194) that it is probably of little importance whether the person's breathing is predominantly abdominal or diphragmatic, predominantly thoracic, or predominantly medial (characterized by activity about the base of the sternum). What seems to be of most importance for almost all speaking occasions is that the speaker have an adequate supply of breath (*exaggerated deep breathing is not required*) and that he be comfortable while speaking. Most persons who have not been specially trained to emphasize the activity of one part of the thoracic mechanism are likely to do pretty well in coordinated participation of all parts of their respiratory mechanism. For the rare individual who does not have adequate breath for normal speech purposes, attention may be directed to an emphasis on either diaphragmatic action and control, thoracic action, or medial action. Our own preference is for diaphragmatic (abdominal) control, because it is easy, effective, and readily discernible. The individual may be directed to breathe while speaking as he or she is likely to breathe when relaxed, unless tightly girdled or belted. On inspiration of breath the abdominal area will be noted to move upward if the person is lying down, or forward if the person is sitting up or standing. On expiration, the abdominal area should pull in. A gradual, controlled pulling in of the abdominal muscles helps to bring about an upward movement of the diaphragm and so to produce a well-sustained, steady vocal tone if the action takes place during vocalization.

It is probably best to minimize or to eliminate entirely breathing characterized by action of the upper chest (clavicular breathing). Such breathing frequently results in a strained humping of the chest and shoulders, and so interferes with easy breath flow. In this awkward and strained position, which is associated with neck and throat tension, proper reinforcement of tone in the resonating cavities becomes difficult so that voice production becomes unnecessarily effortful. It is apparently also more difficult to obtain an adequate supply of breath with "clavicular breathing" so that the speaker finds it necessary to pause for breath more often than with abdominal, thoracic, or medial breathing.

Generally, we do not consider it either advisable or necessary to stress manner of breathing. As a practical matter, we have found that it is usually possible to modify and improve breath use for vocalization without direct attention to the individual's breathing activity. Correction of posture and attention to the initiation and maintenance of proper vocal tones are usually sufficient and effective.

Therapy for Voice Disturbances

The classroom teacher who suspects that one of his students has a voice disturbance should first make certain that he is not imposing a personal preference. Second, the teacher should be certain that no physical condition requiring medical attention is present before any treatment is undertaken. It follows also that if a psychological problem underlies the voice defect, the problem and the child rather than the defect should be treated. With these precautions in mind, the classroom teacher with an understanding of voice production may be of real help to those children with defects of quality, pitch, or loudness of voice. The classroom teacher, as well as the speech clinician, will also do well to bear in mind that despite the best of teachings, not all defects are fully remediable. Sometimes the most apparent defect resists specific improvement, but overall improvement may still be attained if other, not so readily apparent, aspects of voice and speech are trained to the fullest extent. For example, a child with a weakened, soft palate may necessarily speak with a characteristic nasal quality. If this child is helped to articulate clearly, but not pedantically, and to have a wide and flexible pitch range reflective of changes in thought and feeling, the overall impression is likely to be favorable despite the persistence of nasality. Similarly, a child with a high-pitched voice, especially if the child is a boy, may not be able to do much about lowering his fundamental pitch if he is one intended by nature to have a high pitch. Such a child can still be helped if he learns to make full use of his pitch range, and can produce voice that is readily audible and is meaningfully emphatic according to speech content. With these points in mind, several specific suggestions for dealing with particular aspects of vocal deficiency may be considered.

PITCH LEVEL AND RANGE

As indicated earlier, appropriate pitch for an individual should be determined by factors other than either the listener's or speaker's liking for a given pitch range. The other factors are anatomic, including the length and mass of the individual's vocal bands, the relationship of vocal bands to the laryngeal structure, and the size and shape of the other resonating cavities. We are aware that pitch varies inversely as the length and directly as the tension of the vibrating body. Changes in length and tension enable the speak to produce a range of normal or natural pitches that comprise a physically appropriate pitch range.

The production of vocal tones consistent with the intellectual and affective content of speech comprises an appropriate pitch range for speaking.

The natural or "optimum" pitch is that pitch level at which an individual is able to vocalize most efficiently. This is the level at which good quality, loudness, and ease of production are found. For most persons, natural or optimum pitch level is about one-fourth to one-third above the lowest level within the range of pitch levels at which vocalization can occur. It can be found by having the individual intone as low as he can and then having him raise his level a step at a time until he reaches falsetto. If twelve levels are produced, it is likely that level three or four will be the optimum pitch. It helps considerably to use a piano and to match pitch levels with those of the piano in finding total pitch range.

If the child's habitual pitch is found to be more than one level below or above his natural level, it is advisable to train him to initiate voice on his natural level. The same advice, of course, holds for adults. It is well to remember, however, that young growing children have changes in their natural pitch as laryngeal growth takes place. After physiological adolescence, growth changes are not so great, and natural pitch should become pretty well stabilized.

The determination of natural pitch is a point of departure in the production of an adequate and effective pitch range. For most persons voice will be best produced within that part of the pitch range between the natural pitch and one third below the highest pitch. Thus, for a child with a fifteen-level range, pitch levels from five to ten are likely to be produced with good quality and with ease. With training, the child can learn to initiate voice for usual conversational purposes on his natural pitch level, and to use several levels above it for variety, emphasis, and appropriate expression of feeling. There is no objection to the use of a level or two below natural level if the child has a fairly wide range. If the range is narrow, it is probably best to avoid dropping more than one level below natural pitch. The danger of dropping two levels below natural pitch for a person with a narrow pitch range is that an effortful, breathy voice may be produced which may actually be harmful to the speaker.

BREATHINESS

Vocal quality characterized by breathiness results from air "leakage" between vocal bands during voice production. The ultimate of breathiness is intentionally whispered speech. Voiceless consonants are, of course, breathy, and appropriately so. Vowels, however, and voiced consonants should be produced without any obvious breathiness.

Breathiness may result from overrelaxed vocalization with associated partial approximation of the vocal bands. If a person's voice is pitched too low in terms of his natural pitch range, the tension of the vocal bands will be less than optimum, and the voice is likely to be breathy. If a person is suffering from laryngitis, attempts at vocalization are frequently associated with pain because of contact between swollen inner edges of the bands. To avoid or reduce the pain, the speaker is likely to keep his vocal bands in a partially approximated position, and so will speak with breathiness. Figure 10 shows the position of the vocal bands when they are not sufficiently approximated for good voice production, and yet too closely approximated for purposes of normal breathing.

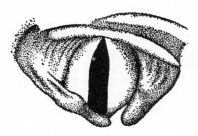

Figure 10. Diagram, adapted from a high-speed photograph, showing vocal bands not sufficiently approximated for good voice production, and too closely approximated for normal breathing.

Courtesy Bell Telephone Company Laboratories, New York.

Sometimes a breathy voice is associated with shyness or timidity. A child who speaks quietly because he is afraid to speak aloud may not bring his vocal bands close enough to vocalize without excessive breathiness. Occasionally a "good" but not necessarily timid child will imitate a teacher's low voice used by him to keep his class quiet. Such a child, in his attempt to speak "low and quiet" may also speak breathily.

There are several reasons for children to avoid breathy voice quality. First, the breathy voice is frequently too low in pitch, and vocalization becomes effortful and unpleasant. Second, breathiness is wasteful in terms of length of phrase in speaking. The child, or the adult for that matter, who speaks with excessive breathiness will need to pause for inhalation more often than would otherwise be necessary. In his attempts to establish normal phrasing, he may speak on residual breath, and his speech efforts will sound strained and be strained.

To overcome breathiness it is frequently necessary to have the child become aware of the difference between a breathy and a normal voice quality. This may be done by having the child place his hand in front of his mouth while saying a sentence such as "My bunny's name is Lanny." Normally, such a sentence, which has no voiceless sounds and only one voiced stop, should be produced with a very minimum of breath felt on the hand placed a few inches in front of the mouth. The child should then be directed to "feel" the breath accompanying a sentence such as "Polly likes to eat thin crackers," which has both stop and fricative sounds and is therefore necessarily produced with accompanying breath. If there is no distinct difference in the child's vocalization of the two sentences, another child whose voice is not breathy should be asked to speak the two sentences while the breathy-voiced child holds his hand about six inches in front of the second child's mouth, and notes the difference.

After the concepts and the feeling of breathiness and nonbreathiness are established, other techniques may be employed to establish normal vocalization. A very simple and often effective approach is to direct the child to speak as if breath were precious and to emit as little breath as possible while talking. Then, for contrast, the child may be instructed to be as breathy as he possibly can, so that the difference can be clearly appreciated.

Another helpful technique is to have the child intone a vowel such as [i] (ee) and to hold the vowel as long as comfortable on a single breath. The vowel [i], because it is relatively tense and high-pitched, is likely to be produced with a minimum of breathiness even by the child who is inclined to be breathy. If this is done successfully, the child may then be directed to intone [ɑ] (ah) and to maintain the sound until he begins to become breathy, or until he needs to inhale. Then he should repeat the effort with a reduced loudness but without obvious breathiness. In this way the child can learn how "quietly" he may speak without becoming breathy. The same technique may be used with a change in pitch rather than loudness so that the child may learn at which pitch level he becomes breathy, and so avoid that pitch level.

Other recommended exercises include saying as much of the alphabet as possible or counting as long as is comfortable on a single breath. When quantity of production becomes the objective, the child is spontaneously likely to conserve breath. As soon as possible, of course, he should be given an opportunity to apply what he has learned in his exercises to reading aloud and conversational speech. Although he should not be interrupted in his normal speaking efforts because of breathiness, the clinician should work out a system of signals to tell the child, when he has concluded his effort, whether he has been successful in his control of breathiness. The teacher, working with the speech clinician, may apply this approach in the classroom situation.

NASALITY

Positive or excessive nasality as a characteristic voice quality, as we pointed out earlier, is associated with a relaxed soft palate during the act of vocalization. In the absence of specific anomaly involving the palate, nasality may occur either because of generally slow or sluggish palatal action or because of specific "retarded" action of the soft palate after the articulation of appropriately nasal sounds. If there is generally sluggish soft palate action, speech as a whole is likely to sound nasal. If there is a limited failure of the soft palate to be elevated quickly immediately following the production of a nasal consonant, the sound or sounds produced after the nasal are likely to be partially nasalized. In the latter case, words such as *me, many, and, among, nine,* and *mine* are likely to be produced as if all the sounds were nasal.

In some cases the excessive nasality appears to be associated with a general expression of lassitude and an air of indifference to the environment. Such children, except possibly in their playground activities, seem to lack the energy for any physical effort, including the elevation of the soft palate. We should not, however, overlook the possibility that the expression of lassitude and apparent indifference may have a physical basis. The contrast in the child's playground behavior may be the effect of strong and specific motivation.

Children who have had their adenoids removed frequently change from having markedly denasal voices to having characteristically nasal voices. This change can be appreciated when we realize that when enlarged adenoids are present, a child does not need to elevate his soft palate very much to obstruct the opening to the nasal cavity. After the removal of the adenoidal tissue, the habit of partial elevation of the soft palate may persist, and nasality may then occur during the production of all speech sounds.

Regardless of the cause of nasality, if therapy is in order it should begin with giving the child awareness of how a nasal voice sounds and, if the child is capable of such understanding, how nasality occurs. The child can easily learn to recognize nasality by having him listen to his teacher intentionally nasalize a sentence such as *The sailor shouted "All aboard!"* or *This is the house that Jack built* and then listening to the same sentences spoken without intentional nasality. Both of these sentences, incidentally, contain no nasal consonants and so provide no temptation to nasalize because of proximity of a sound to a nasal consonant (assimilation).

The child inclined toward nasality may also learn how nasality feels by pinching his nostrils while speaking one of the sentences below. If the child becomes aware of pressure, or a feeling of stuffiness in his nose, or of fullness in his ears, it indicates that breath has entered his nasal cavity that should have been emitted through his mouth.

> Bob took Ted to the zoo.
> Please take care of the kitty.
> The dog chased the bird up the tree.
> Polly likes crackers with cheese.
> Joe played hop-scotch.
> The baby played pit-a-pat.

The same sentences may be used to help the child *see* his nasality. This can be accomplished by placing a cold hand mirror under the child's nostrils while he repeats one of the sentences having no nasal consonants. Clouding of the mirror by the warm air that escapes from the nostrils is visual evidence of positive and inappropriate nasality.

Once awareness is present in a child not organically involved and he is motivated to overcome his nasality, the following techniques may be employed:

Raising the Soft Palate. Have the child stand before a mirror and yawn with his mouth wide open. The child should be directed to note that his soft palate tends to lift up. He should learn how this feels as well as how it looks for the soft palate to elevate.

The child may be directed to blow up a previously stretched balloon. Even if he fails to blow the balloon to a large size, he should feel the action of the soft palate in his attempt.

The child may be directed to say [ɑ] (*ah*) while pinching his nostrils. All sound should come through the mouth, and no stuffiness should be felt. Then the child should be directed to produce a nasalized [ɑ]. The procedure should be repeated with other vowels and for such words as *boy, girl, tree, tall, big, go, bread, hot, skip, stop,* and *dog,* and short phrases such as *go away, pretty girl, big boy,* and *a slice of bread.* If the child is old enough to understand the difference between nasal and nonnasal sounds, he should be encouraged to make up his own list of words and phrases for practice.

Ear Training. The child can be helped to distinguish between appropriate and inappropriate nasality by listening to appropriate articulation of the following pairs of words:

moo	two	an	at	him	hit
me	bee	wing	wig	pen	pet
my	by	I'm	I'll	can	cat
no	go	in	it	bean	beat
may	pay	aim	ape	seem	seat

It may also help if the clinician informs the child that occasionally words in the second column will be intentionally nasalized and the child is to signal when he becomes aware of such nasalization. The clinician with good control, who can turn nasality off and on at will, may go beyond single words to pairs of phrases and sentences.

If a recorder and playback are available, ready use may be made of such an instrument in helping the child to recognize his own nasality. A sentence or two may be recorded by the nasal child and the same material by another child without the defect. The child "in training" may then hear the difference in voice quality between himself and a peer. Later, recordings may be used to help the child recognize improvement in exercises and for parts of readings or conversation. Many children enjoy a chance to do intentionally what they are seeking to improve. Permission "to do the wrong thing" should be given so that the child may practice and so gain voluntary control over nasality. The same approach, of course, is also relevant for other aspects of voice therapy as well as for the improvement of articulation.

General Articulatory Activity. Often the child who speaks nasally will also be one whose overall articulatory activity lacks precision and clearness. For this child, in the interest of improving articulation in general as well as nasality in particular, more precise and energetic articulatory activity is recommended. With increased activity of the lips and tongue, there will also be a reflexive increase in energetic activity of the soft palate. The child should also be instructed to direct all nonnasal sounds through his mouth and to increase the feeling of front-of-the-mouth activity. Words and phrases such as the following might be used in drill work and incorporated into practice sentences and conversational speech.

two	do	pet
treat	tweet	pit
pooh	boo	step
chew	food	slip
tuck	buck	tent
see	saw	spot
lick	tick	tack
bing	bang	stuck

come along	sing a song
take some tea	beat the drum
red rose	don't trip
all aboard	pickled peppers
leave the boat	hit the deck
stay away	broken bones
let's go	pack of sticks

DENASALITY

Some children speak as though they have either chronically stuffed noses or enlarged adenoids that block the entrance of sound into the nasal cavities. These children need to be helped to become aware of adequate nasal resonance when it is required.

Humming with lips relatively relaxed so that a sensation of tickling is experienced is a recommended technique for establishing nasal resonance. Another useful device is the intentional lengthening of nasal consonants. The child may be instructed to hum and then follow the hum with a vowel. Specifically, the exercise might proceed as follows:

1. Hum gently on a sustained breath, first with the sound *m*, then *n*, and then [ŋ]. Repeat each hum three or four times.

2. Begin a hum and then blend with a vowel.

3. Prolong an initial nasal sound and blend with a vowel as in *mmm-a*, and *nnn-oo*.

4. Begin with a lengthened nasal, blend with a vowel, and end with a lengthened nasal as in *mmmannn, nnnoonnn*.

Other exercises might include articulating such words as *me, my, moo, may, meal, nail, now, new, never, nice, sing, long,* and *running* with intentional lengthening of the nasal consonants.

Sentences incorporating words with more than a usual number of nasal consonants should be made and conversation with such words and sentences should be practiced. Whenever possible, the child should be encouraged to make up words and sentences so that he may have the pleasure of creative activity as well as practice.

INAPPROPRIATE LOUDNESS

Most children whose speech patterns are a result of identification with normal adults speak loud enough to be heard. Those who speak with inadequate loudness or with voice louder than the occasion demands reflect either their own personalities or the personalities of the adults with whom they identify. Only in the rarest instances is there an organic basis for either a weak or an overloud voice. The comparatively rare organic causes include hearing loss, weakness of the muscles of the larynx, and weakness of the muscles involved in respiration. Furthermore, it is extremely unlikely that the carrying power of the voice is significantly related to the individual's breath capacity or the manner in which he breathes while speaking. As Van Riper and Irwin (1958, p. 258) emphasize, " So long as sufficient air pressure is engendered below the vocal folds, it does not matter how it is created, at least so far as adequate loudness is concerned. But we must have a greater air pressure to have louder speech." In the absence of organic pathology, the will to be heard is sufficient to supply the energy to provide for the necessary pressure below the vocal folds so that they are closed firmly, held together firmly for an appropriate length of time, and then blown apart from their occluded (approximated) position to produce a vocal tone loud enough to be easily heard.

Occasionally we find children who, because of poor posture, or from anxiety, get in the way of their own efforts of effective breathing for speech. A child with a "caved-in" abdominal area may not be able to breathe comfortably and deeply enough for purposes of speech. Obviously, the slump and the associated cave-in need to be corrected. Similarly, any other postural defect which interferes with adequate air intake and easy control of breath output needs to be corrected. Such correction might well be directed to emphasizing the need for the abdominal area to be relaxed and to "push out" in inhalation and to contract and "pull in" gradually in controlled exhalation.

Another fault found in some children is the attempt to vocalize and speak during inhalation. This fault, in the absence of neuropathology, is usually a result of an anxious effort to continue talking when the child's breath supply has been expended. The creation of awareness of what the child is doing can be established by directing him to do intentionally what he is doing unconsciously. Such a child is also likely to gain from breathing exercises that emphasize abdominal control of outgoing breath.

THE OVERLOUD VOICE

Aside from the possibility of a hearing loss which prevents proper monitoring of the voice as it is being produced, the overloud voice is likely to be a product of imitation or an aspect of the personality of the speaker. Our experience as clinicians suggests that most children who speak too loudly are either imitating their parents or competing with their siblings for attention from their parents. We have had parents come to us with complaints about their children's loud voices. They presented their complaints in our offices in voices loud enough to reach the last row of a 40-row auditorium without electrical amplification. The research of Paul (1951) supports our impression that children of loud-speaking parents themselves speak more loudly than do children whose parents are soft-speaking, or who speak with normal but adequate loudness. Moses (1954), talking as a psychoanalyst interested in voice problems, points out that, on the one hand, fearful people speak fearfully (with voices not loud enough to be easily heard) and that the voice of the authority in our culture, on the other hand, tends to be loud.

Certainly, we are inclined to associate aggression and assertiveness with loud voice (Murphy, 1964, p. 43).

Another possible cause for excessive loudness is the existence of a sensory-neural hearing loss. Such impairment makes it necessary for the speaker to vocalize loudly in order for him to hear and monitor himself. Occasionally we find a child with normal hearing who speaks in a way to suggest nerve hearing impairment. Investigation, however, may reveal that he may have been brought up in a noisy environment, or in competition with siblings who were habitual shouters. The child then may have developed a loud voice in order to be heard and share the attention of his parents. His vocal habits may carry over to relatively quiet, noncompetitive situations.

THE WEAK VOICE

In the absence of organic involvement, we may assume that a weak voice is a reflection either of a timid personality or of the reaction of the individual to a given speaking situation. Most children who are unsure of themselves, or of what they have to say, tend to talk with a weak voice. The voice, regardless of the particular speech content, is also saying " Maybe if I don't talk loudly I won't be noticed, or what I have to say won't be heard, and I will be left alone." Occasionally, however, the weak voice may be the result of imitation, and the inadequate loudness has become habitual. The reproduction of such a voice on a playback is a necessary first step in the modification of this manner of voice production.

A possible organic cause of weak voice is the existence of a conductive hearing loss. Persons with conductive loss, in contrast to those with sensory-neural loss, tend to perceive themselves as speaking more loudly than do their listeners. In general, we recommend that any child whose voice is either inappropriately loud or inadequate as to loudness be checked for possible hearing impairment. There may be some value, too, for the parents to have a similar evaluation.

TREATMENT FOR INAPPROPRIATE LOUDNESS

Except for children whose hearing difficulty impairs their ability to monitor their voices, or who have some other organic basis for either their weak or overloud voice, an adequately loud voice should be attainable for all children. Treatment should include the following aspects: (1) an assessment of the voices of the members of the family and other key persons in the child's environment; (2) an evaluation of the personality and adjustment factors that may be associated with the child's manner of vocalization; (3) an evaluation of the specific situations (e.g., the child's voice in the classroom compared with his voice in play activity) that may be associated with inadequate voice; (4) an evaluation of the overall characteristics of the child's voice, in addition to the degree of loudness; and (5) an objectification of the voice through recording and playback so that the child may hear himself approximately as others hear him.

In many instances, children who have been brought to our clinic for their voice problems have been treated through their parents. We have permitted parents to hear their recorded voices and invited them to accept treatment—*in the interest of their child*. Sometimes we accepted the child for treatment only if the parent or parents accepted concurrent voice therapy. Occasionally, we have encouraged parents to subdue a sibling just enough to give the child concerned a fair chance in the vocal competition. Occasionally, we have had to advise counseling for the parents while the child, *after medical clearance*, was undergoing symptom treatment.

In instances where we felt that an adjustment problem was basic to the voice difficulty, we have recommended treatment by a qualified psychotherapist. Whenever possible, we prefer that the choice of a psychotherapist be made with the help of the family physician. Occasionally we have found that a child's voice problem was limited to the classroom. For reasons that developed out of the relationship between a child and a teacher—and sometimes it is a previous rather than a present teacher—the child had become anxiously concerned about his adequacy as a student. Obviously, in such instances, treatment should be directed at the improvement of the child-to-school relationship rather than to the vocal symptoms.

When, after investigation, we are convinced that there is nothing organically or emotionally wrong with the child who is speaking either not loudly enough or too loudly, direct treatment of the symptoms is in order. As we suggested earlier, an overall evaluation of the vocal characteristics of the child is then undertaken. Our experience suggests that the weak voice is often also a breathy voice, and one likely to be too low in pitch. Often, but not always, we find that the loud voice is apt to be too high in pitch. The first order of the procedure for correcting the degree of loudness is to determine the child's normal pitch range and his optimum pitch. When these are determined (see pp. 304–305), the speech clinician should help the child to become aware of them, to initiate voice habitually at optimum pitch, and to vocalize within the the optimum pitch range. Breathiness, if it is found to be present, should be treated by procedures indicated in the section on breathiness.

Ordinarily, after the procedures outlined and after the child has been made aware of the loudness level of his voice through playback, adequate loudness is attained. Occasionally, however, old habits are maintained and the child's voice, though appropriate in pitch and not characterized by breathiness, is still not appropriate in loudness. If it continues to be weak, procedures such as those listed below should be productive of improvement.

1. Record successively the voice of the weak-voiced child and a peer with adequate voice. Have the child make the comparisons and rerecord until both clinician and child are satisfied with the result.

2. If available, employ visual feedback apparatus so that the child may see when his voice is at the proper level. Most tape recorders are equipped with "magic eyes," which may be so employed. An oscilloscope may serve both to impress the child and to provide him with a basis for visual monitoring. A simpler and more readily available apparatus, though perhaps not quite so impressive, is the raised hand and approving look of the teacher or clinician when the child's voice is at a proper level and the lowered (thumb-down) hand and disappointed (but *not* disapproving) look when the voice level is not loud enough.

3. Emphasis on clarity of articulation with lengthening of the vowels and nasal consonants is often of considerable help. Support for this procedure may be found in the investigation of House and Fairbanks (1953) that overall intelligibility *decreased markedly* when the experimental subjects spoke at reduced loudness levels. By emphasizing clarity of articulation, the child is likely to use greater energy not only for articulatory activity but also for the accompanying respiratory behavior while speaking. The result is a reflexive increase in air pressure below the vocal folds, and a louder voice.

4. The game of *competitive speaking* or "Who can talk loudest in the group without shouting?" may be employed as motivation and play. It may be of help if some of the competitors are encouraged at the beginning of the game to give the weak-voiced participant a chance to be heard. Later on, the erstwhile weak-voiced member should be permitted free and open competition.

5. The need for the child to adjust his voice level to the listener in terms of distance between listener and speaker may need emphasis. A teacher may bring about such an adjustment by asking a child a question when he is standing close to the child and then intentionally moving away from him. Another technique is to have the child stand in front of the room and speak just loud enough to be heard by his classmates in the first third of the room, then in the second third as well, and finally throughout the room. This procedure impresses the child with the need

to change his voice level according to the number of listeners and the distance between himself and the farthest listener.

6. Pretended situations, such as announcing the arrival of a train or plane, giving orders to a military group, or speaking in a crowded and noisy place (a train station or a airport waiting room), can also be useful to help the child to be heard under difficult situations. Artificially competitive noise situations, such as speaking against a masking noise or buzzing noise, may also be used. If these techniques are employed, *care must be exercised that the optimum pitch range is maintained*. We would not want a child to speak loudly at the expense of vocal nodules.

CONTROL OF BREATH FOR SPEAKING

As indicated earlier in our discussion of breathing faults, difficulty in breathing is not a frequent cause of vocal difficulty for the otherwise normal child. We should be alert to see that the children do not attempt to vocalize while inhaling. Vocalization should occur on an easy, controlled exhalation of breath. Because only a rare and occasional child will attempt vocalization on inhalation, we recommend that the teacher who has such a child in his class arrange for him to be given corrective instruction on an individual basis. It is better for most children to do their breathing while speaking without special awareness or consciousness of the action involved.

If a child shows throat or laryngeal effort in speaking, attention might be directed to abdominal control for expiration. Usually such attention serves to distract the child from excessive tension in the upper part of the respiratory mechanism. Other therapeutic suggestions relative to breathing faults were indicated earlier.

Review of Principles for Correcting Voice Defects

1. *Medical clearance is a must* for any child who presents a voice problem and for whom vocal therapy is contemplated. A child who develops a vocal disturbance should be examined by a physician and, if at all possible, by a throat specialist for the detection and treatment of possible physical pathology before consideration is given to voice training.

2. When a child's vocal defects seem to be associated with personality disturbances, referral to a competent counselor or psychotherapist is in order. It should not be overlooked, however, that poor vocal habits may persist after the initial cause is no longer present. This principle holds true for vocal defects of both physical and psychological origin.

3. Often vocal defects are temporary and of short duration and call for patience and understanding rather than active treatment.

4. A voice is a product of the mechanism that produces it. The mechanism belongs to the individual, and the product should be consistent with its features. Neither the professional speech clinician nor the teacher, nor any other person who may influence the child, has a right to decide what kind of voice the child should have. Fundamentally, this decision was made by the way the child was physically endowed. The objective of vocal therapy is to help the child to make the best possible use of his vocal endowment.

5. The classroom teacher, especially if he is respected and liked, has a personal responsibility that his own voice be free of undesirable traits which his children may imitate.

6. Vocal habits, both good and bad, tend to persist. Considerable motivation is necessary to help a child to wish to change his defective voice and to maintain vigilance that changes are maintained.

7. The child with a vocal defect should be helped to become aware of what his defect is like acoustically, and how it feels. He needs to be aware of how his voice sounds and feels when it is at its best. Objective attitudes and objective listening to his own voice and comparing his own voice with others by listening to " on-the-spot " recordings are of help.

8. Often a " negative " approach is helpful. By creating awareness of the nature of the undesirable vocal traits and how they are produced, voluntary control may be established. Thus a child, by intentionally *doing what is wrong*, learns to know what he is doing, and so becomes conscious of what he should not do. By contrast, awareness must be created of the right way to produce voice and to replace the undesirable characteristic with a desirable one.

References and Suggested Readings

ANDERSON, V. A., *Training the Speaking Voice*, 2nd ed. New York, Oxford University Press, Inc., 1961, Chaps. 2 to 5. (A clear exposition of the voice mechanism and principles and techniques for voice improvement. Excellent practice materials for the teacher and clinician.)

BERRY, M. F., and J. EISENSON, *Speech Disorders: Principles and Practices of Therapy*. New York, Appleton-Century-Crofts, 1956, Chaps. 9 and 10. (These chapters include a more advanced and technical consideration of voice disturbances and their treatment than will be found in most of the other suggested readings.)

BRODNITZ, F. S., *Keep Your Voice Healthy*. New York, Harper & Row, Publishers, 1953. (A physician offers suggestions as to how to have a good and "healthy" voice.)

CURTIS, J. F., in W. Johnson, et al. *Speech-Handicapped School Children*. New York, Harper & Row, Publishers, 1967, Chap. 4.

EISENSON, J., *The Improvement of Voice and Diction*, 2nd ed. New York, The Macmillan Company, 1965, Chaps. 2 to 9. (These chapters include a discussion of the voice mechanism and expositions of techniques and procedures for voice improvement. The principles are applicable to school-age children. Practice materials may be used with the older children.)

HOUSE, A., and G. FAIRBANKS, "The Influence of Consonantal Environment upon the Secondary Acoustical Characteristics of Vowels," *Journal of the Acoustical Society of America*, XXXV (January, 1953), 105–113.

MOORE, P., "Otolaryngology and Speech Pathology," *The Laryngoscope*, LXXVIII, 9 (September, 1968), 1500–1509. (This article includes a clear and simple description of normal vocal-fold activity in vocalization.)

MOSES, P. J., *The Voice of Neurosis*. New York, Grune and Stratton, 1954. (A psychiatrist and otolaryngologist describes his approaches to persons with voice problems.)

MURPHY, A. T., *Functional Voice Disorders*. Englewood Cliffs, N.J., Prentice-Hall, Inc., 1964. (A clear introductory consideration of personality disturbances and voice disorders.)

PAUL, J. E., *An Investigation of Parent-Child Relationships in Speech: Intensity and Duration*. Ph.D. Thesis, Purdue University, 1951.

SCHNEIDERMAN, N., "An Investigation of Selected Factors Affecting the Judgment of Pitch Placement of Defective Voices." Unpublished doctoral dissertation, New York University, New York, 1959.

VAN RIPER, C., *Speech Correction*, 4th ed. Englewood Cliffs, N.J., Prentice-Hall, Inc., 1963, Chaps. 7 and 8.

———, and J. V., IRWIN, *Voice and Articulation*. Englewood Cliffs, N.J., Prentice-Hall, Inc., 1958, Chaps. 7 to 13. (These chapters explain voice production and problems related to voice disturbances. Highly recommended for an upper-level consideration.)

WILSON, D. K., "Children with Vocal Nodules," *Journal of Speech and Hearing Disorders*, XXVI (February, 1961), 19–25.

Problems

1. Review the section on the vocal mechanism. From the viewpoint of the production and reinforcement of sound, what musical instrument is most directly comparable to the voice mechanism?

2. Good vocalization is the product of *periodic vibration*. What does this term mean? What kind of human sounds are *complex and aperiodic*? You may consult Curtis (1967, pp. 183–185) for your answer.

3. What are the characteristics of a normal, effective voice?

4. What is the most frequent physical cause of defective voice?
5. Why is puberty often a period of frequent voice disturbance? Why are males more likely to be affected than females?
6. What is the role of identification in the formation of vocal habits?
7. What is nasality? How do you distinguish this characteristic from denasality? How would you check for each?
8. Why is it important that every child who may be considered for voice therapy first be given medical clearance?
9. What is optimum pitch? How would you determine this for a child? Are you vocalizing within your optimal pitch range?
10. What is the evidence that breathing faults are a cause of vocal disturbance?

Chapter 13

Stuttering

General Observations

Except for children with articulatory defects, stutterers, if we accept them as a total special population, present the highest incidence among those who are defective in speech. The incidence is about 1 per cent among children of school age. Thus it is likely that almost every classroom teacher and certainly every speech clinician with more than a year of experience has had some dealings with a stutterer. These, and other professional workers concerned with stutterers, may have shared their perplexities about the children and their aberrant speech. They may have exchanged observations and opinions about a form of behavior that varies in amount and degree of severity. They may have expressed bewilderment about the comparative ease and fluency some stutterers have for brief or long periods of time, and about their sudden relapses. Those who have made private and comparative observations may have noted that fewer adults stutter than do children, but that almost all adults who stutter began doing so when they were children and almost always before adolescence. They may also have noted that relatively few very old adults stutter. And those who have had experience with persons with severe hearing impairments may even have noted an almost total absence of stuttering in this population. All of these observations, and some others we shall soon mention, have been made by professional investigators. They, too, continue to be perplexed about stutterers and stuttering, even though they have strong opinions, if not theories, about the problem.

There is obviously much about stuttering that is still to be learned. We would at the outset like to suggest that if we cease to regard stutterers as a total and "homogeneous" population we will begin to learn considerably more in the near future than in the hundreds of years that we have spent in speculations, critical observations, and even carefully designed investigations. For the moment, however, we will present several observations that have withstood the test of time about persons whose speech is characterized by rhythm and fluency different from most other speakers, who repeat and hesitate, and who prolong sounds, or block on sounds, more than most of us do in our talking. (Later we shall present a "formal" definition of stuttering.)

Accepted Observations About Stutterers

1. There are more stutterers among boys than among girls. Research on the incidence of stuttering shows a ratio of two to 10 males for each female stutterer. Probably an average ratio is four male stutterers to each female stutterer. In a survey in England reported by Andrews and Harris (1964, p. 186), a ratio of four boys to one girl was found among children. However, a ratio of about eight men to one woman was found among adults.*

2. The severity of stuttering tends to be greater among boys than among girls. We are, of course, talking about individuals. We have, in fact, known many severe female stutterers, but not nearly so many—even considering the ratio difference for the incidence of stuttering—as for males.

---

* Harris and Andrews (1964, p. 186) observe, "It is interesting to note that those girls who do stammer appear to have a higher loading of genetic and neurologic predisposing factors." Several references will be made to the Harris and Andrews report. We consider the report of their study of an entire school population of 7,358 children in the nine plus and 10 plus age-range in Newcastle, England, to be of especial significance to our understanding of the background history of stutterers (stammerers) and stuttering (stammering). The terms in parentheses are used by the British, where Americans tend to use *stutterers* and *stuttering*. The Newcastle investigators included speech therapists, psychologists, a psychiatrist, and a statistical analyst. Each stutterer (stammerer) was matched for age, grade, and sex with a normal-speaking child. Eighty-six stutterers were diagnosed by the speech therapist, of whom 80 participated in the complete study. Thus, the investigation had a population of 160 children and their mothers, who were assessed through interviews and standardized test inventories for clinical background, psychiatric evidence, personality traits, and aspects of intelligence.

3. Stuttering tends to be more persistent, to endure for more years, for boys than for girls. This explains the ratio difference noted in our first observation.
4. No stutterer, regardless of the severity of his difficulty, stutters at all times. Almost all stutterers have times when their speech is relatively if not completely free of significant hesitancies, blocks, repetitions, or prolongations. In group-speaking situations, and in singing, stutterers are likely to do about as well as other children.
5. Stuttering is more likely to begin in the nursery, kindergarten, and primary grades than in the secondary grades. It is comparatively rare for a child to begin stuttering after age 12. Andrews and Harris (1964, p. 186) report that 50 per cent of the children in their survey were stuttering (stammering) by age five, and 95 per cent were doing so by age seven. "Onset after the age of 10 is rare."
6. Many young children in the kindergarten and first grade seem to have been on the verge of stuttering without becoming stutterers. They were hesitant and repetitious, but apparently had no awareness of their manner of speaking. By the time these children reached the age of eight or nine, their speech seemed to be "normal" again.

The observations we have just noted are among the relatively few generalizations or "facts" accepted by students of stuttering. Beyond these, there is considerable difference as to the cause of stuttering, and the choice of treatment. We will not attempt to resolve these differences. Instead, we will present several of the more prevalent points of view, and suggest what the classroom teacher can safely do about children who are considered stutterers. We shall also suggest therapeutic approaches that are widely used with some success by speech clinicians in and out of school settings.*

The Nature of Stuttering

From the point of view of overt speech behavior, stuttered speech is characterized by hesitancies, blocks, repetitions, and/or prolongations of sounds in excess of normal. These may be referred to as disfluencies.

---

* One of the confounding observations about stutterers is that a great variety of approaches, some without any apparent rationale, have been used on stutterers with varying degrees of success—at least for a time.

Because many young children of preschool and primary school age have so-called disfluencies which, according to occasion, may occur in as much as 10 per cent of utterance, we should be liberal in our concept of the normal. In addition to disfluencies, the stutterer's voice is likely to be somewhat tense and narrow in pitch range and in modulation. Many children who regard themselves as stutterers also entertain feelings of anxiety and apprehension about some speaking situations or about communicative speaking in general. Some, amazingly, do not!

PRIMARY STUTTERING

Many speech therapists distinguish between two types of stuttering. When the speech symptoms are limited to repetitions, hesitancies, and prolongations, and when these occur without any evidence that the child is aware of them, or does anything to avoid speaking, the child may be characterized as a primary stutterer. Van Riper (1963) considers primary stuttering to be the first stage of the disorder but he does not suggest an inevitable progression to more severe stages (secondary stuttering). He describes the primary stutterer and his speech as

> broken by an excessive amount of repetitions of syllables and sounds, or less frequently, by the prolongation of a sound. He does not seem to be aware of his difficulty. He does not struggle or avoid speaking. He does not seem to be embarrassed at all. Indeed he seems almost totally unconscious of his repetitive utterance. He just bubbles along, trying his best to communicate (Van Riper, 1963, p. 24).

SECONDARY STUTTERING

If speech disfluencies become associated with facial grimaces, tics, or other forms of spasmic movements either of the articulatory mechanism or of other parts of the body that are not ordinarily directly concerned with speech production, we have secondary stuttering. It is usually assumed that the nonlinguistic associates of stuttering arise initially as an effort on the part of the speaker either to delay, distract, or avoid speech, or as a device to "break through" a block that occurs, or which it is feared may occur, in the speech effort. When nonlinguistic, overt, accessory activity takes place, we may assume that the stutterer has become aware of his hesitations, repetitions, blocks, and/or prolongations, and is doing something in an attempt to modify what takes place in his speech, or what he anticipates may take place.

The stutterer with secondary symptoms, in contrast with the primary stutterer, is aware of the nature of his speech. He has begun to respond to himself as an atypical speaker, if not an atypical person. His accessory movements reveal both apprehension of what he may do and struggle against doing it. Sometimes the struggle against doing it precedes the actual articulatory and vocal effort. At other times the struggle seems to interrupt the effort. Usually, at least at the outset, the struggle behavior seems to help the stutterer to begin his speech effort or to resume his interrupted effort. Unfortunately, the accessory movements tend to become incorporated in the overall pattern of the stuttering. In time they constitute merely another factor that the stutterer must try to modify in his fight against stuttering.

Frequently, the breathing of the secondary stutterer shows marked irregularity. Sometimes the stutterer takes a deep breath and then expires most of it before beginning to speak. This, in our judgment, is a breathing mannerism that many stutterers are taught by poorly informed adults who confuse stuttering symptoms with stuttering cause. Occasionally, a stutterer attempts to talk while inhaling. Often stutterers interrupt their speaking to inhale before there is any physiological or speech need to do so. Many stutterers modify the normal inspiration-expiration ratio (a short period of inhalation followed by a considerably longer period for exhalation) so that their inhalation-exhalation ratio is about one to one.

Bloodstein (1960) also argues against the use of the terms primary and secondary stuttering. On the basis of his clinical experience, he suggests four developmental phases or overlapping stages for stuttering, but cautions that in some instances individual children who are regarded as stutterers may skip whole phases. The first three phases are considered by Bloodstein to be most differentiating. The phases are characterized as follows:

Phase 1. The child's difficulty is usually episodic with repetitions the chief characteristic. Prolongations, forcings, and hard contacts and various associated symptoms ordinarily found among advanced stutterers may also be present.

Phase 2. The child's difficulty becomes increasingly chronic, though it may fluctuate considerably in severity. Most of the "stutterings" occur on the major parts of speech. The child now thinks of himself as a stutterer but apparently does not avoid opportunities to speak and ". . . has little or no concern about his stuttering except in severe cases or at moments of unusual difficulty."

Phase 3. The child's difficulties in speaking have begun to become *situational*, in that he has more difficulties, and anticipation of difficulties, in some situations than in others. The stutterer has now an elaborately developed symptomology including devices for postponement, starting, and release. Despite these, he apparently continues to be comfortable about speaking, or at least does not avoid opportunities to speak. Toward the close of phase 3, there begins to be evidence of emotional reactions to his stuttering which, in this respect, signal the fourth stage.

Phase 4. The individual, who may now be quite "grown up," is sensitive about his speech. Many young children, however, may show this sensitivity shortly after the onset of their difficulty. In many instances the individual blocks and is apprehensive that he will block if required to talk. Nevertheless, in most play activities and in noncommunicative speaking, the stutterer is likely to be free of his speech difficulties.

For varying reasons, other authorities do not accept the terms or the implications of *primary* and *secondary* stuttering. Johnson believes that the early disfluencies of children are normal, however frequently and under what circumstances they occur, and does not regard the disfluencies as a first or primary stage of stuttering. His recent investigations reveal, however, that "For the 'stutterers' the median number of repetitions that involved either words or syllables was approximately six per hundred words, and for the 'non-stutterers' the median number was between one and two per hundred words. The median numbers of all other kinds of disfluency were about seven for the clinical group and five for the control group per hundred words" (Johnson, 1961, p. 135).

The Measurement of Stuttering

It is difficult to measure behavior in which the individual who is performing has subjective responses to his own behavior and is reacting at the same time to the responses of others. In this instance the behavior is stuttering. One way out of the dilemma is to be oblivious, or pretend to be, of anything but what can be measured in the behavior. Essentially, this is what the Scale for Rating Severity of Stuttering (Johnson, Darley, Spriestersbach, 1963), developed at the University of Iowa, attempts to do. This scale has been modified and simplified by Andrews and Harris (1964, pp. 281–282) and presents four grades for stuttering (stammering).

The judgment of degree of impairment of communication is one made by listeners. The speaker (stutterer) may feel quite differently about how impaired he judges his communication to be.

Andrews and Harris code the symptoms as *A* for simple repetitions, *B* for prolongations and hard blockings, and *C* for associated facial and body symptoms.

Brutten and Shoemaker (1967, pp. 31–35) postulate stages in the development of stuttering based on their assumption that stuttering is

Scale for Grading Severity of Stuttering (Stammering)*

Grade 0	No stammering
Grade 1	Mild stammer
	Communication unimpaired
	0-5 per cent of words stammered
Grade 2	Moderate stammer
	Communication slightly impaired
	5-20 per cent of words stammered
Grade 3	Severe stammer
	Communication definitely impaired
	More than 20 per cent of words stammered

* Based on Andrews and Harris (1964, page 185).

a conditioned (learned) disintegration of speech behavior. Stage 1 is characterized by predominantly fluent speech with occasional fluency failures which may be the result of adverse (noxious) conditions, but not the result of learning (conditioning). Stage 2 is characterized by an increase in fluency failures and qualitative modification "that are indicative of emotional conditioning." Stage 3 is characterized by "the development of conditioned negative emotional reactions to the act of speaking, the words employed, or the speech produced."

The Iowa Scale of Attitude Toward Stuttering (Johnson, Darley and Spriestersbach, 1963, pp. 265–266, and pp. 283–287) measures the speaker's (stutterer's) attitude toward stuttering on the basis of rating 45 statements about persons who stutter in a variety of situations, e.g., "A stutterer should not plan to be a lawyer." The rater, who may be a stutterer, is asked to indicate his attitude toward the statement by indicating whether he agrees or disagrees with it, and the degree of his reaction—agree, moderately agree, undecided, moderately disagree, strongly disagree.

Associated Speech Defects

We have already mentioned that stutterers frequently have defective voices, which are usually characterized by tension and narrow pitch range. In many cases, also, articulatory defects are present. Sound substitutions among young children, and lisping and lalling, occur more frequently among stutterers than is normal. Often enough to be significant, the histories of stutterers reveal that their speech onset was somewhat slower than for nonstutterers who were not clearly delayed-speech children. It is probably no chance coincidence that recent studies strongly suggest marked similarities in the family background of stutterers, children with retarded language development, and children with defective articulation. Andrews and Harris (1964, p. 191) report that "Late and poor talking and family history together effectively discriminate stammerers from nonstammerers, and as information about these items may be available prior to the onset of stammering one might well identify the non fluent preschool children who are 'at risk' of stammering." This position is not accepted by Johnson, who states:

> . . . practically all children diagnosed as stutterers have spoken for from six months to several years without being regarded as 'defective in speech'; so-called stuttering children are, in general, normal children, physically and mentally (Johnson, 1967, p. 281).

Conditions Associated with Stuttering

We indicated earlier that no stutterer, regardless of the severity of his stuttering, stutters every time he speaks. Even severe secondary stutterers are often free of stuttering, and sometimes even free of anxiety that they may stutter. Parents of stutterers, teachers, and even the stutterers themselves may be aware that they can engage in choral activity without stuttering, that they can talk aloud to themselves with normal fluency, and that they can usually talk to pets or other animals without difficulty. Many stutterers can talk fluently while playing, especially if the talk is on a nonsense level. Some stutterers can talk normally to younger persons and a few can talk to a selected peer or even an adult without difficulty or with less than usual difficulty. Stuttering, then, may be regarded as a situational problem. We have suggested some situations conducive to relatively free-from-stuttering speech. Are there any general situations conducive to stuttering? Recent research suggests an affirmative answer.

Brown (1945), in several studies, found that stutterers tend to have verbal cues or indicators that are related to increased stuttering. These include: initial words in sentences; longer words in sentences; more nouns, verbs, and adverbs than other parts of speech; and accented syllables within words.

Eisenson and Horowitz (1945) found that stutterers had increased difficulty with reading material as the intellectual significance of the material was increased.

Lanyan (1969), however, found that the likelihood of a stutterer having difficulty (stuttering) on any given word depends not on how much information the word conveys but on word length and how much speech (articulatory) production is required to say the word.

Eisenson and Wells (1942) found that stutterers had increased difficulty when they were shifted from choral reading with normal speakers to solo reading and were responsible for communicating what they were reading aloud.

All the above studies and others available in the literature strongly suggests that there are two factors or situations conducive to increased stuttering. These are: (1) awareness that what is to be spoken has intellectual content; and (2) awareness of communicative responsibility for the speech content. It is not surprising, therefore, that Bloodstein (1950), in what might be considered a converse study, found that adolescent and adult stutterers as a group reported that their stuttering was reduced or absent when they felt no need to make a favorable impression and when they did not feel individually responsible for their utterance. This, as we pointed out earlier, is in line with the observations of most teachers who have observed stutterers in their periods of fluency and periods of relative difficulty.

Beyond these linguistic and environmental situations, which tend to be related to the incidence of stuttering, there are other factors that apparently influence speech control. Most stutterers have increased difficulty when they are fatigued. Stutterers tend to stutter more when they expect to stutter than when such expectancy does not exist. On an individual basis some stutterers expect to stutter in special situations or with specific persons more than they do in other situations or with other persons. By and large, these expectancies tend to be confirmed by actual experience. Even when other speech and associated stuttering manifestations are not present, stutterers experience feelings of apprehension and anxiety because of their anticipation of stuttering. The result is that they respond to themselves as if they had stuttered even though the listener-observer may have seen no external evidence of stuttered speech.

The last point suggests an aspect of stuttering that is deserving of consideration. Although what the listener-observer hears and sees may be important in the evaluation of stuttering, *much goes on within the stutterer that cannot be evaluated by anyone but the stutterer.* How he feels about himself when he anticipates the need for speech is important. How much effort and anxiety does the stutterer entertain when he succeeds in controlling his stuttering? Does the stutterer feel better when his speech seems normally fluent than when he hesitates, blocks, repeats, or prolongs his utterances? These are subjective aspects of stuttering of extreme importance to the individual stutterer even though they do not readily affect the response of the listener. If we appreciate this, we can begin to understand why some adolescents and adults who seem to speak without any of the speech and associated mannerisms of stuttering nevertheless regard themselves as stutterers. They do so, we may conclude, because they feel like stutterers, even though they do not overtly behave like stutterers.

Theoretic Points of View as to the Causes of Stuttering

Theories as to why people stutter are numerous and diverse in their points of view. Many theories once influential, if not dominating, have become reduced in importance, not because they have been disproved or discredited but because their proponents have ceased proposing them or have changed their minds. The attempt in this chapter will be to present several current points of view. This will be done with responsible awareness that we are not including many other points of view which, in a larger or more specialized text, might well be mentioned. The points of view that will be considered in this chapter may be broadly classified along the following lines:

1. Stuttering is a constitutional problem. There are physical reasons that predispose a person to stuttering or that make him a stutterer.
2. Stuttering is essentially a learned form of behavior that may happen to anyone.
3. Stuttering is a manifestation of an underlying personality disorder.

STUTTERING AS A CONSTITUTIONAL PROBLEM

The proponents of the theoretical position that there is a constitutional predisposition to stuttering point to research studies to support their stand. Some of the findings suggest that, as a group, stutterers' familial histories include the following incidents as occurring more often than in the population as a whole: (1) more stutterers; (2) more left-handedness; (3) more twins; (4) later onset of speech; and (5) higher incidence of illnesses and traumas that might cause damage to the nervous system. Support for this position comes from some of the investigations of Berry (1939) and Nelson (1939) and more recently from the findings of the Andrews and Harris Survey (1964, p. 101). The last report includes the presence of significant genetic and neurologic predisposing factors and a higher than usual incidence of birth traumas or evidence of subsequent brain injury. In addition, it reports findings of delayed onset of speech and a high incidence of speech and language problems other than stuttering, ". . . but by far the most important predisposing factor is the inheritance from either parent of the genetic predisposition to stammer."

Findings of recent studies by Curry and Gregory (1969) and Perrin (1969) have implications that suggest that stutterers may be different in their neurophysiological organization from nonstutterers. Both investigations employed a special perceptual-listening task (dichotic listening) to compare the responses of stutterers and nonstutterers. The dichotic listening task requires the listener to attend to two different auditory signals presented simultaneously, one to the left ear and one to the right. In essence, the ears of the subject are engaged in competitive listening. Earlier findings indicate an interesting difference in ear-reporting depending upon the nature of the auditory signal. Speech signals such as digits or words when presented dichotically are reported by most subjects as being received in the right ear. Nonspeech signals such as clicks, snatches of melody, and other nonspeech environmental noises are usually reported as being received in the left ear (Kimura, 1967, p. 20). The systematic differences between the ears in dichotic listening are interpreted as reflecting the functional differences between the two cerebral hemispheres, consistent with the fact that each ear has its greatest number of connections with the contralateral hemisphere. Findings have been fairly uniform that when the subject reports differences in perception of auditory signals, speech signals tend to be referred to the right ear (processed by the left and normally dominant hemisphere) while nonspeech signals are referred to the left ear (processed by the right or nondominant hemisphere). These findings occur only in binaural competitive (dichotic) listening tasks. This, of course, is a laboratory technique and not the one that pertains to usual listening situations.

Curry and Gregory (1969) and Perrin (1969) found that stutterers did not make the referrals to the right ear for speech signals along the expected lines. Although there was some variation for individuals, the Curry and Gregory data indicate that taken as a group, "stutterers had smaller difference scores between ears on dichotic verbal scores than did nonstutterers. Seventy-five per cent of the nonstutterers obtained higher right-ear scores on the dichotic verbal task, whereas 55 per cent of the stutterers had higher left-ear scores." Perrin's findings confirmed those of Curry and Gregory.

Specifically, Perrin found that stutterers showed a clear left-ear preference for words and sentences in dichotic reception, whereas nonstutterers showed a right ear preference for such materials. As a group the stutterers were not different from the nonstutterers in regard to their ear preference for vowels and for noises. As a general observation Perrin (1969) notes, "When a hemisphere exerts some control over speech function in the stutterer, it is the right, which is the reverse of that found in normals." We appreciate, of course, that ear preference is contralateral to cerebral control.

Andrews and Harris (1964, p. 191) suggest a psychobiological theory of stuttering along the following lines:

1. In some instances, a predisposition may be sufficient to initiate stammering (stuttering).
2. "Emotional stress at an age when adequate speech function is precarious may result in a disturbance of this balance of speech maturation and so produce a repetition of sounds and syllables characteristic of stammering. In a child with abnormal speech development, this period of vulnerability will be prolonged. If there is sufficient genetic and neurologic predisposition only minor anxieties will be sufficient, whereas if there is minimal predisposition a more severe emotional stress will be required to initiate stammering."
3. Once the involuntary repetitions of sounds and syllables have begun, the child soon learns to anticipate those words and situations that are difficult for him. "It is this anxiety about specific word and situational cues, and its reduction as they are passed, that results in the development of both the severity and complexity of the stammer syndrome."

This position may explain why all children who may have a predisposing background do not necessarily become stutterers. If a child is fortunate and is free of severe illness, physical, and psychological trauma during the developmental stages of speech, he may be reasonably "safe" from becoming a stutterer.

If, however, conditions are less fortunate, and either illness or emotional disturbance upsets the child during the speech-development stage, stuttering is likely to result. In other words, constitutional factors provide a subsoil for stuttering. Stuttering itself is a product associated with the subsoil and the specific environmental, physical, or psychological factors that tend to nurture it.

An interesting psychobiologic view of stuttering is held by Travis (1946, pp. 3–5, and 1957, pp. 916–946). According to Travis, the child who becomes a stutterer starts life with a deviant cerebral mechanism that tends to prolong infantile behavior and so makes for difficulty in adjustment. The stutterer, in his attempts at speaking, is not successful in inhibiting infantile impulses or speech mannerisms. Childish wishes, hates, and fears force their way into the stutterer's expression and become part of the characteristics of stuttering. The stutterer, as he grows older, is torn between the forces that urge infantile expression and the fears of the consequences of such expression. Travis regards the stutter's speech as an unhappy compromise between his drive to express himself and his fear of revealing himself.

In the *Symposium on Stuttering* (Eisenson, ed., 1958), the positions of West and Eisenson are based on the assumption that stutterers are neurologically different from nonstutterers. West's position is highly speculative. Eisenson's position, which will be considered later, does not assume that stutterers are a homogeneous group either in their neurological background or in the factors that are conducive to the disorder.

STUTTERING AS A LEARNED FORM OF BEHAVIOR

The proponents of the point of view that stuttering is a learned form of behavior are, as we might expect, opposed to believing that stutterers as a group are significantly different constitutionally in any way from nonstutterers. Instead, children who stutter are considered to be essentially normal children in regard to heredity, physical development, health history, psychological traits, intelligence, or any other single factor in which the first group of theorists we discussed found important differences. Johnson (1967), a leading proponent of "normality of the stutterer" school, holds that stuttering is a *speech disturbance which can happen to anyone*. How stuttering has its onset and how it becomes established as a reaction to some but not all speaking situations are explained through principles of learning that apply to behavior in general as well as to stuttering in particular.

The early stages of stuttering are explained as resulting from a misevaluation of the disfluencies normal in young children. Young children of preschool age and in the early primary grades are inclined to be repetitious and hesitant when they talk as well as in other forms of behavior. Parents, teachers, or other adults who mistake these disfluencies for stuttering symptoms, and who show concern or anxiety about them, are likely to transmit this attitude to the child. When a child becomes aware of adult anxiety and permits it to affect him, he may approach a speaking situation with an attitude of apprehension. It is not the hesitation or repetition but the speaker's reactions to them and to the reactions of other persons to which he in turns reacts that make the child into a stutterer.

In another publication Johnson (1961, p. 138) explains that:

The problem called stuttering begins, then, when the child's speech is felt, usually by the mother, to be not as smooth or as fluent as it ought to be. There seems as a rule to be a quality of puzzlement mixed with slight apprehension and dread about the mother's feelings. She uses the only name she knows for what she thinks must be the matter with her youngster's speech, and that word is "stuttering"—or, if she has grown up in England or certain other parts of the world, "stammering."

. . . She may not be sure of herself at first in deciding that her child is stuttering, but her use of the word crystallizes her feelings and serves to focus her attention on the hesitations in the speech of her child.

Johnson emphasizes that the mother's feelings and apprehensions tend to become apparent to the child and in time the child "takes from the mother the feelings she has about his speech."

Eisenson (1966) "tested" Johnson's assumption that stuttering is a result of maternal reaction to the child's speech by investigating the incidence of the disorder among preschool and primary-grade children brought up in kibbutzim (communal organizations) in Israel. Children in these settings were cared for by nurse-teachers throughout the day. They saw their parents in the late afternoon and on some holidays. They slept, ate, were trained and taught in cottage facilities by the nurse-teachers. There was no conscious differences in the treatment of the children along sex lines. The incidence and sex distribution for the presence of stuttering in children brought up in kibbutzim were essentially the same as those found in the United States and those reported by Andrews and Harris in England. The total incidence was about 1 per cent, with a sex ratio of about four boys to one girl.

To return to Johnson's position, stuttering may be considered a learned and specific anxiety reaction associated with speaking situations. But stuttering and its consequences seem to be unpleasant and apparently more penalizing than rewarding. Normally, behavior that persists is behavior somehow rewarded. Are there any rewards or pleasant after-effects in stuttering? There are, if we look for them. One of the possible rewards is the attention a child may receive that may not otherwise be available to him. The stutterer may learn to enjoy the intensity of reaction and the disturbance he causes by his speech. If he needs these more than he does normal speech, stuttering is likely to persist. In the classroom, the stutterer may be excused from recitations or win sympathy that he may learn to enjoy. He may become a "special child" and be loath to give up that status. Until he is ready to do so, the child who began to stutter through no fault of his own is likely to continue to stutter. Unfortunately, when the penalties of stuttering begin to exceed the rewards, the habits and attitudes of the stutterer may persist, and many stutterers need help in overcoming them. A few, however, seem able to stop without outside help. These children may have taken an accounting of the assets and liabilities associated with stuttering and have reached a conclusion that became translated into self-modified behavior. Certainly, many experienced teachers know youngsters who stuttered in the early grades and who became normal speakers in later grades without any outside help.

For those who do not or cannot stop, a theoretical explanation for the continuance of stuttering can be made along these lines: The stutterer continues to fear that he will stutter in a given situation, or on a given word. He becomes tense and apprehensive in ancitipation of the situation or word. If, with great effort, he finally manages to speak despite the initial tension and anxiety, he brings about a momentary reduction in the anxiety-tension state. This brief period of relief may be sufficiently pleasurable to reinforce and to perpetuate not only the stuttering but also the entire attitude and pattern of behavior associated with it.

The positions of Wischner (1950) and Sheehan (1958) and Brutten and Shoemaker (1969) represent other learning-theory views to account for the development and maintenance of stuttering. Several conditioning theories and therapies for stutterers based on deconditioning are presented in a monograph edited by Gray and England (1969). Gregory (1968) has also edited a monograph on *Learning Theory and Stuttering Therapy*.

STUTTERING AS A MANIFESTATION OF A PERSONALITY DISORDER

Earlier, in discussing the point of view of Travis, we pointed out that he felt that stutterers were maladjusted persons who became so because of initial constitutional differences. There are many psychologists and psychoanalysts who emphasize the maladjustment and do not appear to be concerned with the possibility that stutterers are constitutionally different from normal speakers. They regard stuttering as a manifestation of personality disorder and are inclined to agree that the stutterer speaks as he does because of some psychological need that is better satisfied through stuttering than through normal speech. Stutterers are likely to be characterized as infantile, compulsive, dependent, ambivalent, regressive, anxious, insecure, withdrawn, or by some other adjective or combination of adjectives consistent with the specific theoretic formulation or bias of the theorizer. For example, the psychoanalyst Coriat (1943) looks upon stutterers as ". . . infants who have compulsively retained the original equivalents of nursing and biting." The equivalents, we might note, are the specific oral characteristics of the stutterer, the way in which he repeats, hesitates, blocks, or prolongs on the sounds he utters or stops himself from uttering.

Glauber also looks upon stuttering as an expression of an underlying personality involvement associated primarily with an "arrest in ego maturation." According to Glauber, "The fixation is manifested in the speech symptoms and in the total personality" (Glauber, 1958, p. 93).

Theorists who believe that stuttering is a manifestation of a personality disorder are able to point to a large number of studies to support their position. The results of many but by no means all of these studies suggest that adolescents and adults who stutter are, on the whole, not as well adjusted as nonstutterers. We might add, however, that seldom do the studies provide evidence to indicate whether the stuttering is the cause of or is caused by the maladjustment. The possibility that the stuttering preceded the maladjustment must be considered by those who look objectively on the overall problem of the stutterer and his stuttering. Murphy and FitzSimons (1960) present a detailed consideration of the position that stuttering is an expression of underlying personality dynamics.

MULTIPLE ORIGIN VIEWPOINTS

The points of view we have just presented has each sought to explain stuttering as having a single cause. Obviously, theories inconsistent with one another cannot all be correct at all times. There is a possibility, however, that each of the theories, and the theorists, is correct at some times—often enough, we would gather, to satisfy himself, but not often enough to persuade those holding opposing or even supplementary viewpoints. Before leaving the discussion of theories as to the cause of stuttering we will consider two points of view of practicing speech clinicians who currently believe that stuttering may have multiple causes. Why any given individual stutters can best be estimated by his individual clinical history and the cause that seems most likely to fit his case.

STUTTERING AS A MANIFESTATION OF PERSEVERATION

Eisenson believes that persons tend to persist in a given mode of behavior even when such behavior is not appropriate, when they are confronted with conditions that call for more rapid change than they are capable of making. The tendency for an individual to resist change, and for a mental or motor process to dominate behavior after the situation that originally evoked it is no longer present, is termed *perseveration*. The perseverating phenomenon is normal for all of us. Most often we experience it when tired, sleepy, or under conditions of pressure or tension. We do the same thing or feel the same way even when we are able to recognize that the cause for the doing or feeling has ceased to exist. So, minutes after we have gotten off a bicycle, we may still feel that we are riding on it. When we are tired, and required to talk, we tend to repeat utterances more often than the intellectual aspect of the situation requires. If we do not become anxious or apprehensive about our normal inclination to perseverate, we are not likely to fear recurring or similar situations because we have perseverated. There are, however, physiological and psychological conditions conducive to more than a normal amount of perseverative behavior. Among these conditions are brain damage, lowered vitality, the aftereffects of physical or mental shock, and emotional tension and anxiety.

According to Eisenson (1958), if an individual is required, or feels that he is required, to speak under a condition conducive to perseverative behavior, the perseveration will be manifest in speech. Unfortunately, the awareness of blocked or repetitive tendencies in speech may increase the individual's apprehension about his speaking and so aggravate the condition initially responsible for the speech perseveration. The result is a generalized reaction toward speaking that transforms what might otherwise be hesitation, block, repetition, or prolongation (perseverating manifestations) into stuttering.

Speech conditions that are associated with a feeling of responsibility are more likely to be associated with perseverative speech than speech that is devoid of responsibility. Communicative language content is also associated with perseveration in speaking. Persons who find themselves pressed by their environment, or by their own inner compulsions, to speak intellectually when they have nothing to say, or are not completely prepared to say what they would like, are likely to perseverate in speech. In general, these are speech situations productive of some degree of anxiety.

It is also possible that some persons with an atypical neurological mechanism are unable to respond with spoken language as rapidly as some speech situations require. In such situations, and for such persons, perseveration in speech tends to occur. These may be the persons with a constitutional predisposition to stuttering (Curry, 1969; Perrin, 1969).

Most stutterers, we know, have periods of relative fluency, and others in which they are normally quite fluent. Such conditions include speaking to animal pets, responding as a member of a group (where communicative responsibility is shared, reduced, or lacking), speaking nonsense intentionally, singing (singing is not really speaking because it is devoid of responsibility either for the formulation of the word sequences or its " communication "), and often the recitation of memorized material. All of these conditions share a common feature—the lack of formulating and the responsibility of uttering a thought, or a *propositional statement* (it may be a question) to which an answer might be expected. Stuttering, unless it is patently of neurotic origin, almost always occurs when a speaker is engaged in propositional talking. It has its parallel with the normal hesitations of nonstutterers who are talking about something of importance, even if only of momentary importance, while they are thinking of how to say it. These are normal hesitation phenomena.

In summary, most stuttering behavior is expressed when the speaker is engaged in propositional or communicative interchange. At such times, either because of an anxiety specific to the situation, or a more generalized anxiety about speaking when there is any degree of communicative responsibility, perseveration in speech tends to occur. Only a neurotic individual who feels that he has a commitment to stutter whenever and to whomever he talks or nontalks, is likely to stutter in many other situations. Normal speakers, and stutterers when not under stress, may engage in normal hesitations. However, despite superficial resemblances, normal hesitations, regardless of who produces them, should not be confused with stuttering.

In essence, according to Eisenson, stuttering as a manifestation of perseveration may take place whenever the speaker finds himself inadequate or unequal to the demands of the speaking situation. The perseverating tendency may have a physiological cause, a psychological cause, or a combination of both.

VAN RIPER'S ECLECTIC VIEWPOINT

In his contribution to the *Symposium on Stuttering* (Eisenson, 1958) Van Riper suggests that he is not as much concerned with the cause or causes of stuttering as with its treatment. Elsewhere (Van Riper, 1963, p. 327), he sums up his position as follows:

> What is a student to believe when so many different explanations exist? Our own resolution of the problem is an eclectic one. We feel that stuttering has many origins, many sources, and that the original causes are not nearly so important as the maintaining causes, once stuttering has started. We can find stutterers who partly fit any one of the various statements of theory and some stutterers who fit several. All stutterers are not cut from the same original cloth. It is important that we know these various explanations because the problems of some of the stutterers we meet can thereby be best understood. The river of stuttering does not flow out of only one lake.

Van Riper states that: "*Stuttering occurs when the flow of speech is interrupted abnormally by repetitions or prolongations of a sound or syllable or posture, or by avoidance and struggle reactions*" (Van Riper, 1963, p. 311). Special emphasis is given to the term "abnormal," implying differences in amount, kind, severity, and situations in which the disfluencies (hesitations, repetitions, prolongations) occur. *Avoidance* and *struggle* rarely characterize the abnormal speech of the early (primary) stutterer. However, they tend to constitute the major aspects of the speech and reaction patterns of the "advanced" stutterer. Although Van Riper's definition of stuttering is descriptive of external and observable manifestations, he is fully aware that "the problem of stuttering cannot be defined entirely by what emerges from the mouth" (Van Riper, 1963, p. 314). So, he notes, there are stutterers who repress or interiorize their difficulties, who are on constant and anxious guard to avoid situations that might be conducive to their stuttering, and who use a variety of delaying techniques, including coughing, stretching, scratching, and nose blowing while, presumably, they prepare to talk. Van Riper also notes that some stutterers (we have also known several) show no overt phonetic or linguistic evidence of stuttering, but are constantly apprehensive that they may do so. In addition he notes that "One stutterer will punish himself masochistically; another, with equal feelings of hostility, will spend his life attacking other people. The particular patterns of emotional reaction shown by different stutterers are due to the particular history each has had" (Van Riper, 1963, p. 314).

Van Riper describes four stages of stuttering which approximate the developmental phases observed by Bloodstein. Stuttering changes its characteristics as it develops. This is important because, Van Riper emphasizes, therapy for the stutterer depends upon the stage of development, the form of expression, of the stuttering. "By treating the beginning stutterer in the same way we would treat an adult, we would almost surely make his stuttering worse" (Van Riper, 1963, p. 327). Van Riper acknowledges that all stutterers do not go through all four developmental stages, and that the beginning and final stages are more clearly defined than those which are intermediate. He does believe that at each stage there are characteristically different forms of outward behavior and different kinds of inner feelings.

Van Riper's Developmental Stages of Stuttering

FIRST STAGE

Those of the child's utterances which are abnormally disfluent (there may be long periods—hours, days, or weeks of normal fluency) consist of short effortless repetitions or prolongations of sounds and syllables. The child seems to show no awareness of his disfluencies, no fear of talking, little or no evidence of frustration and only rarely any indication of even momentary "struggle" behavior. Difficulties appear to be associated with states of excitement, ambivalence (indecision), and with situations that involve strong communicative need. Difficulties are likely to be expressed more often at the beginnings of an utterance than midway or at the end of an utterance. Van Riper considers this stage to be *primary stuttering*.

We interpret the manifestations of so-called disfluency in this stage to be related to the child's progress in language development, in the growth of vocabulary and in syntactic proficiency. The child is literally reaching out and trying to say more that is of consequence to the listener, in a linguistically more mature way. In trying out new formulations he may indeed hesitate and repeat some words and phrases, almost always at the beginning of an utterance. These, as we have noted, are normal hesitation phenomena. He may even repeat some initial syllables. So-called disfluencies, sound and syllable repetitions, though they may occur, are relatively infrequent. We believe, as does Van Riper, that there is a difference that may make for a future difference between hesitation phenomena and disfluencies. Support for this position may be found in survey investigations by Wingate (1962) and McDearmon (1968).*

We would like to add a note on the semantic implication of the term *normal disfluency*. Normal fluency, the authors of this text believe, should allow for some amount of so-called disfluencies. These, as we have suggested, are probably better thought of as normal hesitation phenomena.† There seems to be no reason then to use the term *normal disfluency*, which has negative implications for the speech of a child who is *normally fluent*.

SECOND STAGE

The repetitions, hesitations, and prolongations appear more frequently, and are now incorporated into the tempo and rhythm of syllabic utterance. Speech becomes dysrhythmic; prolongations become accentuated and many repetitions end as prolongations. Only rarely does the child reveal awareness of his disfluencies and in fact look or even announce " I can't say it." However, periods of disfluency may be followed by long periods of relatively fluent speech.

---

* McDearmon found that children who are identified as stutterers by at least one parent have disfluencies in the form of sound and syllable repetition and prolongations. Children who are not identified as stutterers are more likely to have word and phrase repetitions. Tension, even at the outset, may accompany the disfluencies of the children labeled as stutterers.

† Normal hesitation phenomena in adults has been studied by Goldman-Eisler (1964).

Stage 2 is still primary stuttering, but with more cause for concern than stage 1.

THIRD STAGE

Awareness and indications of frustration are the chief added features of this stage. There are more moments of stuttering, and so more moments of frustration and of expressions of struggle behavior. Repetitions are no longer easy and "bubbly," but become forced and more of them conclude with prolongations. Breathing abnormalities become evident, possibly as a manifestation that the child has lost control over normally modified respiration for speech. Facial contortions and tremors, including vocal tremor, may be present.

Van Riper considers stuttering tremor to be of great significance in the development of stuttering. "The stuttering tremor appears when a fixed articulatory posture is suddenly invested with a surge of tension. In this third stage the repetitions tend to terminate in fixed postures or prolongations. Tight closures of the lips, the tongue, or the vocal cords occur and tiny but very swift vibrations appear in these structures as a result of the tension. They are called tremors" (1963, p. 330). Van Riper indicates that when the stutterer goes into tremor he has lost control of his speech musculature, and develops apprehensions related to the words and situations associated with the occurrence of tremor.

Van Riper believes that in the third stage the stutterer begins to invest his energies not just in effort to produce his words but also in behavior to escape from his tremors. Many of the contortions and tic mannerisms that characterize the stuttering of the adult have their origin in this transitional stage. "Whatever is done just before an escape from punishment becomes strongly reinforced" (Van Riper, 1963, p. 331). Presumably, in terms of operant learning theory, if release from tremor is associated with a particular action such as a contortion, and release from tremor becomes the immediate objective of the stutterer, the contortion becomes established as the behavior that follows the awareness of tremor or, for that matter, any other overt manifestation of stuttering.

In the third stage there is reduction in periods of remission from stuttering. Although the child still does not avoid speaking and has not yet determined for himself the feared words and situations that he may later associate with his stuttering, he begins to feel frustrated and may begin to be aware that his stuttering is unpleasant to others. This, Van Riper considers is the frustration stage of stuttering. "It is our impression that the stutterer of constitutional origin lingers longest in the first two stages. Perhaps he is accustomed to inadequacy" (Van Riper, 1963, p. 332).

FOURTH STAGE

This is the stage of full-blown secondary stuttering, in which fear is the covert or internal reaction and avoidance the obvious behavior. The stutterer now fears specific words, communicative situations, and selected listeners. He may also develop general anxiety states and entertain feelings of guilt which may be expressed in hostile behavior, which in turn engenders further feelings of guilt. "All sorts of gradations of fear, anxiety, guilt, and hostility may be found in specific stutterers in this stage, but each of these emotional reactions is usually found in some degree" (Van Riper, 1963, p. 332). Many of the overt characteristics of the earlier stages may persist in stage 4. *Fear and avoidance are additions.* Few stutterers who "progress" to stage 4 are likely to make spontaneous recoveries.

One reason for the poor prognosis of the stage 4 stutterer is the development and discovery of *secondary gains*. Despite all of its penalties, there may be some values in stuttering. The stutterer may use his speech as an explanation acceptable to himself if not to others, of avoiding demanding situations, or persons he may find unpleasant. Stuttering may serve as a defense against the demands of his environment, or against his own conscience. Although most stutterers are likely to reject the presence of secondary gains that may maintain stuttering, Van Riper believes that some secondary gain from stuttering is often to be found in adults.

We have dwelt in some detail on Van Riper's position on stuttering, and in the exposition of the four developmental stages, because we believe that what Van Riper describes is clinically observable. It is consistent with the evidence. Nevertheless, we have known children whose stuttering began with the manifestations of stage 3 but who did not go on to stage 4. We have also known older adults who just quit stuttering, even after exhibiting full stage 4 manifestations for many years. Some secondary stutterers, possibly after self-analysis, may modify their own behavior, perhaps because stuttering, despite its possibilities of secondary gains, may no longer be worth the effort. Though advancing age may not have many privileges, one that remains, if the individual cares to exercise it, is to stop a form of behavior that has outlived its usefulness without need to explain the change to anyone. Such adults may continue to be more than normally disfluent but without the accompanying struggle, tics, and techniques of avoidance.

Therapy for Stutterers

Although the burden of therapy for stutterers is one that should be carried by the professional speech clinician, the classroom teacher is necessarily an important member of the therapeutic team. In the discussion that follows, we will consider the objectives of therapy for the primary stutterer and the secondary stutterer as well as the specific role of the classroom teacher in regard to each.

OBJECTIVES FOR THE PRIMARY STUTTERER

In characterizing the primary stutterer we emphasized that his disfluencies, even though excessive, occur without evidence either of awareness or special effort in speaking. Emphasis in the treatment of the primary stutterer is to prevent him from becoming aware that his speech is in any way different from that of others around him and a cause for concern. Awareness of difference, whether it be of speech or any other form of behavior, arises from observed reactions. A young child will have no way of knowing that his speech is atypical unless some person important to him says or does something to direct his attention to the difference. The child who is disfluent is not likely to compare himself with other children until after some older person has made or suggested a comparison. Disfluencies become something for the child to be concerned about only after he has responded to another person's concern. To prevent awareness and concern, we must somehow control the reactions of persons who may show and so create awareness. Essentially, therefore, the primary stutterer is to be treated through his parents if he is not of school age. If he is of school age, teachers as well as parents become the recipients of direct treatment. The primary stutterer should be given no direct speech therapy nor any other form of therapy that he can relate to his speech. Nothing should be done or said to the child that suggests that his speech is in any way in need of change. If the primary stutterer is to be involved in therapy, it is only to permit the trained speech clinician to observe what possible pressures exist in the child's environment which disturb his speech. For this purpose, a permissive play group is recommended. In a play group it is possible for a clinician to observe conditions conducive to increased disfluency. The clinician's observations are, of course, later discussed with the parents with a view toward modification of comparable home conditions so that pressure and excessive disfluencies can be reduced, or, if possible, eliminated. Some of these specific aspects of treatment, and some of the

information to be given to the parents of the primary stutterer, or o
the child believed by his parents to be a stutterer, will now be considered. Many of these aspects, incidentally, are also relevant for the
classroom teacher.

DISTINGUISHING BETWEEN DISFLUENCY AND PRIMARY STUTTERING

Often parents are unduly sensitized about stuttering because of their
own family history. One or both of the parents may have stuttered or
may still be stuttering. Older children or relatives may be stutterers.
Perhaps the parents are being pressured by their own parents to "do
something" about the child's speech. The parents, understandably
concerned, are "doing something" about what they believe to be stuttering.

A first step in the direction of treatment of the parents is to determine whether the child's disfluencies are within the limits of normal or,
in terms of incidence and situation, in excess of normal. Are we, in
other words, dealing with normal disfluency, which includes some
amount of so-called disfluency, or primary stuttering? Information
is obtained from the parents' description and, if possible, imitation of
the child's speech. The parents are asked to recall when disfluencies
most often occur and when they are least likely to occur. The child's
speech should be observed when talking to his parents, with a special
note made as to whether there is any difference in ease of speaking when
the response is made to the mother or to the father. The child should
also be observed in a play situation when he is away from his parents as
well as in their presence. If the total observed speech behavior adds up
to normal speech flow—normal ease of speech—this should be stated
and explained to the parents. We have found that parents are frequently
able to understand and accept hesitancies and repetitions in speech
when these are compared with hesitant and repetitious nonspeech
behavior. We are usually able to get from parents their observations
that not only their child but most children repeat activities when at
play, that young children enjoy hearing the same song or the same
story repeated many times. We try to make parents realize the normality
of repetitions in all aspects of a young child's behavior so that repetition
does not seem abnormal when it occurs in speech.

We have found effective the technique of recording and playing
back part of the interview held with the parents about the child. In
listening to the playback, parents are able to hear their own hesitations
and repetitions as well as those of the interviewer. If they do not consider themselves stutterers, the parents are then able to compare their

own speech with that of their child in regard to the incidence of "disfluencies." If the parents are disturbed about their own hesitant speech, they should be assured that few if any persons are always fluent, except possibly when they are reproducing memorized material. Even actors, it might be pointed out, have occasional "disfluencies," so that non-professional speakers should certainly be permitted some of their own.

Nothing in the interview with the parents should suggest, by words or manner, that the parents were either foolish or overanxious or in any way exercised poor judgment in coming for help about their child's speech. We believe that parents have a right, if not an obligation, to be concerned. We also believe that each child has his own right not to be concerned about all things that may concern his parents. The child's hesitations, if they are normal in frequency and not excessive for the situation, are among those things about which the child should not be concerned. We think that parents are usually able to appreciate that most disfluencies are normal. Furthermore, we point out that the difference between normal hesitation and stuttering may lie in the matter of awareness and anxiety that young children not indifferent to their parents may get from them. We indicate that frequently stuttering is the sum of disfluency, plus awareness plus anxiety, while disfluency alone is developmentally normal speech behavior.

It is possible that in some instances the child may really be disfluent, more than normally hesitant and repetitive in his speech. The advice, nevertheless, still holds. There is much greater likelihood that a child will reduce this manner of speaking without direct attention being paid to it, than with intervention. The only positive suggestion we would make for "correction" is to observe whether a child is trying to arrive at a new, more mature, and syntactically more complex way of saying something than he did before the occurrence of his hesitations and repetitions. For example, a child at age three might say "Johnny is my brother. Johnny and I go to school together." The same child when he is a year or so older might try to indicate the same meanings with a single sentence formulation such as "My brother Johnny and I go to school together," or "I go to school with my brother Johnny." While trying to figure out the new "grown up" way to say things, hesitations and repetitions, or recall of a part of the sentence, most likely the first part, may well take place. If this seems to be the situation, then the mother or the nursery school teacher should give the child a "model" sentence for him to imitate. The model sentence should not be too obvious or too directly offered. We would suggest that the parent or teacher might take an opportunity to make a parallel statement for the child. If our little Johnny's brother is bright, he will get the idea. If not, no harm will be done.

What we are suggesting has more general implication. We believe that most adults have hesitations in speaking when they try new formulations. Certainly observers of the speech of children may readily note this phenomenon. Most children develop control of new formulations such as imbedded phrases and clauses, e.g., "Mary, my very dearest doll, broke her arm today." While "reaching" for this new formulation, this new way of saying two sentences (thoughts) in one, the child may indeed become somewhat disfluent. So may the child in trying out a "big" word, or the expression of any new "big" thought. Hesitations, repetitions, and even backing up and starting again, are all quite normal for adults. Certainly they should be considered normal for children. To repeat an earlier observation, normal fluency should include an amount of so-called disfluencies which are really normal hesitation phenomena. However, it is possible that in some instances, which we believe include most young children with a constitutional predisposition toward at least primary stuttering, children may be delayed in their ability for syntactic development. Their inner linguistic formulations, and so, of course, their expressions, may be inconsistent with age and intellectual level expectations. So, they have difficulty in "mature" expressions of their thoughts. This is the theme of Bluemel's (1957) *The Riddle of Stuttering*.

INFORMATION ABOUT LANGUAGE DEVELOPMENT AND SPEECH FUNCTIONS

Many parents become anxious about their children's speech because they are either uninformed or misinformed about how speech and language develop in children. They are likely to have some vague notions that children begin to talk somewhere about the time that they begin to walk. Most parents have heard about children who talked reasonably plainly at one year of age and may show disappointment if their own children seem slower. We believe that properly informed parents are likely to be less anxious parents, and so, either in an interview situation or in a larger parent group situation, we inform the parents about the normal expectancies in regard to language development, speech proficiency, and the function served by speech. Among the points we emphasize for parents are the following:*

    1. Every child has his own rate and pattern of language and speech development just as he has his own rate and pattern of physical growth

---

* The teacher or clinician might at this point review Chapter 7 on the development of language in children.

and motor development. A slower than "normal" developmental pattern does not necessarily mean that the child is retarded.

2. Language and speech development are related to some factors over which the child has no control. These include the position and number of children in the family, the linguistic ability and intelligence of the parents, the child's sex, and the appropriateness of motivation and stimulation for the child to talk. A first child tends to begin to talk earlier than a second, and a second earlier than a third. Girls, by and large, talk somewhat earlier and more proficiently than boys. The child who is urged to talk too soon may be more delayed in beginning than the child who begins to talk when he is ready and needs to talk.

3. Attentive and available parents are much more helpful for the development of speech than either anxious or nonavailable parents.

4. Language is not likely to be used unless its use is associated with pleasure.

5. Children should enjoy making sounds before sounds are used as words. Even after children begin to use words they continue to enjoy making sounds even when they have nothing to communicate.

6. Many children do not establish articulatory (speech sound) proficiency until they are almost eight years of age. A young child is entitled to lisp, hesitate, and repeat without being corrected except by good example.

7. Children must hear good speech if they are to become good speakers.

8. Fluency does not become established all at once, if indeed it is ever established. Most preschool children speak with some amount of hestitations and repetitions much of the time. Hesitations and repetitions, even up to 10 per cent of utterance, are not abnormal provided they do not abruptly interrupt the flow of speech. In very young children who are just beginning to speak and in many three- and four-year-olds who are striving for grown-up sentence formulations, so-called disfluencies may exceed 10 per cent of utterance.

9. Absence of speech fluency becomes important and a matter for concern when it is associated with specific recurring situations or events. Parents should note whether the child becomes increasingly hesitant when frustrated, when fatigued, or when talking to particular persons. If the child's disfluencies increase sharply in these situations, control of them, if possible, is recommended. Control may take place either by avoiding the situation or by doing nothing that requires the child to communicate in these situations. By communicating, we mean having to answer questions that call for precise answers. Nothing, however, should be done to give the child a feeling that he is not to speak if he wishes to do so.

Parents should also note whether the child becomes increasingly disfluent when he bids or competes for attention. If this is so, parents should be alert to give the child quick attention when he is normally fluent. This is important so that increased disfluency does not result in greater satisfaction than normal fluency.

Parents should know that children do not always want to say something specific or communicative when they talk. They may wish to use words as once they used sounds, merely for the sake of the pleasure derived from utterance. Adults also do this when they sing nonsense songs or talk nonsense words to their children.

Parents should be on guard to watch how often they unconsciously or consciously interrupt their children. Interruption may produce frustration, and frustration in turn produce disfluency. The child who is brought up to silence himself when an adult wishes to talk may interrupt his speech attempts and become hesitant in fear that he may be talking out of turn.

MODIFICATION OF REACTIONS TO THE CHILD'S DISFLUENCIES

If the child is a primary stutterer or is showing any of the speech characteristics associated with stuttering, it is essential that signs of parental anxiety be kept from him. First, of course, we try to assure the parents that despite our acceptance that the child may be in the first stage of stuttering, the second stage or phase is by no means inevitable. By relieving parental anxiety, we hope to reduce the occurrence of displays of anxiety. Parents are encouraged to listen patiently and without tension when the child speaks. They are instructed not to do or say anything that may be interpreted by the child as a sign that his speech is not acceptable. Among the important *do nots* are the following:

1. Do not permit the child to hear the word stuttering used about his speech.

2. Do not tell the child to speed up, slow down, think before he speaks, start over again, or do anything that makes it necessary for him to think about speaking or to conclude that he is not speaking well.

3. Do not sigh with relief when the child speaks fluently, or look upon him with wide-eyed fear that he may speak hesitatingly.

4. Do not show impatience if the child blocks, hesitates, or repeats.

5. Do not ask the child to speak in situations where disfluencies are likely to occur.

Among the important *positive suggestions* for the parents of the primary stutterer are the following:

1. Establish as calm a home environment as can be achieved. Try

to avoid exposing the child to situations that are overexciting, embarrassing, or frustrating.

2. Encourage the child to talk, but do not demand talking even in situations where the child is usually fluent and at ease.

3. Listen to your child with as much attention as you would like him to show you when you are talking.

4. Speak to your child in a calm, unhurried manner, but not in a way so exaggerated as to be difficult to imitate.

5. Keep your child in the best possible physical condition and check for possible ailments if he suddenly shows excessive hesitations and repetitions.

6. Expect that your child will sometimes begin to say things he cannot finish. If he seems to be groping for a word to complete his thought, offer the word to him. Do not, however, anticipate what he may want to say by completing his thought for him.

7. Do all you can to *make speech behavior pleasurable*. Tell amusing anecdotes and read stories that you know the child enjoys. If you note that at a certain time of day your child has an increase of disfluencies, try to make that the time in which you read to him. This reading has two results. It removes the opportunity for the practice of disfluent speech, and with it the possibility that the child may become aware of his disfluencies. It also affords the child an opportunity to be passively engaged in an enjoyable speech activity.

8. Assure your child, if he asks you whether there is anything wrong with his speech, that you think his speech is just fine. If he tells you that sometimes he has trouble getting words out, make him understand that everybody has such trouble at some time so that there is nothing to worry about. Avoid overexplaining and overtalking your assurance, or your child, as a wise child, may suspect that you do not really mean what you say.

THE ROLE OF THE CLASSROOM TEACHER

Virtually all that has been outlined or suggested as appropriate attitude and behavior for the parents of the primary stutterer may be applied to the classroom teacher. The problem of primary stuttering is one that the teacher is likely to meet in the nursery and kindergarten grades and in the first two grades of school. In these grades the teacher has an opportunity to observe the pressure situations that are conducive to increased disfluencies and to control them in the primary stutterer's behalf. The teacher, by being a patient and attentive listener, can help the child considerably. The child who shows signs of primary stuttering should not be corrected in his articulation or have any other aspect of defective speech called to his attention. The teacher should avoid calling upon the child when he is likely to be disfluent and go out of the way to call upon him when he is likely to speak fluently.

The attitude of calm recommended for the primary stutterer's home should also prevail in the classroom. This applies to all children and to the teacher himself. A teacher, who shows ready anger, ridicules a child for an error, or permits children to ridicule one another, creates an attitude of apprehension. On the other hand, the teacher who accepts error as a normal way of life and indicates that it is better to try even though a mistake may be made, sets a tone which most children will accept with pleasure. If any child responds to a mistake with ridicule, the child should be corrected in a private session.

The teacher should be *generous in his praise of any special abilities shown by the primary stutterer*. If he has no special abilities, praise those that are his chief assets.

If the child has been teased because of his speech, or dubbed a stutterer by his classmates, the teacher should assure him that his classmates are mistaken. The primary stutterer should be told that everyone has the same kind of speech trouble at some time just as all children stumble occasionally when they walk or run. It might help considerably if the teacher, in a not too evident way, does some hesitating or repeating of his own. Beyond this, the teacher should explain to the class that teasing and name-calling are not permitted and that some privilege will be denied to any offending member.

Perhaps the teacher's role can best be summed up in a single directive. Be accepting, permissive, and kind; do only those things to and for the primary stutterer, or any other child in your class, that you would want another teacher to do to and for your own child—or for any child you may love!

OBJECTIVES FOR THE SECONDARY STUTTERER

The secondary stutterer, we recall, is aware that his speech is atypical and has reactions to himself and to his environment in terms of his awareness and evaluation of his speech. Therapeutic objectives, therefore, include a modification of the speech pattern as well as a modification of the attitudes that the stutterer has developed toward himself, his speech, and his environment. How much can be done depends upon the professional resources available to the stutterer and his readiness for making use of the resources. In some instances, little more than superficial treatment of speech symptoms can be attempted. Unfortunately, this is not enough for many secondary stutterers, especially for those who have evident personality maladjustments associated with their stuttering. In some settings, psychotherapy as well as speech therapy is available, and more than speech modification can be attempted in a treatment program. When the family of the stutterer has no financial problem, private help can be sought outside of the school.

Where the secondary stutterer shows no evidence of significant maladaptive behavior or of attitudes requiring modifications, treatment may be limited to the speech symptoms. The assessment of what is needed should be made by a psychologist, speech pathologist, or other professional worker trained in personality evaluation. The clinician, we urge, should undertake the assessment of the patient with an objective attitude without assuming either: (1) that every stutterer, by virtue of his stuttering, necessarily has a personality disorder; or (2) that stutterers need treatment only for their speech symptoms to become wholly normal persons.

There is one basic understanding that must be established with the secondary stutterer if treatment, either for stuttering symptoms or for behavioral maladjustments, is to be successful. The stutterer, at the outset, must accept himself as a person who stutters and is in need of treatment. He must not try to conceal his stuttering or fight against the notion that he is a stutterer. When control over stuttering symptoms is established, and attitudes and behavior modified, the once secondary stutterer can then discard his label along with his speech characteristics and associated traits.

Another area of understanding that stutterer and clinician must establish is one of possible gains or values that may have grown out of stuttering. The stutterer must be helped to ask himself, and to answer honestly and objectively, the question, "Am I getting anything out of my stuttering that I don't want to give up?" If the stutterer realizes that his speech may excuse him from social situations he does not enjoy, from running errands when he prefers to be otherwise occupied, or from preparing for daily recitations because he is not called on in school, he will be in a position to weigh the advantages as well as the disadvantages of his speech defect and be prepared for further therapy. When the stutterer ceases to entertain and never uses stuttering as a ready-made alibi for what he might do, or might have been, except for his speech difficulty, then he has traveled a long way toward achieving the objectives of therapy.

TREATMENT FOR THE FAMILY

Often the parents of the stutterer are in need of counseling if the stutterer is to obtain maximum help from therapy. Earlier we indicated that the stutterer's parental attitudes are frequently characterized by high aspiration, rigidity, and unconscious rejection of the child. If the study of the familial picture shows this to be the case for the individual stutterer, appropriate treatment should be undertaken. Our experience indicates that parental resistance to treatment must be anticipated. Often parents want and expect their children to improve without their active participation in a therapy program. Parents must be made to realize that their participation is essential. The aims of therapy for parents are to give them an understanding about the problem of stuttering in general, their child's stuttering in particular, the relationship of their evaluations and attitudes toward their child's speech, and to reduce their own anxieties and possible guilt feelings about their child's speech difficulty. Parents must be helped to appreciate that stuttering does not disappear all at once. Frequently, in fact, speech becomes apparently worse rather than better in the early stages of treatment.

SPEECH GOALS

The stutterer, as well as his parents, must accept the virtual certainty that stuttering will not stop with the beginning of therapy. The immediate objective for the stutterer is to encourage him to speak more rather than less despite his speech difficulty. While speaking more, the stutterer needs to be helped to take an objective view of his difficulty so that the following intermediate objectives may be attained:

1. A weakening of the forces and pressures with which his stuttering is associated.
2. Elimination of the secondary, accessory symptoms of stuttering.
3. Modification of the form of stuttering so that relatively easy, effortless disfluencies replace the specific blocks, marked hesitations, strained prolongations, or repetitions.
4. Modification of the faulty habits directly associated with speaking such as improper breathing, rapid speaking, or excessive tensions of the speech mechanism.
5. Modification of the attitudes of fear, anxiety, or avoidance associated with the need for speaking or that occur after speech is initiated.

THERAPEUTIC APPROACHES FOR SYMPTOM MODIFICATION AND CONTROL: THE ROLE OF THE SPEECH CLINICIAN

Some of the objectives of an overall therapeutic program for stutterers, regardless of the possible etiology for the individual stutterer's difficulty, should include modification with an ultimate hope of elimination of the major speech symptoms manifested by the stutterer. Although the rationale for the use of the specific approach may vary considerably with the theorist or the clinician, a number of approaches are widely used with a considerable degree of success. We shall review those we have used and which have wide application.

Negative Practice. We have previously referred to the principle of negative practice, an approach in which an individual learns to control a habit he would like to discard by practicing intentionally and purposefully that very habit. For a stutterer this would mean that the clinician will direct him to become aware of his manner of stuttering and to practice one or more of the features of the manner. Thus a stutterer will practice his blocks by imitating his own particular way of blocking. When he learns this technique of self-imitation, he will then be helped to modify his blocks through one or the other approaches we will discuss. Through the technique of negative practice the stutterer is helped to undo by consciously doing what he presumably prefers not to do. This approach may be employed to overcome facial or bodily tics, faulty breathing, or any other mannerism which characterizes the speech behavior of the individual stutterer.

Voluntary Stuttering. This approach in effect helps the stutterer to learn a new, easier way of stuttering so that he can get on with the business of saying what he has to say with a minimum of blocking or spasm. One technique is to direct the stutterer *voluntarily to repeat* the first sound or the first syllable of each word. At first the stutterer may repeat the sound or syllable two or three times, or as many times as he feels necessary before he can complete the rest of the word. The repetitions should be easy and "nonsticky." The stutterer usually finds it easier to engage in voluntary repetition in material he reads aloud while observing himself in a mirror. With practice, the number of repetitions are reduced to the minimum needed by the stutterer to enable him to feel prepared to move along and to finish his utterance. Finally, the stutterer reduces the repetitions to the sounds of the words on which he anticipates he may block. We usually proceed with the stutterer from reading to paraphrasing and then to a conversation that incorporates the words that carried the key ideas in material previously read. Ultimately, the technique of voluntary repetition is applied in free conversation. This technique is particularly useful in group sessions in which stutterers observe how successful the members of their group are in their efforts at voluntary, easy repetition. A good repetition (easy and "nonsticky") is given a positive value; an involuntary repetition earns a minus score.

Prolongation or the intentional *lengthening* of initial sounds that are capable of being lengthened (vowels, diphthongs, and continuant consonants) is another approach to voluntary stuttering. The lengthened sound must be produced in an easy, relaxed manner. The stutterer must use the lengthened sound production as a preparatory set to move into the next sound and so to complete his utterance. The modifications from reading to free speaking may follow the sequence suggested for voluntary repetition.

Easy Articulation. Though clarity of diction may suffer somewhat, many stutterers find it helpful to learn a relatively lax, "nonsticky" manner of articulation. This is especially helpful in the production of stop-plosive sounds. With reduced articulatory tension it may become possible for some stutterers to move from sound to sound without abrupt pauses that suggest mild spasms.

Articulatory Pantomiming. Some stutterers need to be convinced that there are no real difficult sounds but only "bogey sounds" that the individual has somehow come to believe are difficult for him. For such stutterers, initial pantomiming of words or phrases—going through the articulatory activity without uttering the words aloud—may be of considerable help. After pantomiming, the stutterer is directed to add voice and to speak (read or engage in free conversation) what had previously been pantomimed. In the second phase, ease of articulation and moving through the utterance are stressed.

Fake Stuttering. A useful group technique is to have a stutterer imitate a speech feature of another stutterer. Many can do this with considerable success. For those who can, a feeling of control is achieved. Such control may then be used to imitate speech free or relatively free of stuttering mannerisms.

Behavior Modification

A recent approach that has been used with considerable success in the treatment of secondary stutterers is behavior modification or conditioning (reconditioning) therapy. This approach is based on the assumption that behavior, including stuttering, can be explained and modified by the appropriate application of learning principles (Shames and Sherrick, 1963, and Wolpe, 1969a, and 1969b). Wolpe assumes that, regardless of the causes for the onset of stuttering, the stutterer eventually develops a neurotic anxiety about his speech. This anxiety maintains stuttering, and thus must be treated. Specific techniques for the modification of anxiety include encouraging the patient to talk about his feelings, and so reducing their strength. Relaxation based on Jacobson's *Progressive Relaxation* is taught to the stutterer and he is "trained" to assume the posture and recognize the feelings of relaxation. When he shows evidence of tension associated with anxiety, the stutterer is trained to relax voluntarily, so that relaxation replaces the tension state. In effect, the awareness of tension cues a state of relaxation. The stutterer is asked to list anxiety-producing (stuttering-producing) situations in order of severity (hierarchies) for him. Each state is then a subject of therapy.

> When relaxation has become adequate and when the hierarchies are ready, one begins the central procedure, which is to present the weakest scene from a hierarchy to the *imagination* of the deeply relaxed patient for a few seconds, repeating presentations until the imagined item no longer evokes any anxiety at all. At each presentation the weak anxiety evoked by the scene is to some extent inhibited by the relaxation so that at the next presentation its evocation is weaker still, until it is eventually zero. The therapist then proceeds to the next scene, and so on, until the whole anxiety has been dealt with. (Wolpe, 1969a, page 19).

Wolpe observes that almost always there is complete transfer of the anxiety from the imagined situation to the corresponding real-life situation as reported by the patient.

A variety of behavior therapy techniques are based on the general approaches outlined above. Several of these are presented in the monograph by Gray and England (1969). Another behavior therapy approach, more elaborate than the one that we have described, is presented in detail by Brutten and Shoemaker (1967). Most behavior therapists report good success in the modification of stuttering symptoms after relatively few sessions as compared with other approaches. Perhaps the success is related to the readiness of the stutterers to do whatever they need to do to put an end to or at least to reduce the overt symptoms of stuttering. Behavior modification approaches require considerable training for the clinician, however, and we recommend that they not be undertaken without such training.

ULTIMATE OBJECTIVES FOR THE STUTTERER

We should like to be able to recommend that a legitimate, ultimate objective for each secondary stutterer is the establishment of normal speech and a well-adjusted personality. Such a recommended objective, however, cannot be made in the light of our experience with many stutterers. Perhaps a more reasonable and more moderate objective may be speech that is relatively free of the more severe characteristics of stuttering, and a relatively normal adjustment. We should not expect a stutterer, not even one who is having psychotherapy, to become better adjusted than most of his peers because most of his peers have some traits that can stand improvement.

Many stutterers are able to free themselves of most significant aberrant speech symptoms. Some, however, continue to have excessive disfluencies under conditions of fatigue, ill health, or stress. For some, also, it is possible that disfluencies are likely to persist on a constitutional basis. For these, the acceptance of disfluency without accompanying apprehension and struggle behaviour may be all that can be achieved. If this attitude can be established, the characteristics of stuttering that generate from anxiety and apprehension are removed and the overall occurrence of abnormal disfluencies is, therefore, reduced.

THE ROLE OF THE CLASSROOM TEACHER

The task of helping the secondary stutterer toward better speech and the improvement of his adjustment problems are, as we have indicated, primarily for the speech clinician and not for the classroom teacher. There are, however, a number of ways the classroom teacher can be of appreciable help to the stutterer in his improvement program.

The teacher should make note of the class situations that appear to be conducive to stuttering. Unless the child volunteers, he should not be called upon to speak in these situations. If he does speak, the stutterer should not be stopped regardless of the severity of his difficulty. If at all possible, however, the stutterer should be called upon for short replies rather than for ones that require lengthy explanations.

If many children are to be called on during a recitation period, the teacher should call upon the stutterer early. Waiting induces anxiety and anxiety an increase in stuttering. The stutterer should know that participation is expected, but that he will not have to wait anxiously for the moment of active participation.

The teacher should also note the conditions or situations when the stutterer is likely to have least difficulty with speaking and call upon him when these situations are present. For example, if a stutterer can recite memorized poetry without difficulty, he should be given an opportunity to recite. If he can read aloud much better than he can recite impromptu, he should be called upon to read aloud.

The teacher can get considerable information from the stutterer as to both easy and difficult speech situations. In most instances, an understanding can be reached with the stutterer as to his participation in class recitations. We recommend a basic principle to be followed in regard to oral recitations: If the stutterer is exempt from any oral activity, he must compensate by some other form of activity. This may call for additional written work done at home, or for board work done in class. Exemption without compensation gives stuttering a positive value that may be difficult to surrender. The teacher should not become a partner to the creation of gains to be derived from stuttering; neither, of course, should the teacher become part of any classroom attitude that inflicts punishment on the stutterer because of his stuttering.

The teacher should try to reward the stutterer for his fluent speech, but to do so without readily apparent fuss. "Very good, Johnny" is much better than a lengthy response of praise because Johnny has been fluent. If the teacher looks pleased, Johnny is likely to get the idea even without a verbalization of the pleasure. There is a very real danger that a remark intended as a verbal reward may actually backfire and become an implied penalty. For example, "You spoke very well, Johnny" may be interpreted to mean that in most instances Johnny does not speak well, hence the need to point out the occasions when speech is good. As a general procedure, the teacher should try to avoid directing attention to good speech as well as to poor speech. The nature and form of the reward should depend upon the intellectual and emotional maturity of the child. Rewards should be given for good speech as for any other worthwhile performance. They should come quickly and inconspicuously.

The teacher should help to create a classroom atmosphere that will encourage the stutterer to talk. Such an atmosphere exists when any child, whether he stutters, has no defect in speech, or has some form of defective speech other than stuttering, feels free to volunteer to speak without fear of penalty or criticism. It may help to explain to the stutterer's classmates, *at a time when the stutterer is out of the classroom*, how they can be of help. Nothing said to the classmates should suggest that the stutterer is in need of pity or excessive sympathy. Instead, the teacher should emphasize that what the stutterer needs is a group of patient listeners when he talks and opportunities to talk. If the stutterer is excused from any recitations, his classmates should be informed that he is doing other work to make up for it. In this way the classmates will not feel resentful that the stutterer is a privileged member of the group. Rather they will feel that he is a member of their group who has a problem that all are helping to solve by their understanding.

Luper and Mulder (1964, Chap. 8) sum up approaches for the treatment of the stuttering child in a school setting, with special emphasis on the interrelated roles of the speech clinician and the classroom teacher.

Cluttering

Cluttering is usually included among disorders of rhythm and fluency. By some authorities (Weiss, 1964), it is considered a forerunner of stuttering. Yet were cluttering to be designated as an articulatory disorder, or as a language disorder, it would be so based upon verifiable observation. A description of cluttering should indicate why all of these designations might well be correct and why, therefore, it deserves its own classification. We are discussing cluttering at this point in our considerations because of its superficial resemblance to stuttering, from which, nevertheless, it needs to be differentially identified.

Superficially, cluttered speech suggests a torrent of words, poorly or partially articulated, with repetitions of monosyllabic words and first syllables of longer words. It is a "hot potato in the mouth" speech, with morphemes falling where they may. Cluttered speech spurts rather than flows, then stops and spurts again. Behind the speech is the clutterer who, unlike the stutterer at any stage, seems unaware of his perpetrations. Objectively, we may characterize cluttering as repetitious, poorly articulated utterance produced at a rate incompatible with the speaker's ability to speak intelligibly. Part of the lack of intelligibility is the clutterer's loose and poorly organized phrase and sentence structure. These last features make it difficult for a listener to anticipate and so comprehend or guess what the speaker is trying to say. Weiss (1964, p. 24) believes that the clutterer may well be at a loss for the words to express his thoughts. "Because the clutterer is inept at finding the necessary words to express his ideas, his speech is studded with clichés and repetitions of words and phrases." We accept this position, with emphasis on the notion that the clutterer does not really have more than a vague idea of what he wants to say, along with an apparent compulsion to say it.

When the clutterer slows down, both articulation and intelligibility improve. Perhaps when he speaks slowly, at a rate compatible with his neuromuscular system when it operates efficiently, the clutterer also gives himself time to think and to formulate his utterance.

BACKGROUND HISTORY OF CLUTTERERS

Clutterers often present a history suggestive of minimal brain disfunction and minimal brain damage (see Chapter 16). Weiss (1944, p. 51) reports a familial history of speech disorders other than but also including cluttering, especially on the paternal side. He views it, as do we, as a *central language imbalance* (*disorder*) which includes such features as delayed language onset, retarded language development, delayed articulatory proficiency, and vocal monotony. We would add to these characteristics slow development of vocabulary and of syntax. As they grow older, clutterers are likely to have reading and writing difficulties, the latter both for legibility and sentence structure. Behaviorally, and motorically, the clutterer is likely to show impulsiveness, late laterality development, and ambi-nondexterity. The clutterer gives the impression of being a loosely assembled person, awkward, and imprecise.

DIFFERENTIAL DIAGNOSIS: STUTTERING AND CLUTTERING

Most stutterers tend to speak better when relaxed and when paying minimal attention to their articulation. In contrast, clutterers tend to improve when they direct conscious attention to their utterance. Stutterers, especially in later stages, show apprehension and anxiety about their speech, and tend to have difficulties that are directly related to their apprehensions. Clutterers, as we indicated, show a benign unawareness about their speech. With awareness, they tend to improve. Finally, the marked difficulties of clutterers in all language functions, written as well as spoken, distinguish them from most stutterers. Thus, though there is some evidence that stuttering has a familial, constitutional basis, the evidence of such etiology for the clutterer is clear.

CLUTTERING AS A TRANSITIONAL STAGE TO STUTTERING

Whether cluttering is a transitional stage, an early stage in the progression toward stuttering, is a moot point. It is possible that when some clutterers are directed to attend to their speech, they may develop anxieties and frustrations growing out of the awarenesses, and begin to speak like stutterers. Van Riper (1963, p. 326) observes "There are clutterers who do not stutter, stutterers who do not clutter, some stutterers who have cluttered, and some who still do." Thus, though some stutterers may begin as clutterers, most do not show the early characteristics that we have described. However, we have known families that included both stuttering and cluttering siblings and a cluttering father. We have also known individuals who shifted periodically between cluttering and stuttering.

THERAPY

The treatment for clutterers is implied in the differential diagnosis. Clutterers do tend to improve when they slow down and "mind their speech." They also tend to improve by being urged to formulate, to think through in words, before they begin to speak. Unfortunately, in conversational give-and-take we cannot ordinarily preformulate our utterances. Most of us have to learn to *talk as we think*. The best we can do for clutterers is to remind them to slow down, and cue them when their speech begins to accelerate, and becomes unintelligible. These external controls, must with practice become habitual. The clutterer must therefore be taught to observe his listeners for indications that he is talking too rapidly and failing to make himself understood. Rewards in the form of verbal and facial approval by the teacher, the clinician, and the family members when the clutterer does "mind his speech" should reinforce such behavior. Practice in making short announcements before the class, and in therapy sessions with the speech (language) clinician are of help. Finally, we wish to re-emphasize that the clutterer's primary problem is with language. He needs help in verbal expression, both oral and written. He needs, to begin with, to learn to make simple statements simply. He needs to learn to become a slow and considered speaker. Perhaps, if he achieves this, he will enjoy his reputation and maintain it.

References and Recommended Readings

ANDREWS, S. G., and M. HARRIS, "Stammering." in *The Child Who Does Not Talk*, C. Renfrew, and K. Murphy, eds., The Spastics Society Medical Education Association. W. Heinemann Medical Books, London, 1964.

BERRY, M. F., "Twinning in Stuttering Families," *Human Biology*, IX, 3 (1939) 329–346.

BLOODSTEIN, O., "A Rating Scale of Conditions Under Which Stuttering Is Reduced," *Journal of Speech and Hearing Disorders*, XV (February, 1950), 29–36.

———, "The Development of Stuttering: II. Developmental Phases," *Journal of Speech and Hearing Disorders*, XXV (November 1960), 366–376.

BLUEMEL, C. S., *The Riddle of Stuttering*. Danville, Illinois, Interstate Publishing Company, 1957.

BROWN, S. F., "The Loci of Stuttering in Speech Sounds," *Journal of Speech Disorders*, X (May 1945), 181–192.

BRUTTEN, E. J., and D. J. SHOEMAKER, *The Modification of Stuttering*. Englewood Cliffs, N.J., Prentice-Hall, Inc., 1967.

CORIAT, I. H., "The Psychoanalytic Conception of Stuttering," *The Nervous Child*, II (1943), 167–171.

CURRY, F. K. W., and H. H. GREGORY, "The Performance of Stutterers on Dichotic Listening Tasks Thought to Reflect Cerebral Dominance," *Journal of Speech and Hearing Research*, XII (March 1969), 73–82.

EISENSON, J., ed., *Stuttering: A Symposium.* New York, Harper & Row, Publishers, 1958. (Six points of view are presented on the nature of stuttering with suggested therapies generally consistent with the theoretic positions. The contributors are O. Bloodstein, J. Eisenson, I. P. Glauber, J. Sheehan, C. Van Riper, and R. West.)

EISENSON, J., "Observations of the Incidence of Stuttering in a Special Culture," *ASHA*, VIII, 10 (1966), 391–394.

EISENSON, J., and E. HOROWITZ, "The Influence of Propositionality on Stuttering," *Journal of Speech Disorders*, X (March 1945), 193–198.

EISENSON, J., and C. WELLS, "A Study of the Influence of Communicative Responsibility in a Choral-Speaking Situation for Stutterers," *Journal of Speech Disorders*, VII (1942), 259–262.

GLAUBER, I. P., in J. EISENSON, ed., "The Psychoanalysis of Stuttering," in *Stuttering: A Symposium.* New York, Harper & Row, Publishers, 1958, pp. 73–119.

GOLDMAN-EISLER, F., "Hesitation, Information, and Levels of Speech Production," in A. V. DeReuck and M. O'Connor, eds., *Disorders of Language.* Ciba Foundation, 1964.

GRAY, B. B., and G. ENGLAND, eds., *Stuttering and the Conditioning Therapies.* Monterey, California, The Monterey Institute for Speech and Hearing, 1969.

GREGORY, H. H., *Learning Theory and Stuttering Therapy.* Evanston, Illinois, Northwestern University Press, 1968.

JOHNSON, W., *Stuttering and What You Can Do About It.* Minneapolis, University of Minnesota Press, 1961. (The author explains in relatively simple language the implications of research findings conducted under his supervision. He emphasizes the normality of the stutterer and his early speech.)

JOHNSON, W., in W. JOHNSON, et al., *Speech-Handicapped School Children,* 3rd ed. New York, Harper & Row, Publishers, 1967.

JOHNSON, W., F. L. DARLEY, and D. C. SPRIESTERSBACH, *Diagnostic Methods in Speech Pathology.* New York, Harper & Row, Publishers, 1963.

KIMURA, D., "Functional Asymmetry of the Brain in Dichotic Listening," *Cortex*, III (1967), 163–178.

LANYON, R. I., "Speech: Relation of Nonfluency to Information Value," *Science*, 164 (April 3, 1969), 451–452.

LUPER, H. L., and R. L. MULDER, *Stuttering Therapy for Children.* Englewood Cliffs, N.J., Prentice-Hall Inc., 1964. (This book is addressed to public school speech clinicians and emphasizes therapeutic approaches for stuttering children which the authors have found to be practical, operational, and effective.)

McDEARMON, J. R., "Primary Stuttering at the Onset of Stuttering: A Reexamination of Data," *Journal of Speech and Hearing Research*, XI, (September 1968), 631–637.

MURPHY, A. T., and R. M. FITZSIMONS, *Stuttering and Personality Dynamics.* New York, The Ronald Press Company, 1960.

NELSON, S. E., "The Role of Heredity in Stuttering," *Journal of Pediatrics*, XIV (1939), 642–654.

ORTON, S., *Reading, Writing and Speech Problems*. New York, W. W. Norton & Company, Inc., 1937. (A pioneer but still highly relevant consideration of organic factors underlying language disorders.)

PERRIN, K., *An Examination of Ear Preference for Speech and Non-Speech in a Stuttering Population*. Ph.D. dissertation, Stanford University, 1969.

SHAMES, G., and C. E. SHERRICK, "A Discussion of Non-Fluency and Stuttering as Operant Behavior," *Journal of Speech and Hearing Disorders*, XXVIII (February 1963), 3–18.

SHEEHAN, J., "Conflict Theory of Stuttering," in J. Eisenson, ed., *Stuttering: A Symposium*. New York, Harper & Row, Publishers, 1958, pp. 121–166.

TRAVIS, L. E., "My Present Thinking on Stuttering," *Western Speech*, X (1946), 3–5.

TRAVIS, L. E., "The Unspeakable Feelings of People with Special Reference to Stuttering," in L. E. Travis, ed., *Handbook on Speech Pathology*. New York, Appleton-Century-Crofts, 1957, pp. 916–946.

VAN RIPER, C., *Speech Correction*, 4th ed. Englewood Cliffs, N.J., Prentice-Hall, Inc., 1963. (Chapters 11 and 12 present Van Riper's views on the nature, causes, and treatment of stuttering. The writing is sensitive, and the positions taken are highly practical. Strongly recommended for teachers and clinicians.)

WEISS, D. A., "Therapy for Cluttering," *Folia Phoniatrica*, XII (1960), 216–228.

———, *Cluttering*. Englewood Cliffs, N.J., Prentice-Hall, Inc., 1964.

WINGATE, M. E., "Evaluation and Stuttering, Part I: Speech Characteristics of Young Children," *Journal of Speech and Hearing Disorders*, XXVI (May 1962), 106–115.

WISCHNER, G. J., "Stuttering Behavior and Learning: A Preliminary Theoretic Formulation," *Journal of Speech and Hearing Disorders*, XII (December 1950), 324–335.

WOLPE, J., "Behavior Therapy of Stuttering: Deconditioning the Emotional Factor," in B. G. Gray, and G. England, *Stuttering and the Conditioning Therapies*. Monterey, California, The Monterey Institute for Speech and Hearing, 1969 (a).

———, *The Practice of Behavior Therapy*. New York, Pergamon Press, 1969 (b).

Problems

1. Define stuttering. Distinguish between primary and secondary stuttering.
2. What is meant by normal hesitation phenomena?
3. Observe two or three speakers in a conversation. Note evidence of normal hesitation phenomena. How does this differ from stuttering?
4. According to Van Riper, what is the difference between so-called normal disfluencies and primary stuttering?

5. What is the difference between a nonstutterer's "Well, well . . ." and a stutterer's postponement devices?
6. Briefly describe Bloodstein's phases of stuttering and Van Riper's stages of stuttering. How are they the same? How different?
7. Talk to two or three stutterers about their feared word or speaking situations. Are there any common factors?
8. Outline your own theory about the onset of stuttering.
9. Read Joseph Sheehan's essay on stuttering in Eisenson, ed., *Stuttering: A Symposium*. Why does Sheehan regard stuttering as a learned form of behavior? What does Sheehan mean by his observation that stuttering is essentially an expression of an approach-avoidance conflict?
10. What is the evidence to support the position that stuttering is a manifestation of constitutional predisposition?
11. What is the evidence that the predisposition to stuttering may be inherited? What is a predisposition?
12. Read Wendell Johnson's position on stuttering in *Speech-Handicapped School Children*. How does Johnson explain the evidence of the heredity of stuttering on a nongenetic basis?
13. Which of the positions on stuttering presented in this text best reconciles the therapeutic approaches with the onset causes?
14. Suppose a four- or five-year-old child is sent to you by a parent with the complaint that he is a stutterer. How would you go about determining whether the child has "normal disfluencies" or is *normally* expressing normal hesitations and repetitions? What would you tell the parent?
15. Why do most stutterers have less difficulty in reciting memorized material than in explaining or paraphrasing it?
16. What is meant by "secondary gains?" What are some possible secondary gains, other than those mentioned in this chapter, that stutterers may entertain? How would you deal with them?
17. What is conditioning? What is deconditioning? How do they relate to therapy for stutterers?
18. What is meant by "desensitization" for stutterers? Can you give any examples of how you or a friend were desensitized against an anxiety- or fear-producing situation?
19. Why should the treatment of a primary stutterer be directed toward the parent? Outline such treatment.
20. What is meant by "negative practice?" How does this relate to stuttering therapy?
21. Distinguish between cluttering and stuttering.
22. How is the treatment of a young clutterer different from that of a primary stutterer? Of an adult clutterer and a secondary stutterer?

Chapter 14

Speech and Impaired Hearing

It is a rare teacher who has not had some experience with a child with impaired hearing. Most observant teachers may have wondered why some child who earnestly looks as if he is listening, nevertheless fails to understand even a simple direction unless it is accompanied by a gesture, or by some visual material. Little Mary may return to school after a short absence with the residual of a cold, and her ears still feel "stopped up," but the same little girl may continue to have some difficulty in understanding her teacher when the teacher's back is turned, or when the teacher is talking from some place other than the front of the room. If this problem is chronic, there is a fair likelihood that our Mary or our Tom may have a slight hearing loss which becomes aggravated in the event of a cold. The alert and observant teacher should recommend that the child be seen by a school nurse or school physician, if either is available, and confer with the child's family about an examination of the child's hearing by their own physician or by an otolaryngologist or an otologist, medical specialists who are concerned with problems of hearing.

Any teacher who has taught 100 or more different children is likely to have had at least one with some degree of impaired hearing. In some instances the child's articulation was also defective, and perhaps even the extent of his vocabulary and his competence for producing conventional syntactical sentences. Generally, the degree of the hearing impairment will be related to the presence and severity of the speech problems. A child may produce voice that is either lacking in adequate loudness or, less frequently, overloud. Conductive losses, which we will discuss later, are associated with inadequate loudness. In contrast, a nerve (sensorineural) loss is associated with an overloud voice.* We shall expand later on the types of speech problems associated with impaired hearing. First, however, we shall consider briefly some aspects of sound and the reception and perception of speech sound by the hearing mechanism.

Sound and the Speech Range

Sound for our purposes may be considered the result of energy applied to a body capable of vibration in a manner that produces waves (disturbances of air) at a rate and in a manner that makes them perceptible to the human ear. Normal, young persons can hear sounds between 20 to 20,000 cycles per second (cps).† Older persons, those above age 30 or 40, tend to lose hearing in the upper ranges, above 8,000 or 10,000 cps. However, since most of the sounds of speech lie within the range 250–4,000 cps, adults of "middle age" suffer no impairment of hearing for speech.

The decibel or dB is the unit of intensity of sound. Very simply stated, intensity varies directly as the amount of energy applied to the body capable of vibration. However, sounds of different pitch are discernible to us at different intensity levels. This, we believe, is related to the differences in the sensitivity of the endings of the auditory nerve in the cochlea of the inner ear. Thus, we may hear sounds within one part of our pitch range at a relatively low intensity, as compared with sounds within a different part of the pitch range which may be perceived (heard) only at higher intensity levels.

The Hearing Mechanism

THE EXTERNAL AND MIDDLE EAR

The external ear, or pinna, is part of the auditory mechanism which most of us refer to as the ear. Its function is, to a limited degree, to help us to gather in sound. Its function may be enhanced by using a hand to

---

* The relationship of voice disturbances to hearing was briefly considered in Chapter 12 on voice disturbances.

† The letters cps for cycles per second may also be represented by Hz or "Hertz." We prefer to use cps because the letters directly represent the concept of the unit of vibration.

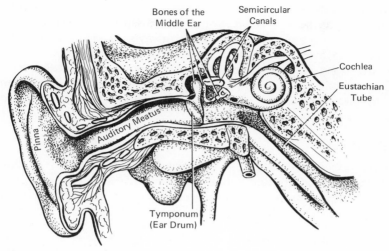

Figure 11. A sectional view of the ear.

cup over the ear. The pinna includes a skin-lined canal leading to the eardrum or tympanic membrane (see Figure 11).

The middle ear is a small cavity on the inner side of the eardrum. The inner ear includes three tiny bones, or ossicles: the malleus (hammer), the incus (anvil), and the stapes (stirrup). The named designations correspond to their resemblance to the objects (see Figure 12).

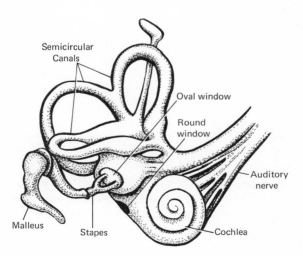

Figure 12. Enlarged representation of the middle and inner ear: the ossicles, cochlea, and semicircular canals.

The malleus is directly attached to the eardrum. The incus constitutes a connection or bridge between the malleus and the stapes. These ossicles are connected but normally *not rigidly fixed* to positions within the middle ear by attachments of ligament and tiny muscles. Thus the ossicles are able to move whenever the eardrum moves, as it does whenever it is stimulated by sound waves (air vibrations). The movements of the ossicles transmit the vibrations of the eardrum from the middle ear to the inner ear.

THE INNER EAR

The inner ear includes (a) the semicircular canals, (b) the cochlea, a snail-shaped structure that contains tiny hairlike structures of varying length, which are in fact the sensitive endings of the auditory nerve, and (c) the vestibule, a connecting area between the semicircular canals and the cochlea.

When air vibrations cause movements of the eardrum, the impulses are transmitted to the stapes which in turn produces movements of the fluid that fills the vestibule. These vestibular-fluid movements stimulate the nerve endings in the cochlea. The stimulations received from the auditory nerve endings are carried by way of the auditory (eighth cranial nerve) to the temporal area of the brain cortex, producing the experience we refer to as sound perception or hearing.*

Hearing Impairment

CLASSIFICATION AND INCIDENCE

Although "functional" definitions of hearing loss will be presented in this section, it is essential to appreciate that the effect of hearing loss is variable. In some instances, what might be regarded as a relatively small amount of hearing loss may be associated with greater impairment of hearing in particular and adjustment in general than a measurably greater amount of hearing loss for other persons. Even among persons born with severe hearing loss, some are able to make considerably better use of a small amount of residual hearing than others. With these reservations in mind, "practical" definitions will be offered.

The *deaf* are those for whom the sense of hearing is so impaired as to have precluded normal acquisition of language learning. Somewhat more broadly, the deaf are those for whom the capacity to hear is so limited as to be considered nonfunctioning for the ordinary purposes of life. Children who are deaf either (1) are not able to learn speech

---

* See the discussion of the speech mechanism in Chapter 5 for the function of the left temporal cortex in the analysis of speech sounds.

through the avenue of hearing; or (2) if their hearing impairment was acquired shortly after "natural" speech was learned, have lost their speaking ability or have become severely impaired in it.

The deaf may be divided into two subgroups according to onset of impairment. The *congenitally deaf* are those who are born without hearing. The *adventitiously deaf* are those who were born with hearing sufficient for the acquisition of speech but later, as a result of illness or accident, suffered severe hearing impairment.

The *hard of hearing* are those for whom the sense of hearing, although defective, is functional with or without a hearing aid. Hard-of-hearing children, although frequently with considerable defects, learned to speak essentially through the avenue of hearing.

Davis and Silverman (1960, pp. 453–454), classify hard-of-hearing children into four groups, based on their average reception for speech. Such reception is usually estimated accurately by averaging the hearing levels for pure tones at 500, 1,000, and 2,000 cps. Class (1) includes those with less than 30-decibel loss for speech; class (2) includes those with hearing levels for speech between 30 and 45 decibels; class (3) includes those with hearing levels between 45 and 60 decibels; class (4) includes those with hearing levels between 60 and 80 decibels. Loss beyond these levels would designate the child as profoundly deaf.

The practical and fundamental criterion for the distinction between the deaf and the hard-of-hearing is *in the manner in which* the child acquires speech. The deaf then include those who require specialized instruction to learn to talk, or to acquire a substitute (visual) system for the normal oral/aural system. The hard-of-hearing are those who learned to speak essentially in the normal developmental manner of hearing children.

Most deaf children are educated in special schools, and many in residential schools. Most hard-of-hearing children are educated in "regular" schools and usually attend classes with hearing children.

INCIDENCE

Estimates of the incidence of impaired hearing in the school-age population vary from about 5 to 10 per cent. Glorig (1959) reports that 3 per cent of a male population between the ages of 10 and 19 were found to have a hearing loss of 15 decibels or more. This figure is based on a sample of approximately 400,000. Davis and Silverman (1960, p. 416) recognize that there is considerable variability in estimates of hearing loss. They say, "Our best estimate is that 5 per cent of school-age children have hearing levels outside the range of normal . . . and that from one to two of every ten in this group require special educational attention."

The 1969 report of the Subcommittee on Human Communication and Its Disorders to the National Institute of Neurological Diseases and Stroke (1969, p. 15) include an estimate of hearing loss in the United States. According to the report, about 250,000 children of school age have hearing losses of sufficient severity to impair their communication ability and their social efficiency. Approximately 40,000 are deaf.

TYPES OF HEARING LOSS AND RELATED SPEECH IMPAIRMENTS

Conductive Loss is associated with external or middle ear abnormalities that impede the transmission of energy (vibratory energy producing sound) to the middle ear. Abnormalities may include an accumulation of hardened wax (cerumen), the presence of a foreign body, and structural malformations such as an incomplete canal, or an exceedingly narrow ear canal. The external ear may be inflamed by disease processes that may affect other skin surfaces. Except for the structural abnormalities, the resultant hearing loss is likely to be temporary, that is, lasting only as long as the abnormal condition persists.

Middle ear involvements include conditions that impair the vibratory-transmissive functions of the ossicles, infections of the middle ear, which are often associated with upper respiratory disease (the common cold), or excessive fluid, often associated with inflammation in the middle ear, and enlarged adenoidal tissue growth in the area of the nasopharynx.

Because most conductive losses are the result, fortunately, of temporary pathologies, most children with such impairments are likely to have normal speech. Chronic involvements may be associated with an inadequately loud voice. This, as we suggested earlier, may be the result of the child's hearing his own voice louder than he is able to hear the voices of other speakers. He assumes, therefore, that he is speaking loudly enough to be heard, even though he may barely be audible to others. This interesting phenomenon takes place because the child with conductive loss hears himself through the vibrations produced by his vocalization by way of the bones of his head. If his inner ear is normal, the nerve endings will respond to these vibrations. However, the child's hearing of himself is not modified by the vibrations that normally would also come to him through air vibration by way of his external and middle ears. The child with conductive loss also hears the voices of others as less loud than they sound to normal ears.

Denasality is also likely to characterize the voice and the nasal consonant sound production of the child with respiratory infections or with enlarged adenoids. Speech, as far as articulation in general is concerned, is likely to be unaffected in children with conductive loss of hearing.

Sensorineural Hearing Loss. This results from involvements of the inner ear or those of the eighth (auditory) nerve. Reception and perception (discrimination) of sound is impaired. Such losses, especially if they are congenital or had their onset before speech was acquired, are associated with vocal, articulatory, and linguistic defects. If the nerve involvement is severe, the child may make little or no sense out of the speech to which he is exposed because he will have difficulty in the analysis of the complex sounds that constitute speech. Usually, high-pitched sounds, including those that comprise most of the consonants of speech, are within the range of impaired hearing. Voice and vowel sounds, if produced with sufficient loudness, are usually heard and perceived. The child may speak excessively loudly in order to hear himself, may produce vowels acceptably but have difficulty with consonants, especially the high-frequency sibilants and the velar plosives, which are not readily visible. He may confuse voiced and voiceless cognate sounds. If the child's impairment is severe and he cannot readily hear functional words (prepositions, conjunctions, articles)—which normally are not given much emphasis in running speech—or grammatical markers (plurals, tense endings), his verbal productions may also be characterized as ungrammatical or agrammatical. He will, therefore, be linguistically deficient.

Some bright children who are apt in visual speech (lip) reading, which they may learn without direct teaching, may have good comprehension of speech, and may themselves have fairly good articulation. Children not apt in visual reading may have severe difficulty in comprehending speech. With the usual reservation for the exceptional child, the severity of speech and language impairment is generally directly related to the severity of the sensorineural loss.

Mixed Hearing Loss. This combines the impairments of conductive and nerve loss. The cause is the existence of both conductive (transmissive) and sensorineural pathology. In effect, the child with such combined pathology will have difficulty in receiving a sound signal as well as difficulty in analyzing (perceiving) those signals that—however weakly —are received. Unless the conductive condition is chronic, the speech characteristics of the child will be related to the factors associated with sensorineural loss.

MEASUREMENT OF HEARING LOSS

Hearing loss is objectively measured in terms of decibels. A decibel is a unit of power or physical intensity. From out point of view, we may consider a decibel the minimum unit of intensity necessary for us to appreciate a difference between the loudness of sounds.

The pure-tone audiometer is widely used as an objective instrument for measuring possible hearing loss. The pure-tone audiometer is an electrical instrument designed to produce a number of tones of discrete or individual frequencies at intensity levels that can be controlled. Most modern pure-tone audiometers cover the frequency range between approximately 125 and 12,000 cycles (Hz) per second. Many audiologists in their examinations, however, do not consider it necessary to go beyond 8,000 cycles. On a pure-tone audiometer the weakest sound that can normally be heard is considered as zero decibels.

Losses are measured in terms of the normal threshold of hearing for tones at specified pitch levels and are stated in decibels. The following tables suggest how we would evaluate the results of a pure-tone audiometric examination. We should always bear in mind, however, that many factors other than the "objective" amount of hearing loss enter into the effect of the loss for the given individual.

Proposed Classes of Hearing Handicap*

Average Hearing Level (American Standard) for 500, 1000 and 2000 cps in the Better Ear**

dB	Class	Degree of Handicap	At Least—	But Less Than—	Ability to Understand Speech	
0						American zero (A.S.A. standard)
	A	Not significant		15 dB	No significant difficulty with faint speech.	
15						"Low fence"
30	B	Slight	15 dB	30 dB	Difficulty only with faint speech.	
45	C	Mild	30 dB	45 dB	Frequent difficulty with normal speech.	
	D	Marked	45 dB	60 dB	Frequent difficulty with loud speech.	
60						Educational deafness
	E	Severe	60 dB	80 dB	Can understand only shouted or amplified speech.	
80						"High fence"
	F	Extreme	80 dB		Usually cannot understand even amplified speech.	

* Eagles, Hardy and Catlin (1968). This table is based on the recommended classification of the American Academy of Opthalamology and Otolaryngology. The term "low fence" refers to the exclusion of "minor deviations and is the point at which impairment is considered to be significant." The term "high fence implies that the impairment is functionally total. The range between the two "fences" is 64 dB wide.

** Whenever the average for the poorer ear is 25 dB or more greater than that of the better ear in this range, 5 dB are added to the average for the better ear.

We strongly recommend Newby's (1964, pp. 104–105) observation as to the need for assessing functional hearing as well as the results of pure-tone audiometry. Says Newby:

> Although the audiogram yields important information concerning the rehabilitative needs of patients, it is most valuable when the information it conveys is combined with the results of clinical speech audiometric tests, which measure directly a patient's ability to hear and understand speech. After all, the measure of the handicap of a hearing loss is how one's communicative ability is affected. Whereas predictions of how communication is affected can be made from the pure-tone audiogram with some certainty, actual measures of the communicative ability can be derived through speech audiometry.

IDENTIFICATION AUDIOMETRY

Identification audiometry is a term to signify the application of appropriate hearing test procedures leading to an initial discovery of a hearing loss.* In the ordinary school situations, a screening test rather than a complete audiometric examination is likely to be given as the first step in the evaluation of a child's hearing. An early and still widely used screening device is the fading-numbers test. A recorded voice is played back and listened to through earphones, either by a single child or by a group of children. The usual recording is of a sequence of numbers, which fade out at the end of the sequence. The results provide information *under the conditions of testing* about the intensity levels at or above which a selected speech sample—a sequence of numbers—can be heard. Unfortunately, as Newby (1964, p. 207) points out, a fading-numbers test is not an accurate indicator of a child's ability to hear normal running speech. The test does have a merit as a rough screening device that permits relatively quick assessment of the hearing of many children.

Another technique that permits screening of children on a group basis is the Massachusetts Hearing Test.† This is a pure-tone rather than a speech-hearing test which was devised to permit screening testing of as many as 40 children at one time at three critical frequencies within the range of normal speech. The usual frequencies tested are 500, 4,000, and 6,000 cycles. Each of these frequencies is presented at sensation

---

* See "Identification Audiometry," *Journal of Speech and Hearing Disorders,* Monograph Supplement, 9 (September, 1961) 9–20.

† This and other testing techniques specially suitable in the school situation are described in some detail in Chapter 8 of H. Newby's *Audiology* (New York, Appleton-Century-Crofts (1964). See also J. J. O'Neill, *The Hard of Hearing* (Englewood Cliffs, N.J., Prentice-Hall, Inc., 1964), Chapter 4.

(loudness) levels of 20, 25, and 30 decibels, respectively. Responses are ordinarily entered on a prepared test blank and consist of a "Yes" or "No" to indicate whether the child who is being examined does or does not hear the spurt of pure-tone sound produced by the test instrument. An audiometrist signals the individual child or children when the response to the sound is expected. According to a prearranged plan, the audiometrist may not always present a tone and signal for a response. Through this procedure some "No" responses are expected and such entries should appear on each test blank.

Another approach for screening employing pure-tone audiometry is the *sweep test*. This testing is done with a pure-tone audiometer, and results are obtained in a very few minutes. In sweep testing the dial is set at a critical point, with allowances made for the room and the "free-floating" noise in the surroundings. The most usual setting is 15 decibels. The examiner then "sweeps" through the frequency range. The child is instructed to signal whether or not he hears the tone produced at each frequency.

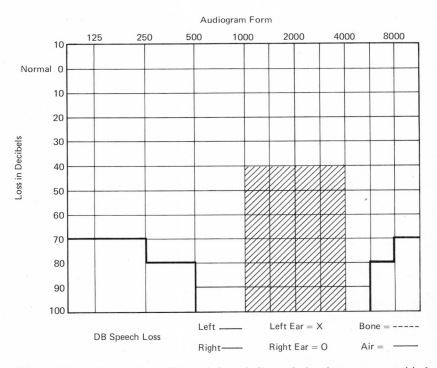

Figure 13. Audiogram Form. The shaded area indicates the hearing range most critical for the reception of speech.

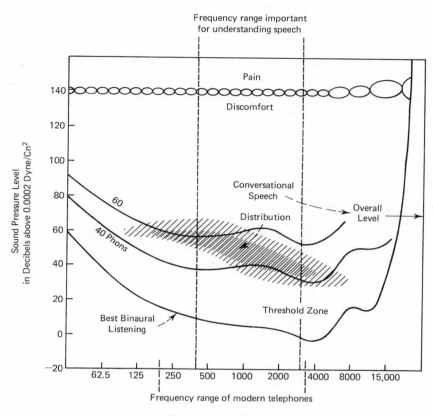

Figure 14. The Speech Area. Speech is a mixture of complex tones, wide band noise, and transients. Both the intensities and the frequencies of speech sounds change continually and rapidly. It is difficult to measure them and logically impossible to plot them precisely in terms of sound pressure levels.

A recent addition to screening tests utilizing standard audiometric equipment (pure-tone audiometry) and headsets is described by Hollien, Wepman, and Thompson (1969). Up to 40 children at a time can be screen-tested in about 15 minutes. This test can be administered by a classroom teacher, a school nurse, or any trained adult. The frequencies employed are 500, 1,000, and 4,000 cps (Hz); the hearing levels used are 35, 25, and 20 dB. ASA standards are used.

As the name suggests, screening tests have as their purpose the singling out of individuals who may have significant losses of hearing at the time of the testing. Final evaluations should include more thorough individual pure-tone testing as well as speech testing through speech audiometry. In addition, of course, an otological examination should be routine.

In many public schools the responsibility for discovering hearing loss among the children has become an integral part of the overall health conservation program. The development of this aspect of the detection and treatment of children's health needs has received considerable impetus from the availability of instruments and techniques for assessing hearing loss that can easily be used in school settings.

School hearing conservation programs have two fundamental purposes. The first is the earliest possible detection of hearing loss so that children, whenever possible, may be referred for medical treatment in the hope that in many instances permanent hearing impairment may be prevented. The second is to provide for the special needs— educational, speech, and audiological—of children whose hearing may not be directly subject to improvement but who can be helped to conserve and make maximum use of their hearing capacities.

Responsibility for the actual assessment of hearing loss varies considerably among school systems. Many large school districts conduct their own hearing testing and conservation programs. Some smaller school districts may contract for hearing services with professional agencies or audiology clinics associated with colleges or universities. In some school districts audiologists or audiometrists are engaged whose responsibilities include the assessment of the children's hearing throughout the grades.* In many schools, including those in which there are organized audiological services, the detection of possible hearing loss continues to be the responsibility of the classroom teacher or the school nurse. The nurse may note a child's difficulty in hearing in her routine examination of the children. The classroom teacher, however, has a daily opportunity to detect whether a child, habitually or occasionally, seems to have difficulty in hearing. The child who frequently misunderstands directions, or who asks that questions directed to him be repeated, or who looks blankly at the teacher talking to him or to the class should be checked for possible hearing loss. The teacher should also watch for the child who seems to hear only when spoken to from one side of the room but fails to hear what is said when spoken to from the opposite side. Some children unconsciously turn their heads to favor the better

---

* As of 1961, 28 state health departments employed one or more speech and hearing consultants as part of their programs ("Identification Autiometry," *Journal of Speech and Hearing Disorders*, Monograph Supplement 9 (September, 1961, p.6). In 35 states, departments of public instruction are charged with responsibility for health examinations, including hearing testing, for the children enrolled in the public schools (*ibid.*, p. 46).

ear. If these habits and manifestations are associated with poor articulation and with voice production inappropriate in quality and loudness, hearing loss should be suspected. Additional significant signs are poor coordination, poor balance, occasional dizziness, and complaints of earaches and of running ears. A child suspected of hearing loss should be referred to the school physician for further examination. If the school has no physician, the possibility of the child's hearing loss should be discussed with the principal and, of course, with the parents, and then referred to a physician.

Therapy for the Child with a Hearing Impairment

HEARING AIDS

Many children whose hearing losses range from moderate to severe are able to get considerable help from a properly fitted hearing aid. The decision whether a hearing aid is needed should be made by the otologist, a medical specialist. The actual fitting of the hearing aid may be done either by the otologist or a properly trained audiologist.* Although many individual factors enter into the usefulness of hearing aids, experience indicates that for children hearing aids are usually indicated when the hearing loss is between 35 and 70 decibels in the pitch range most important for speech. This range is roughly between 200 and 4,000 cycles (ASA standard). For children with more severe hearing losses, exceeding 70 decibels in the pitch range, the help to be derived from a hearing aid is limited. In some instances, only the awareness that there is noise and activity about is made available to the user. This may be important, however, in preventing the child from feeling isolated by inner silence if a hearing aid is not used. To be able to anticipate that someone is about to enter a house because a doorbell ring is heard is often considerably better than to be caught by surprise, or to fail to answer a doorbell because it is not heard.

If a hearing aid is indicated, training in its care and proper use is in order. Such training may be provided by the otologist or by the audiologist associated with a medical center, college, or university speech and hearing clinic.

It is important to appreciate that a hearing aid does not serve to give the user normal hearing in the same sense that properly fitted eyeglasses give most users essentially the equivalent of normal vision.

---

* Many college and university clinics, as well as medical centers, provide services for the selection of hearing aids.

The hearing instrument is, as its name suggests, only an aid. It helps the user to make more complete use of the amount of hearing he has. If the hearing loss is moderate rather than severe, and the individual learns the proper use of his aid, he can approach normal hearing. If, in addition, he learns lip reading and is attentive to his speaker, he comes closer to a complete understanding of oral speech. For the severely deaf, lip reading is of greater importance than for those with moderate hearing loss. The hearing instrument has more limited use, but together with lip reading it can still be a significant aid.

SPEECH AND HEARING THERAPY

Proper medical attention may help many children as well as adults to conserve whatever hearing they have. Proper speech and listening training should help them to make the maximum use of their hearing and to conserve the quality and intelligibility of their speech.

The school-age child with a moderate or greater hearing loss and with skill in lip reading is often able to continue his education in a class with normal-hearing children. This should be the desired goal for all children with hearing loss. We may be encouraged by the accomplishment reported by Wedenberg (1951) to the effect that two young children who had 99 per cent bilateral loss of hearing were nevertheless able to speak spontaneously and to interpret speech through their ears after several years of intensive auditory training.

The hearing therapist helps the child to make maximal use of his residual hearing as well as of his hearing aid, if one is used. In addition, the child is made aware of all the aspects of sound production so that tactile as well as auditory and visible cues are recognized and utilized. In this way the child not only becomes more completely responsive to how other persons speak, but also responds to his now speech with greater awareness. The result is better articulation, better voice, and improved intelligibility. In working with the school child, specific instruction is correlated with academic subject matter. The vocabulary of a new subject is introduced and becomes the core of the speech and hearing instruction.

Newby summarizes the goals of an auditory training program as follows (1964, p. 313):

> The objectives of the auditory training program are, first of all, to persuade the child to accept the hearing aid, and then for him to learn to operate it so effectively that he will never want to be without it. As in any kind of educational training, the procedure is from the known to

the unknown, from the simple to the complex. The emphasis must always be on teaching the child to use his hearing and his vision together. Thus auditory training should not be taught separately from speech reading, and while the comprehension of speech is being taught emphasis must also be placed on helping the child to improve his own speech.

THE ROLE OF THE CLASSROOM TEACHER

As indicated earlier in our discussion of hearing loss as a cause of delayed speech, the classroom teacher can do much to help the child with impaired hearing to live with others successfully. He can help the child to attain a sense of social competence and to accept the fact that he can live normally in his school environment. The hard-of-hearing child is apt to withdraw from others, to live within himself. The teacher can draw him into group living. By giving him duties and helping him to accept responsibilities, the child can be made to feel that he is a necessary member of a group whose participation is important to himself and to his classmates. Again, as with other handicapped children, the teacher can help the child with a hearing loss to accept it and himself and to minimize its potentially impairing influences.

The teacher can aid the child in developing language abilities by encouraging him to converse with others, and by motivating him to use speech and to take his part in the classroom activities. He can make sure that the child's experiences are fairly broad in nature. In addition, the teacher can encourage him to take part in playground activities and to read widely.

The teacher can help the child to appreciate and understand what goes on in the classroom in several ways: (1) by making sure he is seated where he can best see and hear the speakers in the room; (2) by permitting the child to move around the room as he finds it necessary in terms of his hearing; (3) by making certain that the light is on the speaker's face so that the child can see the face; (4) by speaking naturally but clearly and perhaps somewhat louder than might otherwise be necessary when the child with a hearing loss is at a distance from him; (5) by using gestures regularly, so that they will help the child in the understanding of language (one hard-of-hearing child said, " Miss Wilson is easy to understand; she talks with her face and her hands."); (6) by emphasizing what he is teaching by writing on the blackboard; and (7) by remembering to watch the child for signs of lack of comprehension and recalling that when repetition does not help, rephrasing the material often does.

References and Suggested Readings

BERRY, M. F., and J. EISENSON, *Speech Disorders*. New York, Appleton-Century-Crofts, 1956. (Chapter 19 includes a discussion of hearing loss, associated speech symptoms, and therapy.)

DARLEY, F. L., ed., " Identification Audiometry," *Journal of Speech and Hearing Disorders*, Monograph Supplement 9, (September, 1961).

DAVIS, H. and S. R. SILVERMAN, *Hearing and Deafness*. Holt, Rinehart, & Winston, Inc., 1960. (A lucidly written survey of research, including some of their own investigations, on problems of hearing.)

EAGLES, E. L., W. G. HARDY, and F. CATLIN, *Human Communications*. Washington, D.C., U.S. Dept. of Health, Education and Welfare, 1968.

GLORIG, A., "Hearing Conservation Past and Future," *Proceedings of the Working Conference on Health Aspects of Hearing Conservation*, Supplement to the Transactions of the American Academy of Ophthalmology and Otolaryngology (November-December, 1959), 24–33.

HOLLIEN, H., J. M. WEPMAN, and C. L. THOMPSON, "A Group Screening Test of Auditory Acuity," *Journal of School Health*, 39, 8 (1969), 583–588.

KEASTER, J., in W. JOHNSON, *et al.*, *Speech-Handicapped School Children*, 3rd ed. New York, Harper & Row, Publishers, 1967. Chap. 8.

MYKLEBUST, H., *The Psychology of Deafness*. New York, Grune and Stratton, 1960. (A study of deafness and its psychological implications.)

NEWBY, H. A., *Audiology*, 2nd ed. New York, Appleton-Century-Crofts, 1964.

O'NEILL, J. J., *The Hard of Hearing*. Englewood Cliffs, N.J., Prentice-Hall, Inc., 1964.

Subcommittee on Human Communication and Its Disorders. An Overview, Washington, D.C., National Institute of Neurological Diseases and Stroke. U.S. Dept. of Health, Education and Welfare, 1969.

VAN RIPER, C., *Speech Correction*, 4th ed. Englewood Cliffs, N.J., Prentice-Hall, Inc., 1963.

WEDENBERG, E., "Auditory Training of Deaf and Hard-of-Hearing Children," *Acta-Oto-Laryngologica*, Supplementum 94, Stockholm, 1951.

Problems

1. Why is it not advisable to assess the effects of hearing loss solely in terms of the percentage of loss below normal hearing?
2. Distinguish between the deaf and the hard-of-hearing.
3. What are the most frequently used nonobjective techniques for detecting the presence of hearing loss?
4. Define or explain each of the following: (a) cps or Hz, (b) decibel, (c) pure tone, (d) audiometer, (e) audiogram, (f) sweep test, (g) hearing aid, (h) residual hearing.
5. Does a hearing aid give the same assistance to its user as properly fitted glasses do for most persons with visual impairment? Justify your answer.

6. What does *identification audiometry mean*? Describe three techniques commonly used in identification audiometry.
7. Why does Newby (1964) recommend testing for functional hearing, as well as pure-tone audiometry, in the assessment of hearing loss?
8. What specifically can the classroom teacher do for the child known to have a hearing loss?
9. What is the implication of age and acquisition of speech in relation to an acquired hearing loss?
10. What are the characteristic speech defects of a child with sensorineural hearing impairment?
11. How are children with hearing loss educated in your school district?
12. What are the objectives of an auditory training program?

Chapter 15

Cleft
Palate

A facial cleft* is any opening in the oral cavity, lips, or nasal cavity which may be caused either by developmental failure (prebirth), or accident or disease at or following birth. The vast majority of facial clefts are developmental failures. That is, during the embryonic state of fetus, there was a failure of parts of the facial area to fuse and develop normally. Facial clefts may involve the palate as a whole, or be limited to parts of the hard or soft palate. Clefts may also involve the upper gum ridge (alveolar process), the upper lip, and one or both of the nares (the passageway from the nostril to the nasal cavity). Extensive clefts may involve any two or more of the parts of the oral cavity or upper lip. An insufficient palate, though not technically an oral cleft, is believed to be associated with the anomaly. An insufficient palate is one which does not have a normal amount of soft palate. The uvula may be missing or be shortened, and part of the soft palate anterior to the uvula may be smaller than is normal.

Although the specific cause of congenital facial cleft is not known, there is little doubt that heredity plays an important role in its etiology. Other factors that may be associated with congenital facial clefts are believed to be the diet and health of the mother and intrauterine pressure on the developing fetus.

---

* We are using the term *facial cleft* to comprise what is frequently included in the terms *cleft lip* and *cleft palate*.

INCIDENCE

The incidence of facial cleft varies somewhat according to geographic distribution. Surveys record ranges from one in about 600 to one in 1,000 in the population. Probably a moderate estimate is that one child in 750 is born with some form of facial cleft that will require special care and training. Among cleft-palate children the likelihood is that there will be more boys than girls.

VOICE AND ARTICULATION CHARACTERISTICS

From the description of the inadequacy of the mechanism, the speech difficulties are readily discernible. In the speech of the child with a palatal cleft all sounds pass directly into the nasal cavity where normal oral reinforcement is not possible. Therefore, all the vowel sounds are nasalized and most of the consonants have nasal characteristics. For example, [b], [d], and [g] take on the characteristics of [m], [n], and [ŋ]. Other articulatory difficulties are obvious. The plosive sounds [p], [b], [t], [d], [k], and [g] are defective because they are emitted nasally rather than orally. The fricatives [f], [v], [s], [z], [ʃ], [ʒ], [θ] and [ð] are also defective, because the air stream coming through the mouth cannot be adequately controlled.* Because s and z require the direction of an air stream down a narrow channel, they are likely to be the most seriously affected of the fricative sounds. Other distinctive traits include frequent inhalation and considerable use of the glottal stop, particularly before vowels. The resulting speech of a child with a severe cleft-palate condition may be a series of snorting sounds.

Westlake and Rutherford (1966, p. 30) make an interesting observation in regard to the sound substitutions made by young cleft-palate children. They point out that normal children tend to substitute [w], [f], [t], [d], [b], [θ], (th), and [tʃ] for the sounds they are unable to make. In each instance, the sound substituted is one that requires articulatory adjustments similar to the appropriate sound. Thus, we may say that normal sound substitution is close to the required sound and the articulation, and the child with "infantile" speech is moving toward his target. In contrast, cleft-palate children produce substitutes that are quite different from the correct ones. " More than half of their

---

* D. Counihan, ("Articulation Skills of Adolescents and Adults with Cleft Palate," *Journal of Speech Disorders*, XXV, May 1960, 181–187) found that a group of 45 cleft-palate speakers between the ages of 13 to 23 misarticulated the sounds z, s, sh [ʃ], ch [tʃ], and j [dʒ] more than 40 per cent of the time. The investigation also revealed that more than one half of the subjects had poorer articulation than the average five-year-old normal child.

substitutions are glottal stops and pharyngeal fricatives. These sounds, in addition to the [m], [n], and [ŋ], and nasal emissions, account for three fourths of cleft-palate substitutions." Thus, the cleft-palate children are far from the target sounds in their defective articulation.

RELATED PROBLEMS

Certain facial mannerisms are frequently associated with cleft palate. Some children seem to engage in nasal twitching; others look as if they are habitually sniffing. The alae, the winglike structures of the nose, constrict; this constriction compensates for the failure of the nasal port to close.

The child with a facial cleft faces a variety of problems. One of the first that he is likely to encounter is difficulty in feeding, with some possible consequences of poor nutrition. As he grows older, he frequently has dental conditions that require orthodontia. His teeth may fail to erupt, or they may grow in an irregular alignment. He tends to suffer from the effects of colds, with chronic infection of his nasal areas and of the Eustachian tube. These may produce conductive hearing loss. Pannbacker (1969) found that about two thirds of a population of 103 cases of cleft lip and cleft palate (60 males and 43 females) had hearing losses of 15 dB or more on audiometric assessment. However, cases with cleft lip alone, and those with congenital palatal insufficiency, did not have "socially significant audiological defects." Based on their review of the literature, Westlake and Rutherford (1966, p. 18) state: "All researchers agree that there is a high incidence of hearing loss in the cleft-palate population."

LINGUISTIC COMPETENCE

Although we are inclined to think of the cleft-palate child as one whose primary difficulties are with voice and articulation, recent evidence suggests that language competence as a whole may be delayed or improficient in many such children. In a population of 107 cleft-palate children between the ages of two and 15, Morris (1962) found an overall below-age-level expectation of language skills based on standardized test measurements. These included the Ammons Picture Vocabulary Test and the vocabulary subtest of the Wechsler Intelligence Scale for Children. In addition, mean length of sentence used and structural complexity of sentences were also below age-level expectation.

Smith and McWilliams (1968) assessed the linguistic abilities of 136 cleft-palate children ranging in age from 3.0 to 8.11. The population included 86 males and 50 females. Of these 71 had both cleft lip and cleft palate, 46 had cleft palates without cleft lip, and 19 had cleft lip alone. Smith and McWilliams used the Illinois Test of Psycholinguistic Abilities (ITPA) as their investigative instrument. They compared the standard age scores for the nine subtests of the ITPA with the scores for their experimental population. "The data revealed that cleft-palate subjects manifest a general language depression with particular weakness in vocal expression, gestural output, and visual memory. Moreover, in the samples studied, there was a tendency for language weaknesses to become more marked as age increased." It is interesting to note that both male and female subjects with cleft lip alone showed relative weaknesses in motor expression and visual memory, and generally similar linguistic profiles to the children with cleft palate.

Another factor deserving study and consideration in determining the therapeutic needs of the cleft-palate child is his intellectual development. A carefully conducted control study by Goodstein (1961), in which the Wechsler Intelligence Scale for Children was used to assess the intellectual status of cleft-palate children and a matched group of children without cleft palate, indicates that there are significant differences in intelligence levels between the two groups. An appreciably larger percentage of the cleft-palate children fell in the categories of dull normal, borderline, and mentally defective intellectual classifications than did the control children.* The latter group of children tended to distribute very much according to the expected intellectual classification levels. This study points to the need for the individual assessment of the intelligence of the cleft-palate child as well as the related need to adjust the therapeutic program so that the objectives, materials and rate of progress are realistically geared to the child's intellectual capacity.

Westlake and Rutherford (1966), after reviewing some of the literature on the intelligence of cleft-palate children, suggest that one of the reasons for the somewhat lower intelligence test scores may be in involvements, such as hearing loss, that are associated with or etiologically related to the clefts. They conclude (Westlake and Rutherford, 1966, p. 17) that "present information gives little reason for assuming that a person with a cleft is more likely to have a lower I.Q. than any other person." This observation is consistent with the general position taken by Westlake and Rutherford that cleft-palate persons vary individually as much as persons without cleft, and that generalizations are to be avoided in favor of intensive study of the individual who may have a facial cleft.

---

* Though there were more cleft-palate children in the lower intellectual classifications, the children were also represented in the upper classification.

THERAPY: SURGICAL

The first step, if possible, is repair of the oral mechanism to the fullest extent that can be achieved for life processes and speech. The first step, may in fact be a series of steps taken over a period of years, through infancy and childhood. The primary goal of surgery is to provide the cleft-palate child with the best possible functioning of the palate and the vocal mechanism as a whole. A secondary but exceedingly important goal is cosmetic, to do whatever can be done to make the child as good-looking and as normal in appearance as possible.

A variety of procedures are used to close the palate, to lengthen it if possible, and to provide an oral cavity that will serve both the functions of articulation and reinforcement (resonance). Often, as we have indicated, the teeth need to be arranged or rearranged, or dentures provided when this is not possible.

Usually the repair of extensive facial clefts requires a series of operations. Since surgical repair of facial clefts is a highly specialized area in medicine, most of the work is done in fairly large medical centers. Surgeons must not only make the oral cavity adequate for the present but must also predict how future growth will be affected by the surgery.

Descriptions of some of the surgical procedures are presented in Westlake and Rutherford (1966, pp. 79–82), and Berry and Eisenson (1956, pp. 316–323).

PROSTHETIC APPLIANCES

In some cases the surgeon may advise against an operation, for he may wish the child to be older or to be in better health before he operates. The surgeon may feel that the fissure is so great that the available tissue cannot cover it. He may recommend that the child go to a prostho-dontist, a dental specialist, for an obturator; this is an apparatus used to take the place of the palate of the individual. It is usually made of plastic and conforms to the arch of the hard palate. An obturator for the entire palate includes a tailpiece for the soft palate and a bulb at the end around which the pharyngeal wall is constricted. The obturator must be fitted carefully. Although it must be tight, it cannot close the passage completely. The back part of the obturator and the throat are closed by the action of the muscles of the upper portion of the throat. Thus the nasal port is shut off from the oral cavity. The aids should be light and comfortable. They are usually placed in the mouth when the child is young. The prosthodontist makes adjustments as the mouth grows. In some cases, this method of closing the palate is impossible because of the insufficiency and lack of flexibility of the remaining palatal tissues.

COOPERATION OF ALL SPECIALISTS

The treatment of the child with a facial cleft may require long and continuous cooperation and coordination of services. The speech clinician, surgeon, orthodontist, psychologist, and prosthodontist must work together carefully and well. They must have a fairly intimate knowledge of one another's goals and their methods of achieving them. The classroom teacher must work with the specialists and understand their work.

SPEECH CORRECTION

Muscle Strengthening. The speech clinician must help the child to make maximum use of the oral cavity musculature as modified either by the surgeon or by the prosthodontist. Objectives should include making the oral musculatures stronger and more flexible so that they may be used more adequately for speech. Control of breath and the prevention or reduction of leakage of breath into the nasal cavities are the primary goals. This may be accomplished through "blowing exercises." The gentle, sustained blowing of a feather, a ping-pong ball, a candle flame, or a paper butterfly helps to improve the child's ability to direct his breath stream outward toward the front of his mouth, and so to increase oral resonance when application is made to speech production. Swallowing, sucking through a straw, and yawning are also of some help in strengthening the soft palate and throat muscles. Young children may enjoy the interesting noise effects of blowing through the teeth of a comb against which a piece of tissue paper is fixed. A more musical result may be obtained from playing a harmonica.

It must be emphasized, however, that all of these exercises are merely token indicators of what a child may be able to do in non-speech activities. A child may be able to achieve complete success in blowing exercises and yet not be able to control his velum in a manner and at a rate necessary to avoid nasality while speaking. In the final analysis, what matters is how a child with a repaired cleft, or one with an oral prosthesis, uses his mechanism for intelligible and, if possible, appropriate nasal reinforcement. Of the two, *intelligibility should be the primary objective.*

Visualizing Palatal Movement. Actual movement of the palate and the oral mechanism as a whole can now be visualized by means of X-ray photography, taken while the patient is talking. Perhaps the best technique is that of X-ray motion pictures (cinefluorography) which is now available in many medical centers. Information derived from such films enables the clinician to know what needs to be done to improve palatal action and to counteract the tendencies of a person with repaired cleft to use inappropriate movements in his articulatory efforts. It may be possible to see as well as hear the differences when the child speaks slowly and when he speaks at what may be a normal rate of utterance, but not an optimum rate for this child. However, X-ray photography is not always available, so that other less sophisticated methods may need to be used. Simple devices include long bits of light feather glued to the end of a tongue depressor or, perhaps better, an ice cream stick. Placed under the nostrils, the feather should respond to the emitted air. If the air is inappropriately emitted, the clinician and child have a visual cue for this misfunction. Westlake and Rutherford (1966, p. 91) also suggest the use of a small plastic rectangular box, fashioned so that an open space on one of the shorter ends fits against the upper lip so that the nose may extend into the area of the box. Air escaping from the nostrils will cause the feather or paper to move about in the box. Westlake and Rutherford (1966, p. 91) realistically observe that "all these methods are difficult to use with young children, many of whom seem diabolically driven to make the papers fly instead of trying to speak without moving them." We would suggest a counterdiabolic procedure by directing the child alternately to make things move and to talk without producing such movement. This is an application of the principle of negative practice in learning!

Improving the Vocal Quality. Careful ear training and voice training often reduce the excessive nasality. We are not sure how excessive nasal resonance is produced, although we do know that it occurs when the opening of the nasal cavity is too large as compared with the opening of the mouth cavity. The clinician will strive for a satisfactory acoustic balance of nasal and oral resonance. Thus, if the child speaks with a "tight" (hypertensive) oral musculature and a small oral opening, he should be helped to change to the use of a more relaxed and larger mouth opening.

Correcting Articulatory Defects. Although excessive and inappropriate nasality is the primary problem of most cleft-palate children, constant attention should be paid to improving articulation. Recent investigations indicate that cleft-palate speakers with intelligible articulation are likely to be judged as having less nasality than do cleft speakers with poorer articulation (Van Hattum, 1958).

The speech clinician must help the cleft-palate child to improve his overall articulatory efforts. Exercises should be directed at increasing the child's mobility and control of jaw, lip, and tongue movements.

In some instances a hearing loss may increase the difficulties of the cleft-palate child. Impaired hearing may account for the misarticulation of some of the sounds. If the hearing loss is moderate or severe, the use of a hearing aid may be indicated.

The clinician first teaches the sounds that are easiest for the child. For example, *h* is usually fairly easy to teach. Some of the later sounds he attacks are *k*, *g*, *s*, and *z*. Since *k* and *g* involve the soft palate and since the stream of air for *s* and *z* needs very careful control, these four sounds are difficult for the child with a cleft palate. In many instances, there is a persistent tendency for sibilant sounds to be emitted nasally. Considerable effort and time are needed to overcome this tendency.

THE ROLE OF THE CLASSROOM TEACHER

The classroom teacher must augment the efforts of the clinician. He realizes that the degree of normalcy of the child's speech will depend on the condition of the mechanism after its repair and on speech training, motivation, intelligence, and interest. At times the teacher is the liaison between the clinician and the home. He and the clinician advise the parents that the training period for correcting the child's speech may be long and that the work will be hard. They explain to the parents how they can be of assistance to the child.

The teacher helps the child to carry over the work from the correction class into everyday speech. The teacher promotes such activities as creative dramatics, in which the child may sell newspapers on the corner or popcorn at the ball game. This activity gives the child practice in the use of the acceptable speech that he is acquiring.

A child with a cleft palate must learn to adjust to his difficulty. The feeling that he has about his difficulty is often more important than the defects themselves. The attitude of his parents and teachers influences his evaluation of the difficulty. One child with a minor cleft, and who has intelligible speech, may be anxious and concerned, while another with a serious cleft, running from the teeth ridge through to the uvula and with badly distorted speech, may be much less disturbed. The child must feel accepted as he is. When he knows that he is understood and respected, he "feels good." The teacher, by accepting him as he is, by helping him succeed, can make him feel adequate. Often the teacher must work hard to help him achieve a feeling of adequacy because of the effects of his home environment.

Parents sometimes unconsciously reject the child with a facial cleft.

They may be a little ashamed of him. In such instances the teacher's attitude is very important. If the teacher accepts the child as he is, if he promotes satisfactory activity in which the child finds enjoyment and success, the child will be helped to modify his attitudes toward himself.

Other parents are overprotective; they are unduly concerned about the child. As a result of this concern, they may be overly indulgent. The teacher, therefore, may need to compensate for the parents' over-solicitude. The teacher should not let feelings show and should not impose unnecessary limitations. The child with a facial cleft should be expected to perform according to his intellectual capacity. Allowances should be made only on the basis of hazards to health.

References and Recommended Readings

ANDERSON, V. A., *Improving the Child's Speech*. New York, Oxford University Press, Inc., 1952. (Pages 224–233 include a description of cleft palate speech and suggestions for treatment.)

BERRY, M. F., and J. EISENSON, *Speech Disorders*. New York, Appleton-Century-Crofts, 1956, Chap. 14.

GOODSTEIN, L. D., "Intellectual Impairment in Cleft Palate," *Journal of Speech and Hearing Research*, IV (September 1961), 287–294.

McDONALD, E. T., and H. KOEPP-BAKER, "Cleft-Palate Speech," *Journal of Speech and Hearing Disorders*, XVI (March 1951), 9–19. (This article includes a discussion of how to achieve a balance between oral and nasal resonance.)

MOLLER, K. T., C. D. STARR, and R. R. MARTIN, "The Application of Operant Conditioning Procedures to the Facial Grimace Problem," *Cleft Palate Journal*, VI (July 1969), 193–201.

MORRIS, H. L., "Communication Skills of Children with Cleft Lips and Palates," *Journal of Speech and Hearing Research*, V (March 1962), 79–90.

PANNBACKER, M., "Hearing Loss and Cleft Palate," *Cleft Palate Journal*, VI (October 1969), 50–56.

SMITH, R. M., and B. J. McWILLIAMS, "Psycholinguistic Abilities of Children with Clefts," *Cleft Palate Journal*, V (April 1968), 238–249.

SPRIESTERSBACH, D. C., and D. SHERMAN, eds., *Cleft Palate and Communication*. N.Y., Academic Press, 1968. (A high level scientific approach by ten contributors to the multiple aspects of cleft palate).

VAN HATTUM, R. J., "Articulation and Nasality in Cleft Palate Speakers," *Journal of Speech and Hearing Research*, I, (December 1958), 383–387.

VAN RIPER, C., *Speech Correction*, 4th ed. Englewood Cliffs, N.J., Prentice-Hall, Inc., 1963, Chap. 13. (Van Riper has excellent illustrations for types of cleft palate. He discusses the psychological and social problems of persons with cleft palate which he believes are often as severe as for many stutterers.)

WEST, R. M., and M. ANSBERRY, *Rehabilitation of Speech*. New York, Harper & Row, Publishers, 1969, pp. 89–104.

WESTLAKE, H., and D. RUTHERFORD, *Cleft Palate*. Englewood Cliffs, N.J., Prentice-Hall, Inc., 1966. (A study guide for the understanding of the problems of persons with cleft palate. Emphasis is on the individual with cleft palate and the need to determine therapy based on his special problems.)

YULES, R. B., and R. A. CHASE, "Pharyngeal Flap Surgery: A Review of the Literature," *Cleft Palate Journal*, VI (1969), 303–308. (The authors indicate that there is a lack of available criteria for determining when the pharyngeal flap procedure should be used.)

Problems

1. What are the types of facial clefts? What are the chief causes?
2. What is meant by the term "cosmetic problem?" What can be done to avoid or minimize such a problem in cleft-palate children?
3. Contrast the positions of Westlake and Rutherford and Van Riper (see references) on the psychological and social implications of a facial cleft for a child or an adult.
4. What problems, other than speech, are often associated with cleft palate?
5. The voice of the cleft-palate child, even after repair, is often excessively nasal. Why?
6. Why is it especially important to ameliorate any hearing loss that may be associated with cleft palate?
7. One of the new surgical procedures for reducing nasality is called the "surgical flap." Check the literature for a description of this operation and the circumstances that indicate when it is the procedure of choice.
8. Why is the strengthening of the oral musculature important in the therapeutic program for a child with cleft palate?
9. What should be the primary objective in speech training for a cleft-palate child?
10. What are the most frequent articulatory errors made by young cleft-palate children? How are these errors different from those made by most young children?
11. Describe some techniques that may be used by clinicians to help them, and their cleft-palate children, to visualize excessive nasal emission?
12. What is a prosthetic appliance? When is its use indicated for persons with cleft palate?

Chapter 16

Brain Damage and Brain Dysfunction

In this chapter we shall consider the implications of brain damage for the acquisition and development of speech. Three groups, whose syndromes are by no means always clearly defined, will be discussed. These groups are the cerebral-palsied, the "minimally" brain-damaged (minimal brain dysfunction), and the congenitally aphasic (dyslogic) children.

The Cerebral-Palsied: Definition and Problems

In a narrow and literal sense the term *cerebral palsy* refers to motor involvement (palsy or paralysis) on the basis of brain damage. The motor involvement may vary in type or degree and may include obvious severe paralysis, motor weakness, and/or motor incoordination. It is usually possible to relate the nature of the motor disability with localized pathology in the brain. However, in some instances, pathology and manifest impairment are not easily associated.

In a broader sense, cerebral palsy refers to several conditions that are associated with the cerebral pathology, but not necessarily specific to the motor impairments. Perhaps it would be more accurate to say that many cerebral-palsied individuals have such impairments as hearing loss, visual difficulties, other sensory difficulties such as the

393

integration of sensory stimuli, perceptual and intellectual decrement, and related behavioral problems. These involvements, which all too often occur multiply among the cerebral-palsied, underlie general learning disabilities and specific difficulties in the comprehension of speech and in acquiring and developing language proficiency, both oral and written. We should note and emphasize that many individuals who are known to have congenital brain damage, and who have manifest motor involvements are entirely free of any associated impairments. Thus we cannot stress the point too strongly that for any child, regardless of whether motor or sensory involvements are evident, a complete assessment of potential abilities as well as limitations is in order. High-level intelligence and high-level potential achievement are definitely represented among the population of the frankly cerebral-palsied.

INCIDENCE

Figures as to the incidence of cerebral palsy vary considerably according to criteria. The incidence would be high if the collector of the data assumes that the existence of any of the conditions mentioned above is presumptive evidence of cerebral palsy, or if the condition cannot be attributed to some other specific cause. Behavioral disturbances, especially of the "acting out" variety, are perhaps all too frequently considered to be associated with brain damage. The incidence is likely to be considerably lower if the investigator demands clear-cut positive evidence of brain damage, such as would satisfy a pediatric neurologist who might be concerned with "hard-sign" indications of neuropathology. Psychologists, and neurologists as well, who view the assessment of perceptual and cognitive functioning as an extension of a neurological examination, would stress the significance of findings of perceptual impairment (the failure to derive meanings from sensory imput) and impairment of intersensory integration as evidence of brain damage, even when motor disabilities are minimal. Investigations along this line are reviewed in monographs by Birch (1964) and Allen and Jefferson (1962). A conservative estimate of the incidence of cerebral palsy is about three per 1,000 of population (Altman, 1955, and McDonald and Chance, 1964, p. 2). Interestingly, this incidence may be somewhat higher in the 1960's than in previous decades because many children who are now surviving the conditions that make them cerebral-palsied would have died in the first half of the century. We may hope, however, that immunization against measles and rubella may reduce this incidence sharply in future years.

CAUSES OF CEREBRAL PALSY

The causes of cerebral palsy are, unfortunately, both numerous and varied. By definition, whatever the specific cause, it must be one that damages or retards the development of one of the centers of the brain that is involved in the production and control of motor activity. There is also a high incidence of sensory defects, predominantly hearing and vision, as well as mental retardation. These impairments are associated with pathologies of the cerebrum, cortical and subcortical, in the cerebral palsied.*

The major causes of cerebral palsy include developmental maturational failure beginning in the embryonic stage. In many instances, such failure is associated with illness incurred by the mother during the early months of pregnancy. Rubella, or German measles, is high among such illnesses. Trauma affecting the brain, associated with the mother's prolonged labor or precipitous labor, is also one of the more frequent causes. Any condition that cuts off or sharply reduces the oxygen supply to the child's brain and that occurs immediately before, during, or after the child is born may cause cerebral palsy. Such conditions include maternal hemorrhaging, a tightened umbilical cord around the child's neck, an injury that occasionally, but fortunately rarely, may result from forceps delivery, or cerebral hemorrhaging of the child from unknown causes. Prematurity (babies born before full term and weighing less than five pounds) is high among the conditions associated with cerebral palsy. Even after the child has survived his first hazardous journey through the mother's birth canal, he may incur damage to the brain from head trauma or from some infectious involvement that produces brain damage.

Although all causes of brain damage cannot be specifically related to the type of cerebral palsy a child may have, certain etiological correlates are recognized. External trauma to the brain (head injury that affects the brain) is likely to produce spastic cerebral palsy. Anoxia (a cutting off or sharp reduction in the supply of oxygen to the brain) tends to be associated with athetoid cerebral palsy. In the embryonic state, the stage of the development of the child's central nervous system may be affected by the illnesses of the mother.†

---

* See Crothers and Paine (1959) for medical considerations. A brief summary of the pathology of cerebral palsy may be found in Brown (1967, pp. 376–378).

† McDonald and Chance (1964, Chapter 2) present an excellent brief review of the neurophysiology and etiology of cerebral palsy.

Disturbances Related to Cerebral Palsy

Many cerebral-palsied children have multiple handicaps usually associated with the basic brain damage. On the physical side these handicaps include epilepsy and impairments of hearing and vision. Many children also show considerable mental retardation even when allowances are made for the inadequacy of the test instruments. In addition, there are often subtle disturbances in perceptual ability, such as the ability to recognize and reproduce forms and appreciate spatial relationships. This impairment interferes with the children's learning potential and with their attempts at adjusting to their physical environment.* Another area of difficulty is emotional stability. Many cerebral-palsied children are disturbed children. Some of the disturbances arise out of a reaction to their multiple handicaps. Others arise out of the reactions of the parents and siblings to the cerebral-palsied children, and theirs in turn to their parents and siblings. Perhaps an even greater cause of emotional disturbance may be attributed to the frequent failures in attempts at communication, which may have the unfortunate result of allowing quick and chronic frustration to become an established mode of behavior.

INTELLIGENCE AND EDUCABILITY

Intelligence. Until very recently, testing instruments used for estimating the intelligence of cerebral-palsied children have had severe limitations. Most tests used were initially standardized on populations that did not include a significant number of children with motor handicaps or the other handicaps often associated with cerebral palsy. Tested by such instruments, the cerebral-palsied population showed a large incidence of mental retardation. Fortunately, there are now several instruments available that require little or no verbalization and call instead for relatively gross motor actions in the test situations. Such tests enable us to make a more adequate estimate of the intelligence of the cerebral-palsied. These tests include the Ammons Full Range Picture Vocabulary Test, the Revised Peabody Vocabulary Test, the Revised Columbia Mental Maturity Scale, and Raven's Progressive Matrices. The results

---

* See Cruickshank's discussion of the multiple-handicapped child (1970, pp. 3–12) for an explanation of these factors; also the discussions by C. Kennedy and L. Eisenberg in Birch (1964, pp. 13–26 and 61–76).

obtained from surveys employing these tests suggest that there is probably less mental retardation among the cerebral-palsied than was earlier reported. There is little question, however, that the incidence of mental retardation is considerably greater among the cerebral-palsied than among the population at large. Estimates as to the amount of mental retardation range from 25 per cent to more than 50 per cent.

While becoming aware of the intellectual limitations of many of the cerebral-palsied, we should not overlook the important fact that intellectual genius is also present in this physically handicapped group. Taken as a whole, all levels of intellectual capacity are represented among the cerebral-palsied, as they are among the population at large.*

Educability. Because many cerebral-palsied children have multiple handicaps, including mental retardation, a large percentage of the children have been classified as uneducable. Many are "trained" in resident institutions rather than in schools. Of late, increasing numbers of cerebral-palsied children are being educated in special classes in regular public schools. Private schools specializing in the treatment of the handicapped are also accepting the cerebral-palsied and giving them the benefit of improved understanding and teaching techniques. A majority of cerebral-palsied children have sufficient intellectual capacity for education along with the nonhandicapped in the normal classroom situation. Many of these children, however, will require special attention from the speech clinician as well as understanding from the classroom teacher.

Therapy for the Cerebral Palsied

THE CEREBRAL PALSY TEAM

For children with more than minimum or residual cerebral palsy, a program of training calls for the cooperation of a team of professional specialists. Included in the team are the physician, the psychologist, the social worker, the physical therapist, the occupational therapist, the teacher, and the speech clinician.

The physician or physicians must estimate to what extent the child's neurological involvements may affect his learning. Frequently, an orthopedic surgeon is called upon for recommendations as to how classroom equipment or home furnishings are to be constructed or adapted to the child's needs. The orthopedic surgeon's advice is also needed in

---

* Allen and Jefferson, in their manual on the *Psychological Evaluation of the Cerebral Palsied Person* (1962) describe tests and suggestions for the modification of procedures needed in the assessment of the cerebral-palsied.

matters relating to the improvement of motor abilities and the prevention of physical disabilities.

The physical therapist, working with the physician, strives to improve
the child's performance in coordination and motor activity. Specific
therapeutic measures may be employed which may help the child to
learn how to control his speech musculature so that a proper degree of
relaxation and synergy of movement is achieved. Such therapy prepares
the cerebral-palsied child for the work of the speech clinician.

The occupational therapist functions as an observer of the child's
motor activity and trains the child specifically in "occupational" skills.
Essentially, the occupational therapist supplements the work of the
physical therapist.

The psychologist, through testing and observation, makes an appraisal
of the intellectual capacities and the present and potential abilities as
well as the disabilities and limitations of the cerebral-palsied child.
Recommendations as to the child's educability and type of education
are made by the psychologist. Periodic reappraisals are made so that
objectives and goals may be changed according to the manner and rate
of the child's development.

The social worker investigates the home situation of the cerebral-
palsied child. He obtains information about the child's home and the
attitudes of the parents and other key members in the household. In
addition, the social worker helps to adjust the members of the family
to their problem in relationship to the child and in the interest of the
child.

The speech clinician evaluates the child's speech problems and trains
him to improve his communicative skills. Speech disabilities are found
in 50 to 75 per cent of cerebral-palsied children. Some of the disabilities
can be considerably improved; others can be modified only slightly.
Realistic goals must be established that are consistent with the child's
sensory and motor abilities and intellectual capacity. Progress, it must
be recognized, is often slow and amounts of improvement are not likely
to be discerned on a day-to-day basis.

SPEECH THERAPY*

Specific speech therapy for the cerebral-palsied child with speech
disabilities must be adapted to the child in terms of his involvements.
If a child has a hearing loss, speech signals must be intensified. This

---

*See McDonald and Chance (1964 Chap. 6) for a detailed consideration of the
language and speech problems of the cerebral palsied.

can be accomplished through the using of a speaking tube or through the use of amplification and headset earphones. For many cerebral-palsied children, an overall program would include the following:

1. Relaxation and voluntary control of the speech musculature. Often much of this work has been accomplished through the training given by the physiotherapist.

2. The establishment of breath control for vocalization and articulation. Many cerebral-palsied children breathe too deeply or too shallowly for purposes of speech. Frequently children attempt to speak on inhaled breath. For most cerebral-palsied children, a normal length of phrase is not to be expected. Short, uninterrupted phrasing is a more modest and more possible achievement. Devices such as blowing through a straw, the " bending " of a candle flame, and the moving of ping-pong balls on flat surfaces and up inclined planes are helpful in establishing breath control.

3. Control of the organs of articulation. Considerable exercise is needed to establish directed and independent action of the tongue and to overcome the frequently present tendency of the cerebral-palsied child to move his jaw as he attempts to move his tongue. Children enjoy such exercises as licking honey from their lips, or reaching for a bit of honey or peanut butter placed on the upper gum ridge. A lollipop held outside the mouth for licking provides a sweet objective for the tip of the tongue. The child should be shown what he does by observing himself and the speech clinician in a mirror.

4. Work on individual speech sounds. The sounds most frequently defective are those that require precise tip-of-the-tongue action. These include *t, d, l, n, r, s,* and *z*. Intense auditory stimulation, even if the child has no significant hearing loss, often helps him to become aware of what he is expected to produce. Sound play, calling for repetition of sounds the child can produce, may give him a feeling of accomplishment in the early stages of speech training. For many children, normal proficiency of articulation may not be expected. The production of " reasonable facsimiles " of sounds so that speech, though defective, is intelligible, is frequently all that we have a right to expect.

5. Incorporation of sounds in words and phrases. Many cerebral-palsied children have considerable difficulty in making the transition from the production of individual sounds to connected speech. Abrupt stops are frequent, especially when words include stop plosive sounds or others that call for rapid articulatory action. The child should be encouraged to keep his sounds moving, to keep his articulation in action, even if there is a resultant lack of precision in the effort as a whole. Articulation must, of course, be coordinated with breathing and vocalization.

The Classroom Teacher's Responsibility for the Cerebral-Palsied Child

Because the cerebral-palsied child may look different, because frequently he is unable to participate in many of the activities of other children, because his family may have been oversolicitous, or may have unconsciously rejected him, he is apt to have difficulty in adjusting to a group. When the teacher accepts his infirmity, is casual about it, but still demands from him standards within his reach and performance within his capabilities, the teacher is doing the child a real service. If the teacher does not let his sympathy show but accepts the child in a friendly fashion with cheerful affection, the child's adjustment is made easier. The child should participate in such regular classroom activities as going on visits. The teacher should consider the cerebral-palsied child just another member of the group who enjoys and likes living with his classmates, and should provide new experiences that give adequate scope for his abilities and energies.

Cerebral-palsied children speak better when relaxed. They do better when they have confidence in themselves and their abilities. When they are anxious or frustrated, they have more difficulty with their speech. When the teacher can help the child to feel that he is making a contribution to group living, and that he is accepting and carrying through responsibilities for successful group activity, he is assisted in attaining a feeling of "belongingness" with his classmates and a feeling of security in this particular environment. The teacher gives him frequent opportunities to relax. At times the teacher or children may make things easy for him physically; for example, his seat may be moved to a particular spot that is more readily accessible for the current activity. Whatever is done should be done in as casual a manner as possible so that no attention is attracted to the activity and the cerebral-palsied child will be able to feel comfortable rather than self-conscious.

Brain Damage Without Apparent Motor Involvement

Many brain-damaged children are not obviously cerebral-palsied. Some have such minor motor involvements that they are not suspected of having incurred brain damage until they are of an age when language comprehension and the acquisition of speech are normally expected. These children, as we indicated earlier, are often problems and puzzles to themselves, their families, and their teachers. The reasons for this perplexing state of affairs should become clear in the discussion that follows.

The Concept of Minimal Brain Dysfunction

During recent years, and increasingly since the 1960's, teachers and clinicians have been confronted with the terms *minimal brain damage* and *minimal brain dysfunction*. The second term assumes the presence of the first, but not on the basis of the " hard signs "—the physiological, and structural alterations that many neurologists require as evidence of brain damage. In brief, the child with minimal brain dysfunction is not frankly (obviously) cerebral-palsied. He does not have clear and unquestioned indications of sensory and motor impairments, or of aberrant reflexes, that are the " hard-sign " indications of brain damage. Neurologists, psychologists, and teachers who do accept the concept of minimal brain dysfunction do so on the assumption that there are relationships between brain functioning and dysfunctioning, and behavior. So, they agree:

> we must accept certain categories of deviant behavior, developmental dyscrasias, learning disabilities, and visual motor perceptual irregularities as valid indices of brain dysfunctioning, They represent neurologic signs of a most meaningful kind, and reflect disorganized central nervous system functioning at the highest level. To consider learning and behavior as distinct and separate from other neurologic functions echoes a limited concept of the nervous system and of its various levels of influence and integration (Clements 1966, pp. 6–7).

THE SYNDROME OF MINIMAL BRAIN DYSFUNCTION

The term *minimal brain dysfunction* refers to a combination of manifestations (syndrome) present in children who are of near-average, average, or above-average intelligence. These manifestations, all of which are not necessarily present for any given child, include problems of attention and memory, impulsivity, mild motor disabilities (awkwardness, delayed laterality), perception, conceptualization, and speech and language development. These children are *perceptually* and *intellectually inefficient*, so that they do not meet the expectations for educational achievement based on their intelligence test scores, especially for those scores derived from " nonlanguage " or performance inventories. Often, in fact, they present problems in learning during the school years, and so become identified. They are often among the " under-achievers," especially in the language subjects—reading, spelling, and often arith-metic as well. Their thinking tends to be concrete and ego-oriented and they may have difficulty with abstract conceptualization and abstract language. Occasionally, however, some children show surprising flashes of insight as well as an ability to appreciate the abstract. Thus, they may be inconsistent and puzzling performers who show wide day-to-day variations in their accomplishments. For a detailed testing of the sympto-matology of the child with minimal brain dysfunction see Clements (1966, pp. 11–12).

Developmental Aphasia (Dyslogia) and Brain Damage

In a literal sense, *aphasia* means without language or without speech. However, the term aphasia and aphasic are used by professional persons concerned with problems of language related to brain damage as desig-nations for language impairments that were acquired at a stage after language was established. These include impairments in the compre-hension and production of spoken as well as written language. The terms may also be used for a child who incurs damage and language impairment following accident or disease of the brain (encephalopathies). Fortunately, the young child, up to the age of early adolescence (12 to 14 or so) has such great plasticity of the brain and such great reorgani-zational and recuperative capacity that recovery and resumption of language functioning may ordinarily be expected. Exceptions are found, however, among children who incur bilateral or profuse damage of the cerebrum.

In our earlier discussion of minimal brain damage and minimal brain dysfunction we anticipated our consideration of the child whose impairments are so severe as to make him essentially nonverbal. We shall use the terms *developmental aphasia, congenital aphasia*, and *dyslogia* synonymously to designate such a condition in the child.

DEVELOPMENT APHASIA (DYSLOGIA) AND BRAIN DYSFUNCTION

Children who are born with brain damage because of a prenatal condition, or who have incurred brain damage as a result of a birth injury or a cerebral pathology before the age at which speech usually begins, are frequently severely retarded in their speech onset and development. Often, even after these children begin to speak, articu-lation, voice, and vocabulary development are impaired. In very severe cases, usually associated with damage to both hemispheres of the brain, even the comprehension of language may be severely and sometimes completely impaired. It is likely that most of these children who do learn to understand speech also suffer from an appreciable degree of mental deficiency, and others from hearing loss with or without mental deficiency. Our own experience with brain-damaged children leads us to believe that, where hearing loss and mental deficiency are not complicating factors, language learning may be delayed but is usually established by age four or five. In most cases where hearing and intelligence are relatively normal, language is learned and speech, however defective, is usually established by the time the child has reached school age.

There are, however, a small group of children with slow maturation of the central nervous system, who, because of minimal brain damage and considerably more than minimal brain dysfunction, do not "spontaneously" acquire speech. These children must be taught directly what most children acquire naturally—by listening, identifying, and finally by imitating and then creating on their own an infinite number of utterances they could not possibly have learned through imitation. These children are *developmentally* or *congenitally aphasic* or *dyslogic* (without language). Following are some critical differences that distinguish this child from his speaking as well as his nonspeaking age peers.

1. The developmentally aphasic (dyslogic) child has perceptual difficulties related to one or more sensory modalities, but primarily for the perception of those auditory events that constitute the sounds of speech. (See Eisenson (1966) and (1968) for an exposition of this point.)
2. The dyslogic child is often slow in developing laterality. At the age of five or even later he may not have established a preferred hand or foot or an eye or an ear. Often associated with this developmental lag is confusion in directional and spatial orientation.
3. Inconsistency of response is almost a universal characteristic of the dyslogic child. A response made to a situation on one occasion may not be made on a succeeding occasion. A response that may be completely appropriate when first made may simply fail to be made on successive occasions.
4. Morbidity of attention is associated with inconsistency of response. Occasionally the dyslogic child may become so completely absorbed with the situation to which he is attending that he cannot shift his attention to new situations, despite the intensity of a new stimulus. Thus, loud noises may be ignored, or at least are not immediately able to compete for attention with what is

already concerning the child. In contrast with this compulsive and persistent manner of attending to a situation, the dyslogic child may sometimes have such fleeting attention as to seem to be reacting to everything, and adequately to nothing.

5. Associated with inconsistency of response and morbidity of attention is lability of general behavior. The dyslogic child may behave excessively and exhibit uncontrolled emotionality because of seemingly trivial disturbances. If the child is disturbed at all, he is disturbed a great deal. Along with emotional lability there is accompanying hyperactivity. The child may suddenly change from being relatively docile to being active beyond easy control.

6. A characteristic feature of the language development of the dyslogic child, aside from the initial retardation, is unevenness of ability. Even after this child begins to use language, he does not show the expected increments or the "ordered" pattern by which most children increase their linguistic abilities for day-to-day communication. Many dyslogic children learn to say a few words at intervals far apart, but may during these periods have a normal or better than normal increase in their comprehension vocabularies. They may show parallel disparities in learning to read and write. The result may be that even after the children are in the mid-primary grades, their educational achievements are so uneven as to cause considerable concern to their teachers, their parents, and to themselves. They are often painfully slow in achieving an integrated pattern of development with those features that go together and that are ordinarily found together.

The features we reviewed of the developmentally aphasic child may be understood in terms of the impaired efficiency of their neurological mechanisms. The overall effects of the cerebral differences in this brain different child is to aggravate any sensory impairments they may have—some have slight to moderate degrees of hearing loss—and to reduce their perceptual and intellectual potentials. Functionally, these children do not hear as well as audiometric results would suggest they should be able to hear. Otherwise stated, they do not hear as proficiently as nonbrain-damaged children do with the same amount of "objectively measured" hearing. Similarly, and more generally, they often function considerably below the upper limits of their mental potential. They disturb easily, and have very good cause for such reactions.

Clinical Assessment. For the brain-damaged dyslogic child such an assessment should be made only by highly competent specialists. This child is not easy to diagnose into a clear-cut category. He often responds, or fails to respond, in the manner of a deaf child. Sometimes he seems to respond with the slowness and limited understanding of a severely mentally retarded child. Often he behaves as if he were emotionally disturbed. It is essential, therefore, that a team of clinicians, including a physician and, if possible, a neurologist, an audiologist, and a psychologist, make the assessment. It may well be that a given child may have brain damage and hearing loss, and his general lability may be a reaction to his own impairments. Even when language learning is proceeding, he, as well as his teachers and parents, may be responding to his uneven abilities with repeated frustration.

The most severely developmentally aphasic children do not have enough language when they reach school age to enter regular classes. In some school districts they may be accepted in special classes for aphasic or neurologically handicapped children. Usually they need prior training to be prepared for such classes. Such training is now offered in clinics or in medical or educational centers here and abroad. Approaches that have been found useful emphasize speech-sound discrimination, visual stimulation in association with oral language, sequencing of visual materials and of oral language presented more slowly and in smaller units than in normal speech utterance, and the direct teaching of syntax. We have found that many preschool developmentally aphasic children do well by an almost exclusively visual approach that introduces arrangements of pictures to tell something (visual semantic sequencing), which later becomes associated with oral language. Essentially, the child learns that utterances, whether visual or audible, have "law and order," out of which sense and meanings are derived. By approaching the child primarily through his visual and less impaired modality, which incidentally and importantly permits him to look as long and as often as he needs to derive meaning from his input, the notion of representation and symbolization becomes established. Thus, many children begin to be able to read on a primer level before they are able to do much talking.

Programs for congenitally aphasic children are now being developed at the Institute for Childhood Aphasia at Stanford University. Programs with a different emphasis and orientation have been published by Barry (1961) and McGinnis (1963).

Therapeutic Approaches. Such approaches to improve the speech and language impairments of the school-age dyslogic child should be shared by the language clinician and the classroom teacher. Many dyslogic children continue to need specialized help—either ancillary to regular class teaching or, as we have indicated, in special classes—throughout the primary grades, and some even beyond this level. If the child has made sufficient progress to be attending grade school, he still requires the additional therapy that is a product of understanding and patience. The classroom teacher may help the child to work to his maximum level of ability by motivation that is timed to the child's periods of best effort. The dyslogic child, more than most, needs encouragement, because he is never quite certain what he may expect of himself. In the absence of severe sensory or motor disability, many, if not most, dyslogic children may be helped to achieve at least a normal level of overall proficiency. Care must be exercised that the child not be pushed too hard, or urged too soon, as he begins to acquire language and learn how to behave in a world of linguistic symbols. With good timing, and with an educational schedule geared to awareness of his labile inclinations and his intellectual limitations, the teacher and clinician can equalize their demands and his abilities so that proficiencies may develop despite an early unevenness in developmental patterns.

References and Recommended Readings

ALLEN, R. M., and T. W. JEFFERSON, *Psychological Evaluation of the Cerebral-Palsied Person*. Springfield, Illinois, Charles C. Thomas, Publisher, 1962.

ALTMAN, I., "On the Prevalence of Cerebral Palsy," *Cerebral Palsy Review*, XVI (1955).

BARRY, H., *The Young Aphasic Child*. Washington, D.C., Alexander Graham Bell Association for the Deaf, 1961.

BERRY, M. F., and J. EISENSON, *Speech Disorders*. New York, Appleton-Century-Crofts, 1956, Chaps. 15–18.

BIRCH, H. G., ed., *Brain Damage in Children*. Baltimore, The Williams & Wilkins Company, 1964. (Includes a selective annotated bibliography on brain-damaged children.)

BROWN, S. F., in W. JOHNSON et al., *Speech-Handicapped School Children*. New York, Harper & Row, Publishers, 1967.

CLEMENTS, S. D., *Minimal Brain Dysfunction in Children*. NINDB Monograph 3. Washington, D.C., U.S. Department of Health, Education, and Welfare, 1966.

CROTHERS, B., and R. S. PAINE, *The Natural History of Cerebral Palsy*. Cambridge, Harvard University Press, 1959. (An authoritative medical presentation of cerebral palsy, based on a review of 1,800 cases.)

CRUICKSHANK, W. M., *Psychology of Exceptional Children and Youth*. Englewood Cliffs, N.J., Prentice-Hall, Inc., 1970.

CRUICKSHANK, W. M., F. A. BENTZEN, F. H. RATZEBURG, and M. T. TANNHAUSER, *A Teaching Method for Brain-Injured and Hyperactive Children*. Syracuse, Syracuse University Press, 1961. (A detailed description of the educational implications of a pilot study with hyperactive, brain-damaged children.)

CRUICKSHANK, W. M., and G. M. RAUS, *Cerebral Palsy: Its Individual and Community Problems*. Syracuse, Syracuse University Press, 1955.

DE HIRSCH, K., "Studies in Tachyphemia, IV: Diagnosis of Developmental Language Disorders," *Logos*, IV (1961), 3–9.

EISENSON, J., "Perceptual Disturbances in Children with Central Nervous System Disfunctions and Implications for Language Development," *British Journal of Disorders of Communication*, I, 1 (1966), 21–32.

EISENSON, J. "Developmental Aphasia: A Speculative View with Therapeutic Implications," *Journal of Speech and Hearing Disorders*, XXX, 1 (February 1968), 3–13.

McDONALD, E. T., and B. CHANCE, *Cerebral Palsy*. Englewood Cliffs, N.J., Prentice-Hall, Inc., 1964.

McGINNIS, M., *Aphasic Children*. Washington, D.C., Alexander Graham Bell Association for the Deaf, 1963.

PERLSTEIN, M., *Cerebral Palsy*. National Society for Crippled Children and Adults, Chicago, December, 1961. (This is a booklet in the *Parent Series*, in which a medical authority on cerebral palsy provides answers to questions parents might ask about their cerebral-palsied children.)

STRAUSS, A. A., and W. C. KEPHART, *Psychopathology and Education of the Brain-Injured Child.*, Vol. II. New York, Grune and Stratton, 1955. (An exposition on differential diagnosis and educational approaches for brain-damaged children.)

United Cerebral Palsy Society, *Seven Essentials in Educational Planning for Children with Cerebral Palsy*. New York, The Society Program Division Bulletin 2, February, 1955.

Problems

1. Children now referred to as being cerebral-palsied were once generally referred to as spastics. Why is the term cerebral-palsied more appropriate than spastic?
2. What are characteristics of the chief types of cerebral-palsy conditions?
3. Why are many cerebral-palsied children multiply handicapped? What are the most frequent types of handicaps?
4. Why is it difficult to be certain about the intellectual assessments of cerebral-palsied children?
5. Is it reasonable to believe that all cerebral palsied children can achieve normal speech? Justify your answer.
6. Can a cerebral-palsy condition be acquired by an adult? Justify your answer.
7. What is meant by *minimal brain dysfunction*? What are the arguments for and against this concept?
8. What does the term *perceptual dysfunction* imply?
9. Compare an obviously (frankly) cerebral-palsied person with one designated as having minimal brain dysfunction and so presumably

minimally brain damaged. What are some similarities? What are some essential differences?

10. What does the term *emotional lability* signify when applied to the brain-damaged child?

11. What is developmental aphasia (dyslogia)? In what respects does the developmentally aphasic child resemble the one with minimal brain damage?

12. Why may it be said that a developmentally aphasic child often shows maximal brain dysfunction and minimal brain damage?

13. What is the rationale for approaching the developmentally aphasic child through his visual modality?

14. Why is the developmentally aphasic child described as one who is perceptually and intellectually inefficient?

15. What is the difference between hearing impairment and auditory perceptual dysfunction?

16. How would you go about establishing a differential diagnosis for the developmentally aphasic child and one who may be either mentally retarded or severely impaired in hearing?

Indexes

Subject Index

Author Index